Prentice Hall Advanced Reference Series

Computer Science
DUBES AND JAIN   *Algorithms for Clustering Data*
SHERE   *Software Engineering and Management*

Engineering
FERRY, AKERS, AND GREENEICH   *Ultra Large Scale Integrated Microelectronics*
JOHNSON   *Lectures on Adaptive Parameter Estimation*
MILUTINOVIC   *Microprocessor System Design GaAs Technology*
WALRAND   *Introduction to Queueing Networks*

Science
BINKLEY   *The Pineal: Endocrine and Nonendocrine Function*
CAROZZI   *Carbonate Depositional Systems*
EISEN   *Mathematical Methods for Biology, Bioengineering, and Medicine*
FRASER   *Event Stratigraphy*
WARREN   *Evaporite Sedimentology*

Prentice Hall Endocrinology Series

Mac E. Hadley
Series Editor

BINKLEY *The Pineal: Endocrine and Nonendocrine Function*

FORTHCOMING BOOKS IN THIS SERIES (*tentative titles*)

BENSON, BLASK, AND LEADEM *Prolactin*

BITTMAN AND JONASSEN *Neuroendocrinology of Reproduction*

GUILLETTE *Comparative Endocrinology of Vertebrate Reproduction*

HADLEY *The Melanotropins*

HAZELWOOD *The Endocrine Pancreas*

MCNABB *Thyroid Hormones*

MEIER *Chronoendocrinology in Vertebrates*

PANG *Hormones in Calcium Homeostasis*

PICKERING, SWANN, AND WAKERLY *Hormones of the Posterior Pituitary*

RAO, KELLER, AND TOBE *Comparative Invertebrate Endocrinology*

TIMIRAN AND QUAY *Hormones and Aging*

TSUI *Endocrine and Immune Interactions*

The Pineal: Endocrine and Nonendocrine Function

Sue Binkley

Temple University

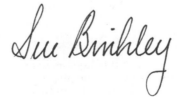

PRENTICE HALL, Englewood Cliffs, New Jersey 07632

Library of Congress Cataloging-in-Publication Data

Binkley, Sue Ann (date)
  The pineal.

  Bibliography: p.
  Includes index.
  1. Pineal body. I. Title. [DNLM: 1. Pineal Body—
physiology. WK 350 B613p]
QP188.P55B494 1988   591.1'42   87-18734
ISBN 0-13-676181-X

Editorial and production supervision: Gloria Jordan
Interior design: Natasha Sylvester
Cover jacket design: 20/20 Services, Inc.
Manufacturing buyer: S. Gordon Osbourne

Prentice Hall Advanced Reference Series
Prentice Hall Endocrinology Series

© 1988 by Prentice Hall
A division of Simon & Schuster
Englewood Cliffs, New Jersey 07632

Printed in the United States of America
10 9 8 7 6 5 4 3 2 1

ISBN 0-13-676181-X 025

Prentice-Hall International (UK) Limited, *London*
Prentice-Hall of Australia Pty. Limited, *Sydney*
Prentice-Hall Canada Inc., *Toronto*
Prentice-Hall Hispanoamericana, S.A., *Mexico*
Prentice-Hall of India Private Limited, *New Delhi*
Prentice-Hall of Japan, Inc., *Tokyo*
Simon & Schuster Asia Pte. Ltd., *Singapore*
Editora Prentice-Hall do Brasil, Ltda., *Rio de Janeiro*

Dedicated to

Ed and Ann Lingenfelter

Contents

Foreword   **xiii**

Preface   **xv**

1 INTRODUCTION   **1**

   1.1 Introduction   1
   1.2 Possible Roles of the Pineal   2
   1.3 Early History of Pineal Research   4
   1.4 Circadian Rhythms: A Unifying Theme   8
       References   10
   1.5 A Note on Terminology   10

2 METHODS USED TO STUDY THE PINEAL   **12**

   2.1 Introduction   13
   2.2 Location and Dissection of the Pineal   13
   2.3 Anatomical Methods   15
   2.4 Surgical Methods   17
   2.5 Pharmacological Methods   21
   2.6 In Vitro Techniques   23
   2.7 Indole Assays   26
   2.8 Enzymes   30

2.9   Environmental Lighting   32
References   32

3   PINEAL ANATOMY   35

3.1   Variation   38
3.2   Gross Anatomy   38
3.3   Histology   39
3.4   Ultrastructure   40
3.5   Vascularization   50
3.6   Innervation   51
3.7   Pineal Recess   53
References   53

4   PINEAL BIOCHEMISTRY   55

4.1   Indoleamines   55
4.2   Nonindoles   63
References   68

5   PINEAL REGULATION BY LIGHT AND DARK   70

5.1   Interaction of Light and Circadian Clocks   70
5.2   Daily Cycles   72
5.3   Photoperiod   73
5.4   Constant Light and Constant Dark   75
5.5   Refractory Period and Rapid Plummet   79
5.6   Resetting   82
5.7   Light Quality   82
5.8   Photoreceptors   82
References   84

6   NEURAL AND ENDOGENOUS CONTROL OF PINEAL FUNCTION   86

6.1   Variation in Regulation   86
6.2   Neural Pathway and Consequences   88
6.3   Pineal ß-Receptors   90
6.4   Second Messengers   94
6.5   Intrapineal Control   94
6.6   Systemic Catecholamines   97
References   98

7   MAMMALIAN PHOTOPERIODISM   100

7.1   Introduction   100
7.2   The Role of Circadian Rhythms   102

7.3   Seasonal Reproduction in Hamsters:
The Role of Light   104
7.4   Seasonal Reproduction in Hamsters:
The Role of the Pineal   105
7.5   Melatonin Replacement   106
7.6   The Melatonin Hypothesis   108
7.7   Other Considerations   110
7.8   Nonseasonal Reproduction   112
7.9   Nonreproduction   113
      References   113

8   CIRCADIAN RHYTHMS   116

8.1   Introduction   116
8.2   Surgery   117
8.3   Melatonin Replacement   121
8.4   Eyes   123
8.5   Pineal and Ocular Cycles   124
      References   125

**9   OTHER FUNCTIONS OF THE PINEAL
AND MELATONIN   128**

9.1   Introduction   129
9.2   Color Change   129
9.3   Interactions with the Eyes   134
9.4   Electrophysiology and the Pineal   137
9.5   Thermoregulation   139
9.6   Behavior   142
9.7   Hypertension   143
9.8   Endocrine System   143
9.9   Summary   149
      References   150

**10   PINEAL HORMONE SECRETION
AND ACTION   156**

10.1   Introduction   157
10.2   Hormone Secretion   157
10.3   Target Tissues and Cells   162
10.4   Mechanism of Action   168
       References   171

**11   OTHER SUBSTANCES THAT MAY BE
IMPORTANT TO THE PINEAL   175**

11.1   Introduction   176
11.2   Arginine Vasotocin   176

11.3 Hypophysiotropic Hormones 180
11.4 Other Pineal Factors 180
References 182

12 PINEAL FUNCTION IN HUMANS 185

12.1 Introduction 185
12.2 Anatomy 185
12.3 Biochemistry 189
12.4 Physiology 191
References 199

13 DEVELOPMENT AND AGING 203

13.1 Introduction 203
13.2 Embryonic Development 204
13.3 Neonatal, Preweaning, and Posthatch
Development 207
13.4 Puberty 212
13.5 Aging 214
References 216

14 COMPARATIVE PINEAL ENDOCRINOLOGY: MAMMALS 221

14.1 Vertebrates in General 222
14.2 Mammals 225
References 236

15 COMPARATIVE PINEAL ENDOCRINOLOGY: BIRDS, REPTILES, AMPHIBIANS, FISH, AND NONVERTEBRATES 242

15.1 Introduction 242
15.2 Birds 243
15.3 Reptiles 247
15.4 Amphibians 250
15.5 Fish and Lampreys 251
15.6 Nonvertebrates 254
References 254

16 PERSPECTIVES 262

16.1 Introduction 262
16.2 The Pineal as a Photoreceptor 264
16.3 The Pineal as an Endocrine Gland 264

16.4 The Pineal as a Neuroendocrine
      Transducer   264
16.5 The Place of the Pineal in Endocrine
      Hierarchies   265
16.6 The Role of the Pineal in Clocks   265
16.7 The Pineal as a Calendar   271
      References   281

17 EPILOGUE   284

17.1 Introduction   284
17.2 Anatomical Relationships   285
17.3 Biochemistry   286
17.4 Regulation   287
17.5 Clock Function   288
17.6 Calendar Function   289
17.7 Output Signals and Targets   289
      References   289

GLOSSARY   291

ANNOTATED BIBLIOGRAPHY   295

INDEX   301

Foreword

The volumes representing the Prentice Hall ENDOCRINOLOGY SERIES are intended to supplement other more general texts currently used in typical endocrinology courses. Each volume completely covers a particular subject and provides additional information on a topic generally treated in less detail in a general endocrinology textbook.

Written by authorities in their respective fields of endocrinological research, the texts are particularly useful in graduate seminar-type courses where often a specific subject is chosen to be covered in depth. Each text should also prove useful to scientists and medical professionals interested in an in-depth coverage of a particular aspect of endocrinology, and they will also find the up-to-date references particularly useful.

The field of endocrinology can generally be divided into two areas: comparative endocrinology and human endocrinology. The latter topic is usually very clinically oriented, whereas the former is generally concerned with a broad coverage of the endocrine system of a diverse group of animals, including invertebrates. It is obviously difficult to incorporate these diverse coverages into any one volume, and therefore the individual texts comprising the series will sometimes reflect a particular emphasis, clinical or comparative, whatever the particular interest of the author. Many of the volumes in this series will, however, provide a broad coverage of a particular topic.

Besides those volumes that will cover a classic topic in endocrinology, the series also hopes to deal uniquely with topics not generally available to readers of general endocrinology texts. Volumes presently contracted for and in preparation include: The *Melanotropins, Hormones in Calcium Homeostasis, Hormones of the Posterior Pituitary, Comparative Invertebrate Endocrinology, Chronoendocrinology in Vertebrates, Comparative Endocrinology of Vertebrate Reproduction, Thyroid Hormones, Endocrine and Immune Interactions, The Endocrine Pancreas, Prolactin, Hormones of the Adrenal Cortex.*

Mac E. Hadley
University of Arizona

Preface

This book is about the pineal,[1] a small central body in the brains of most vertebrates. The pineal mediates responses to environmental light and dark, and in some species it is a "biological clock" for daily cycles. The gland is involved in synchrony of physiological cycles with time of day and time of year. Time cues are derived from the environmental lighting, either directly by the pineal or indirectly via the eyes. The pineal has a role in interpreting seasonal changes in day length, and especially for seasonal control of reproductive functions.

The purpose of this book is to provide an introduction to the pineal. It is intended for an audience of senior undergraduates, beginning graduate students, and for anyone interested in the ways light and time organize physiology.

The scope is the environmental endocrinology of the pineal and its hormone, melatonin. It is introductory rather than advanced, and comprehensive rather than detailed. It requires minimal background of the reader as opposed to a symposium volume, which demands a fuller knowledge of its user.

Chapters 1 to 4 review the history of pineal research, describe the methods used to study the pineal, and outline the gland's anatomical and biochemical features. Chapters 5 to 9 deal with pineal functions and regulatory mechanisms, including photoperiodic and circadian

[1]See Section 1.5 on terminology and the use of *pineal* as a noun.

rhythms. As noted in Chapter 5, regulation of the pineal by light and dark was worked out first in rats and chickens. Mammalian photoperiodism was classically studied using the reproductive system of the hamster, and so this system is the cornerstone of Chapter 7.

Our understanding of the pineal's role in circadian rhythms derives from research with birds, so those studies make the largest contribution to Chapter 8. Chapter 9 deals with a potpourri of interesting pineal-related functions such as skin color change and the function of melatonin in the eye. Chapters 10 and 11 focus on the pineal hormone, melatonin, and other substances such as arginine vasotocin that may be related to pineal function. Chapters 12 to 15 cover the comparative endocrinology, development, and aging aspects of the pineal. Chapters 12, 14, and 15 cover the pineal on a species-by-species basis, which should help achieve an understanding of the specialization that occurs in pineal physiology and which is central to an understanding of its function. The final two chapters provide some models and perspectives for viewing the data that has been presented as well as notes on the current status of pineal research and possible future directions. An annotated bibliography lists books on the pineal, and the references in these books plus the references at the ends of the chapters virtually comprise the entire pineal literature.

I thank Karen Mosher for assistance in proofreading the manuscript. Michael Bouldin and Karen Mosher assisted in the preparation of the line drawings. Dr. H. R. Tatem provided the CAT scan and radiograph showing the location of the human pineal, and Drs. John McNulty, Marcia Welsh, and Moira Cioffi made the photomicrographs that show pineal anatomy. Drs. Mac E. Hadley, Milton Stetson, George Brainard, John McNulty, George Vaughan, Mary K. Vaughan, Bea White, Mark Rollag, Charles Ralph, and Russel Reiter provided helpful advice, suggestions, and information. Special thanks are due editorial staff members at Prentice Hall (Ken Tennity, Gloria Jordan, and Elaine Luthy). The author is grateful to Regulatory Biology of the National Science Foundation and to Endocrinology of the National Institutes of Health for the financial support of her research which led to this volume.

Sue Binkley
Temple University

1

Introduction

1.1 Introduction

Knowledge of the pineal, like that of other biological structures, has progressed from speculative to concrete information. As in other areas of science, this progress resulted from technological advances such as improvements in microscopy and the invention of chemical assays. It was also facilitated by the explosion of interest in and funding for science that occurred in the second half of the 20th century. Most of all, progress came from the imaginations of scientists who dedicated their professional lives to the study of the pineal.

At the same time, there was a conceptual obstacle to understanding pineal function: the gland was sometimes viewed as a vestigial remnant of the evolutionary process, a structure lacking modern

1

function. Removal of the pineal (pinealectomy) from experimental animals did not result in death and effects of pinealectomy were not immediately apparent. Without drastic and clear effects of pinealectomy, discovery of the functions of the pineal became a longstanding problem in the field. A breakthrough came with the realization that pineal functions depend on time of day and environmental lighting. Early investigations that did not take these conditions into account created confusion.

Though we now know much about the organ, the story of the pineal is still incomplete. Research continues apace. Pinealologists continue to address questions: What are the details of pineal cellular structure? How does the pineal perceive light? What are the targets of melatonin? What molecules comprise the catalogue of pineal substances? What are the practical uses for pineal knowledge in agriculture and human health? What is the importance of the pineal in biological clockworks?

1.2 Possible Roles of the Pineal

A number of general roles have been suggested for the pineal gland over the years based on anatomical observations, studies of function, and studies of biochemistry [1, 3, 4, 11, 12, 17, 18].

1.2.1 Photoreceptor

Photoreceptors are anatomical structures that are capable of detecting light. Pineal glands of some species contain structures that remind scientists of the anatomy of retinal photosensory cells. Moreover, in amphibians and reptiles, the pineal is near an eye-like structure in the dorsal center of the head (the "third eye"). Electrical responses to light or dark can be measured in pineal glands of some animals. Isolated pineal glands from some species are light sensitive. The case for pineal light reception is thus strong for some species.

1.2.2 Endocrine gland

Endocrine glands are classically considered to be ductless glands that secrete hormones (molecules that act as chemical messengers) into the bloodstream. The pineal seems admirably suited to act as one of these glands as it is highly vascularized and ductless. When it was learned that the pineal synthesized a molecule, melatonin, that could be found in the bloodstream, melatonin became the primary candidate for a pineal hormone. The fact that extracts of pineals lightened the color of pigment cells (e.g., melanophores) in skins in some lower vertebrates provided one possible target tissue.

1.2.3 Transducer

Some endocrine organs receive neural signals from nerve tracts from the brain and respond by secreting their particular hormones into the bloodstream; these organs have been called *neuroendocrine transducers*. One example is the median eminence of the hypothalamus, which responds to brain signals by secreting small peptide hormones into the hypophyseal portal veins. A second example is the adrenal medulla, which releases epinephrine into the blood in response to signals from sympathetic nerves. The pineal is a third example. The pineal is innervated by the *nervi conarii*. When the brain signals the pineal, melatonin is produced and released into the blood.

The concept of neuroendocrine transduction has been extended to include the fact that some pineals convert light-dark information into hormone signals. The pineal can be a *photoneuroendocrine transducer*. It is not yet clear, however, whether this term should be reserved for those pineals that are themselves light sensitive, or whether it can be used more broadly to include the pineal glands whose light information is relayed indirectly from the eyes.

1.2.4 Biological clock

Biological clocks are cellular components that possess timing ability in an organism. The pineal is a biological clock (although, it should be noted, it is not the only biological clock) in some species because it is capable of self-sustained oscillations in vitro. The oscillations may be *circadian rhythms*. (Circadian rhythms, as we shall see in Section 1.4, are biological cycles that continue to oscillate in constant conditions with periods close to 24 hours. A daily change that coincides with a daily change in light and dark or temperature, but that does not persist in constant conditions, does not satisfy the criteria of all investigators for use of the term *circadian*.) Light-dark information is used to "set" the biological clock. Periodic secretion of a hormone (e.g., melatonin) provides a means for the pineal gland to send time signals to other parts of the body.

The pineal clock appears to be important for measuring nightlength (scotoperiod) and daylength (photoperiod); the measurement of either defines the other since the two must add up to 24 hours. As a yardstick is used to measure dimension, so the pineal gland may provide the standard against which the lengths of light and dark are compared, thus acting as a "timestick."

1.2.5 Regulator of regulators

The pineal gland may enhance or inhibit the production or secretion of hormones from other endocrine glands. For example, there may be a pineal-hypothalamus-pituitary-gonad axis, a hierarchy in which one gland controls another with the pineal gland at the apex. The advantage of such organization is that it permits amplification; that is, a small number of molecules secreted by the initial receptor organ can result in a "cascade" of sequential, ever-increasing, cellular responses.

1.3 Early History of Pineal Research

Most of the information in this book is derived from "data" collected in experiments; that is, there is tangible evidence (e.g., photographs, numbers, graphs) that can be examined, analyzed, and criticized. Repetition of experiments by several investigators increases the credibility of a given piece of evidence. However, there is another story, and that is about the scientists themselves, the detectives who followed leads to dead ends or who made observations leading to new discoveries. This book is not intended as a chronicle of pineal scientists, but some history will be touched on here to show that interest in the pineal did not originate in the last decade but extends back through time.

Those who have written of pineal history have not only provided a chronology [21], but also divided it into epochs of understanding [1, 11, 12]. Professor Kappers [12] divided the scientific advances in pineal research into three eras; and Professor Altschule [1] suggested four historical periods. Kappers' first time frame, like Altschule's, includes "superstitious notions," pre-Cartesian and post-Cartesian ideas, the discovery of the pineal, and early suggestions as to its possible function (300 B.C. to the end of the 19th century). The second era, "preliminary studies," was ushered in by technical advances in microscopy; during this period there were anatomical investigations of pineal comparative anatomy, embryology, and histology (first half of the 20th century); this era also included early studies involving pinealectomy. In the third era (Kappers) or third and fourth eras (Altschule), anatomical investigations continued, but knowledge of pineal physiology (function) resulted from advances in biochemistry and pharmacology (second half of the 20th century). The pineal was functionally linked to other structures of the body and its own mechanisms were studied. A key to unlocking pineal function was the recognition that environmental light and dark were important. Brainard [2] identified the period from 1954 to 1965 as the "decade of transformation" when "the pineal gland was demonstrated to be an active neuroendocrine transducer in contrast to a functionless vestige as earlier proposed."

1.3.1 Discovery of the human pineal

Credit for discovering the human pineal has been accorded to an Egyptian anatomist, Herophilos (325–280 B.C.), and an Alexandrian

physiologist, Erasistratus [9, 10]. Herophilos and Erasistratus assigned the pineal a "tap" or "sphincter" function. In this valvular
function, the pineal regulated the stream of "pneuma" or "spiritus" or
"vital spirits" from the third to the fourth ventricle of the brain
whence it might be changed into "animal spirits" for the transport by
hollow nerves [9, 10, 21]. This idea, the "pre-Cartesian superstition"
that the pineal was a "memory valve" [1], can be said to have
persisted into the present time since there have been suggestions that
the pineal regulates the flow of cerebrospinal fluid.

The pineal derived its name through the efforts of Galenos (Galen of
Pergamon, A.D. 130–200). According to Zrenner [21], he was the first
to write of the pineal and describe its location. He considered the
structure to be a "gland," separate from surrounding brain structures.
In the human, the pineal has a "pine cone" shape so it was called
conarium (*konarion, konareion, soma konoeides*). The Latin word for
pine cone was *pineale*. The gland has also been called the *cervical
body*. The pine cone comparison also persists in the name given to the
nerves that enter the pineal, the *nervi conarii*. The pineal is also
called the *epiphysis* (or *epiphysis cerebri*). The word *epiphysis* (a
combination of *epi*, meaning "upon," and *phesthai* meaning "to
grow") refers to the location of the pineal, at the top of, or lying over,
the brain in many organisms. The term *epiphysis* contrasts with the
term *hypophysis*, which refers to the pituitary and its location beneath, or lying under, the brain.

Galen ascribed to the pineal the role of a lymph gland. This idea
was challenged by scientists during the Renaissance in Europe (14th,
15th, and 16th centuries) when many aspects of anatomy, medicine,
art, and religion were freshly examined. Berengario da Carpi
(1460–1530) introduced the idea that the pineal filtered the cerebrospinal fluid in the brain. The extensive vascularization of the pineal
was recognized by Andreas Vesalius Bruxellensis (1514–1564). Fran-
castor (1483–1553) noted that the pineal was an unpaired organ in
the center of the brain. For this reason it became a candidate for the
locus of coordination of information from the paired sensory organs
(presumably the eyes and ears), and was termed the *sensorium com-
mune*.

It was a natural consequence of this thinking, then, that Descartes
(1596–1650) perpetrated the idea that the pineal gland was the "seat
of the soul." The Cartesian view was

> That there is a small gland in the brain in which the soul exercises its
> function more specifically than in its other parts. We have also to bear in
> mind that although the soul is joined to the whole body, there is yet in the
> body a certain part in which it exercises its functions more specifically than
> in all the others. It is a matter of common belief that this part is the brain,
> or possibly the heart—the brain because of its relation to the senses, the
> heart because it is there that we feel the passions. But on carefully

examining the matter, I seem to find evidence that the part of the body, in which the soul exercises its functions immediately is in no wise the heart, nor the brain as a whole, but solely the innermost part of the brain, viz. a certain very small gland, situated in a midway position, and suspended over the passage by which the animal spirits of the anterior cavities communicate with those of the posterior cavities, in such fashion that its slightest movements can greatly alter the course of those spirits; and reciprocally that any change, however slight, taking place in the course of the spirits can greatly change the movements of this gland. [4]

The Cartesian pineal was capable of movement, it coordinated visual images, it gave a place for imagination, it was the site of consciousness, and it seated common sense. In *De L'homme* Descartes described and drew diagrams for a pineal role in sleeping and waking and the direction of the pineal by environmental light information perceived by the eyes. [5].

However, the Cartesian view was disputed [21] and the pineal was made jest of. Thomas Gibson called attention to genital analogies that Galen had applied to the pineal region:

The first is Glandula pinealis, or Penis; because it representeth the Pine-nut, or a Man's Yard. It is seated in the beginning of that Pipe, by which the third and fourth ventricles are united. Its basis is downwards, and its apex or end looks upwards. It is of a substance harder than the Brain, of a pale colour, and covered with a thin Membrane. This Gland des Cartes thinks to be the primary seat of the Soul, and that all animal operations draw their origine from it. But Bartholin has sufficiently confuted that opinion; for it seems to be but of the same use as other Glands, and particularly the Glandula pituitaria placed near it, viz. to separate the Lympha from the Arterial blood; which Lympha is resorbed by the Veins (or it may be by Vasa lymphatica) as was shown from Dr. Lower. Near to this on both sides of this third Ventricle four round bodies appear. The two upper are lesser, and are called Testes; the two greater are lower and are called Nates. The chink betwixt the Nates is called Anus. (quoted in [8])

However, even today, we recognize parallels between the Cartesian view and our modern understanding of the brain.

In the mid-18th century, psychosis was correlated with pineal calcification, a view disputed in 1779 by Morgagni: "[Calcification] has been found with madness and without it also, yet I would not have you forget there is not any one disorder wherewith it is so frequently to be join'd as with madness" (quoted in [1]).

1.3.2 Anatomy

Improvements of microscopic techniques sparked examination of most of the tissues of the vertebrate body. The comparative anatomy, histology, and embryology of the pineal were subjects of investigation

[1, 11, 12, 13]. The pineal gland was recognized as "photosensory" (Studnicka 1905) and secretory, and its associations with the "third eye" (parietal or frontal organs) of lower vertebrates were recognized. Most important, in 1898, links between the pineal and human reproductive function were made—Gutzeit (1896) described a boy with prematurely mature external genitalia and teratoma of the pineal region, and Heubner (1898) correlated premature puberty with pinealoma in a boy. Marburg (1909) coined terms for premature development of the sex organs associated with a pineal tumor—*pubertas praecox* and *genitosomia praecox*. He further suggested that the syndrome was due to underfunction of the pineal and that the pineal might normally act to inhibit reproduction in children. In conjunction with these ideas the pineal gland was called *Keuschheitsdruse*, the "chastity gland." Foa's (1912) removal of the cock's pineal organ with subsequent enlargement of the comb and testis seemed to prove the idea, but Foa's study has not been repeated with modern techniques.

1.3.3 Physiology

The modern era of pineal research opened about 1954 with the publication of a review of pineal literature by Kitay and Altschule [13] and continues to the present. In this era, anatomical research continued. Bioassay advances and biochemical assays allowed the assessment of quantities of pineal molecules. In 1917 McCord and Allen had noticed that pineal extracts lighten the color of frog skin [3]. A landmark in the biochemistry of the pineal was the isolation of a possible pineal hormone in 1958 by Lerner, Case, Takahashi, Lee, and Mori. The hormone was an indole molecule, and it was named *melatonin* because pineal extracts lightened melanophores. The project for the identification of melatonin consumed some quarter million bovine pineal glands.

About 1960 there was the realization (from work showing that light affected reproduction) that the pineal was regulated by light [7]. Proof of this came with the discovery (by Fiske, Bryant, Putnam) that constant light reduced (about 25%) the weight of rat pineals after 9–10 weeks and with evidence (of Quay) that constant light altered pineal morphology in mice.

In the early 1960s, this discovery was buttressed by observations that pineal indoleamines showed daily variations, and by the finding that pinealectomy abolished dark-induced diminution in size of hamster testes [3, 9]. Explaining these events with melatonin and/or pineal peptides has been a subject of research since that time. In 1968, Gaston and Menaker established the pineal as a biological clock by showing that pinealectomy abolished perch-hopping rhythms in sparrows. As summarized by Brainard [2], there were two formulations that shaped the course of pineal research:

First, they [Wurtman and Axelrod] termed the pineal a "neuroendocrine transducer"—an organ which converts a neural signal concerning environmental information into an endocrine signal which acts on distant parts of the body. . . . Secondly, Wurtman and Axelrod promoted the "melatonin hypothesis" that proposed melatonin to be the hormone which is secreted from the pineal in response to environmental lighting and which is responsible for the observed pineal-gonadal effects.

1.4 Circadian Rhythms: A Unifying Theme

There is a unifying theme for understanding pineal physiology. The parts played by time of day and environmental lighting are key factors in appreciating the place of the pineal in the overall organization of vertebrate physiology. Factors that affect the pineal are time of day, season of year, occurrence of light and dark, and duration of light and dark.

1.4.1 Daily and seasonal cycles in the environment: The input

There are a number of parameters (e.g., temperature, humidity, and barometric pressure) that vary on daily and seasonal bases and are correlated with the earth's rotation and axis angle with respect to the sun. The most precise of such variables is the timing of light and dark. Environmental lighting can provide precise time cues for a daily "clock" (dawn and dusk) and "calendar" (annual waxing and waning of day and night length).

The pineal may be involved in the detection of light and dark in a number of ways: (1) directly via photoreceptor cells in the pineal, (2) via neural signals from the retinas of the lateral eyes, (3) via signals from the "third eye," and (4) via signals from as yet unidentified extraretinal light receptors (ERRs).

1.4.2 Circadian rhythms: The action

Most organisms, in addition to being able to detect light, have rhythms that are about 24 hours in length and that persist when the organisms are kept in constant conditions (constant darkness and temperature). (See, for example, Fig. 1.1) These rhythms, called *circadian rhythms* because they are "about a day" in length, are timed by environmental cues. Since almost all organisms can detect light, and since the signals are precise, it is not surprising that living things have made use of environmental light and dark changes to "set" their "biological clocks." Certain single cells have circadian rhythms, and there are also structures that have been identified as possible "pacemakers" in multicellular organisms. The pacemakers are structures whose rhythms synchronize or provoke other rhythms in an organism. The suprachiasmatic nuclei of the hypothalamus of vertebrates, the

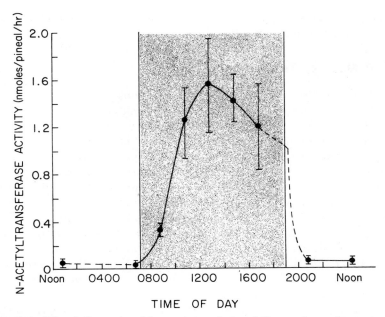

Figure 1.1. The daily cycle of the activity of pineal N-acetyltransferase in rats kept in LD 14:10. The enzyme exhibits peak activity in the dark that can be 30 times or more the light levels [14]. The measurement was of ^{14}C-serotonin N-acetylated per gland per hour. (Plotted from data tabulated in Klein, Reiter, and Weller [15] replicating the 1970 discovery by Klein and Weller [14].

optic lobes of cockroaches, and the eyes of sea slugs are candidates for pacemakers. The pineal may also act as a pacemaker or may be subservient to other pacemakers; in this case the pineal may relay time information to still other rhythmic or nonrhythmic organs. The pineal produces melatonin on a nightly basis from serotonin due to a vigorous rhythm in the activity of a pineal enzyme. In some species, other structures, such as the retina, are also capable of nightly melatonin synthesis.

1.4.3 Endocrine interactions: The output

The pineal was among the first endocrine organs found to have prominent daily changes in hormone production. This finding stimulated investigations of daily cycles in other hormones and we now know that most endocrine function is organized on a daily basis [16]. The pineal may function, via rhythmic melatonin production, to stimulate or synchronize rhythmic changes in other endocrine glands. Endocrine glands may not be the only "targets" of the pineal. The brain and other nonendocrine structures could receive time signals from the pineal by responding to melatonin. Melatonin rhythms are found in humans as well as in animals, so that the pineal is part of the human endocrine system [19].

1.5 A Note on Terminology

The student who explores beyond this book will find that various terms are used for the pineal, including *pineal gland, pineal body,* and *pineal organ.* Dictionaries identify *pineal* as an adjective; however, your author uses it as a noun to avoid confusion since all four terms refer to one structure. This usage was chosen for the following reasons: (1) many (but not all) dictionaries list other endocrine glands—pituitary, thyroid, adrenal—as nouns as well as adjectives; (2) *pineal* appears as a noun in verbal and written usage; (3) using *pineal* as a noun eliminates the problem of whether to call it a "body," "gland," or "organ" (the same structure is designated by all these terms); and (4) using *pineal* as a noun appeals to parsimony because it saves space and words. The astute reader will note that the dictionary definition cited at the beginning of the chapter is from a volume that is more than a decade old [20]; however, it was the most scientifically enlightened that has been brought to the author's attention—because it listed functions. Some current dictionaries do not ascribe a role to the pineal. There is a difference of usage with regard to pronunciation. Most dictionaries indicate pronunciation as pin̄ ē ăl (short "i"); however, some investigators refer to it as pin ē ăl (long "i"), presumably a reference to the origin of its name from the shape resemblance to pine cones.

The word *melatonin* is less controversial; its pronunciation and part of speech (noun), like its chemical structure, are a settled matter. Some authors, however, find it difficult to let the word stand alone and generally use it in a phrase, such as "melatonin levels." The word *melatonin* seems short enough (and is used throughout this book). Nonetheless, diverse abbreviations for melatonin (M, MEL, or MT) are starting to appear in the literature. Melatonin, like the pineal, has not escaped unfortunate associations: the hormone was recently referred to as the "Dracula of hormones" because of its nighttime synthesis [6].

REFERENCES

1. Altschule, M. 1975. The four phases of pineal studies. In *Frontiers of pineal physiology,* ed. M. Altschule, pp. 1–4. Cambridge, Mass.: MIT Press.
2. Brainard, G. 1978. Pineal research: The decade of transformation. In *The pineal gland,* ed. I. Nir, R. Reiter, and R. Wurtman, pp. 1–20. J. Neural Transmission Suppl. 13. New York: Springer-Verlag.

3. Czyba, J., C. Cirod, M. Curé, and N. Durand. 1964. Sur les corrélations épiphyse-testiculaires chez le hamster doré (*Mesocricetus auratus Waterh.*). *C. R. Soc. Anat.* 131:324–333.

4. Descartes, R. 1649. Les Passions de l'âme. In *Body and mind in western thought*, ed. J. Reeves, pp. 293–294. New York: Penguin Books, 1950.

5. ———. *Treatise of man (De l'homme)*. French text with English translation and commentary by T. S. Hall. Cambridge: Harvard Univ. Press, 1972.

6. Dracula of hormones. *Newsweek*, November 25, 1985, pp. 94–95.

7. Fiske, V. 1975. Discovery of the relation between light and pineal function. In *Frontiers of pineal physiology*, ed. M. Altschule, pp. 5–11. Cambridge, Mass.: MIT Press.

8. Gibson, Thomas. 1763. *The anatomy of human bodies epitomized*. London: A. & J. Churchill.

9. Hoffman, R., and R. Reiter. 1965. Pineal gland: Influence on gonads of male hamsters. *Science* 148:1609–1611.

10. Kappers, J. 1960. Innervation of the epiphysis cerebri in the albino rat. *Anat. Rec.* 136:220–221.

11. ———. 1965. Preface. In *Structure and function of the epiphysis cerebri*, ed. J. Kappers and P. Schade, pp. ix–xv. Progress in Brain Research 10. Amsterdam: Elsevier.

12. ———. 1981. A survey of advances in pineal research. In *The pineal gland I: Anatomy and biochemistry*, ed. R. Reiter, pp. 1–25. Boca Raton, Fla.: CRC Press.

13. Kitay, J., and M. Altschule. 1954. Preface. In *The pineal gland: A review of the physiologic literature*, pp. v–viii. Cambridge, Mass.: Harvard Univ. Press.

14. Klein, D., and J. Weller. 1970. Indole metabolism in the pineal gland: A circadian rhythm in N-acetyltransferase. *Science* 169:1093–1095.

15. Klein, D., R. Reiter, and J. Weller. 1971. Pineal N-acetyltransferase activity in blinded and anosmic rats. *Endocrinology* 89:1020–1023.

16. Krieger, D., ed. 1979. *Endocrine rhythms*. New York: Raven Press.

17. Reiter, R. 1981. The mammalian pineal gland: Structure and function. *Amer. J. Anat.* 162:287–313.

18. ———. 1984. Preface. In *The pineal gland*, ed. R. Reiter, pp. v–vi. New York: Raven Press.

19. Vaughan, G. 1984. Melatonin in humans. In *Pineal research reviews II*, ed. R. Reiter, pp. 142–201. New York: Alan R. Liss.

20. *Webster's New Collegiate Dictionary*. 1975. Springfield, Mass.: G. & C. Merriam Co.

21. Zrenner, C. 1985. Theories of pineal function from classical antiquity to 1900: A history. In *Pineal research reviews III*, ed. R. Reiter, pp. 1–40. New York: Alan R. Liss.

2

Methods Used to Study the Pineal

"In estimating melatonin concentration . . . we obtain the greatest accuracy and precision when the melatonin concentration to which the tadpoles are subjected ranges from 0.1 to 2.5 ng/ml. Samples for the assay are diluted accordingly. The following is a stepwise protocol for the assay.

1. In a volume of 2 ml, samples of melatonin solution, standards, and unknowns appropriately diluted, are measured into disposable 15-ml polyethylene beakers . . . and placed on a white background under illumination.
2. For each sample, 10 light-adapted . . . tadpoles are selectively captured with a blunt medicine dropper, drained of excess tadpole growth medium on nylon mesh, and transferred to the sample to be assayed.
3. The time at which each group of 10 tadpoles is placed in the test sample is recorded. The tadpoles remain in the sample under bright (white fluorescent) illumination for exactly 30 minutes.
4. After 30 minutes . . . the melanophores in a triangular area between the eye and mouth on the left side of the head are "read" . . . an appropriate stage number is assigned according to the Hogben index."

C. Ralph and H. Lynch [21]

2.1 Introduction

Methods used to study the pineal gland have been the methods that are commonly used in the field of endocrinology: histology, surgery, hormone replacement, organ cultures, cell cultures, hormone isolation, hormone assays, and enzyme assays. Progress has resulted especially from application of these techniques in protocols that paid attention to time and environmental lighting.

The timing is important in protocols for pineal experiments both for the treatments and for sampling. For example, a series of time points (time series, time profile, time sequence) for a hormone or enzyme can be sampled in either of two ways. First, the time points can be obtained sequentially, one after another (e.g., one every 2 hours at 2 A.M., 4 A.M., . . . midnight, 2 A.M.). To obtain 24-hour or longer profiles entails investigative personnel in the laboratory around the clock. Second, the time points can be obtained from populations of animals adapted to light-dark regimens that are artificially staggered one from the other (e.g., with 6 LD 12:12 cycles with lights-on times at midnight, 4 A.M., 8 A.M., noon, 4 P.M. AND 8 P.M., a 24-hour series with points at 2-hour intervals can be obtained by sampling the six populations at two convenient points, noon and 2 P.M.). In addition to consideration of time of day and lighting, the length of time of a treatment in days or weeks is important. For example, it takes 10 weeks or so for hamster testes to regress in short photoperiods, and it takes 8–14 days for most rhythms to entrain to light-dark cycles.

2.2 Location and Dissection of the Pineal

Location and dissection of the pineal is somewhat dependent upon species. However, once the gland is found in one species (e.g., rat or chicken where it is large and accessible), it is more easily located in another.

2.2.1 Location

The pineal is an unpaired organ usually found in the midline of the brain occupying the space formed at the point where the cerebral hemispheres and cerebellum meet (Fig. 2.1). In most species the gland is a distinct organ, separate from the brain. It usually has a club-shaped top, which often ends at the meninges beneath the top of the skull. Often, if the meninges are pulled off, the pineal comes off with them; in fact, some brain atlases and brain anatomy figures lack a pineal gland because it was removed with the meninges. The association with meninges is so close (e.g., in sparrows), that a piece of meninges must be removed with the pineal during pinealectomy to

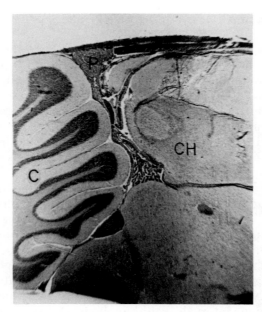

Figure 2.1 Section through the brain of a sparrow to illustrate the location of the pineal (*P*), the cerebellum (*C*), and the cerebral hemisphere (*CH*). The pineal runs from just beneath the skull and meninges with a long stalk extending to the choroid plexus region.

avoid leaving a pineal remnant and to ensure complete pinealectomy. The pineal extends by a stalk to the choroid plexus, which is usually recognized as a knot of blood vessels. The pineal is usually well vascularized and in some species, such as the sparrow, is recognized by the convergence of large venous sinuses that surround it. Heavy vascularization sometimes obscures the gland; in such species the pineal is more easily located by finding it first in a freshly killed animal so that bleeding does not interfere with dissection. Gross dissection of pineals reveals variation among species, (1) in location of the club of the gland (whether it is just beneath the skull and meninges or is deeper), (2) in length and thickness of the stalk, (3) in blood supply, and (4) in association with meninges.

To recapitulate, imagine that we can see through things, and are looking at the pineal from a point above the center of the top of the head of an animal such as a chicken or rat. We would see each of the following in turn: (1) a layer of feathers, scales, or hair; (2) a layer of skin (the scalp); (3) a layer of bone (the central point of skull, which directly overlies the pineal, is conveniently marked in some species by a convergence of sutures); (4) a layer of meninges (the top of the pineal may be visible if it abuts the meninges), and (5) the left and right cerebral hemispheres and the cerebellum. The uppermost pineal (surrounded by blood vessels) is located at the point where these last three structures converge and the stalk descends downward (away from the viewer) among them toward the choroid plexus.

2.2.2 Dissection

The dorsal approach permits the rapid dissection (less than 1 minute per pineal) which is required for some procedures (e.g., enzyme assays). The dissection of the pineal of a 3-week-old chick is typical of the general method used. The chick is decapitated, and then the skin of the head is pulled forward to expose the upper surface of the skull. The stump of the spinal cord (which is white and shiny) is located in the head, and a sharp point of a pair of scissors is inserted about halfway into the brain through the cord and its canal. The scissors are turned to the right, and a cut is made through the skull and brain about 0.5 cm to the right of the midline. The scissors are turned to the left without withdrawing them, and a second cut is made about 0.5 cm to the left of the midline. The flap of skull is deflected forward exposing the brain. In the chick, the meninges and pineal generally stick to the skull flap and the pineal, which is about 2 mm in diameter, can be plucked from its site with a watchmaker's forceps.

The dissection of the pineal of a young or adult rat is similar to that for the chick. In contrast to the dissection of the chick pineal, the rat pineal often remains in the brain portion of the head when the flap of skull is deflected forward. The gland (1–2 mm in diameter) may be visible at the top of the brain. If not, it is found by gently separating the cerebral hemispheres and cerebellum. Some animals have long stalked pineals (the stalk of the rabbit pineal is about 0.5 cm long). Some pineal glands, such as that of the sparrow or frog, are tightly bound to the meninges. Very small pineals may require the use of a dissecting microscope or jeweler's loupe for dissection.

2.3 Anatomical Methods

The pineal gland, partly because of its small size, has been a candidate for most of the traditional methods of anatomical examination [25]. In those pineals (e.g., adult human) in which concretions occur, they may be an obstacle in making sections; some investigators have decalcified pineal tissue before making sections to address this problem.

2.3.1 Light microscopy

Pineal sections to be studied by light microscopy (LM) are prepared using standard histological techniques: fixation with formalin, Bouin's solution, or glutaraldehyde; wax or plastic embedding; sectioning with a microtome or ultramicrotome; and staining (e.g., with hematoxylin-eosin). Most pineals are small and present few technical challenges. However, some pineals (e.g., those of humans) contain calcium concretions. These concretions can be as large as sand grains and present problems in sectioning. To retain pineal relationships with surrounding structures, the gland can be studied in situ. A block of tissue containing pineal and surrounding brain tissue can be dissected and studied. However, this cannot always be done since skull removal may disrupt the anatomy, so decalcification of skull must be done to permit sectioning through a block that includes skull, brain, and pineal.

2.3.2 Electron microscopy

Transmission electron microscopy (EM, TEM) is used to obtain higher magnification of sections of tissue than that permitted with LM. The orientation of the pineal (front, back, left, right, top, stalk) can be maintained by dissecting the gland from a block of tissue in the fixative (glutaraldehyde). The gland is treated with osmium tetroxide, embedded in plastic, sectioned on an ultramicrotome, and observed with a transmission electron microscope. Scanning electron microscopy (SEM), which is used to visualize surfaces, has been valuable for examination of pineal surface anatomy, vasculature, and concretions.

2.3.3 Histochemistry

Histochemical studies have a common goal: to localize biochemicals to anatomical sites (e.g., cell types or organelles). The art of histochemistry is, then, to find a way of detecting these molecules in sections of tissue. The chromatic properties of stains may be used for identification of chemical reactions (or series of reactions). Often a precursor, or reactant molecule, is supplied by the investigator and the cellular location of a visible product made from that reactant is possible.

A special case of histochemistry used for the pineal gland has been fluorescence histochemistry. Monoamines—norepinephrine, epinephrine, dopamine, DOPA, serotonin, melatonin—can be visualized in sections of pineal glands [17]. Typically, dissected brains are frozen in liquid nitrogen. A block of the frozen tissue is cut out and freeze-dried. Then the block of tissue is sectioned. Sections of freeze-dried tissue are exposed to gaseous formaldehyde. The reactions produce fluorescent molecules called the *fluorophores*. The location of the fluorophores (which reflects the location of the monoamines) is observed with a fluorescence microscope or a light microscope equipped with special lamps and filters for fluorescence micro-scopy. These microscopes supply light of particular wavelengths (e.g., 410 nm for catecholamines) which cause the molecules to emit visible light (e.g., at 480 nm). Noradrenaline characteristically has a green fluorescence, and serotonin has a yellow fluorescence. Fluorescence microscopy can be combined with electron microscopy so that the structures that contain the fluorophores can be identified. From the characteristic excitation and emission spectra, the identification of the molecules can be made by techniques of microspectrofluorometry. Variations in the techniques used for tissue preparation sometimes include perfusion of the animals (e.g., with paraformaldehyde and glyoxylic acid), which promotes fluorescence intensity of the different molecules.

Yet another means of detection of molecules (e.g., peptides and proteins) in sections is immunohistochemistry. This method is de-pendent on the production of an antibody of the molecule which may be present in the pineal cells.

2.3.4 Autoradiography

In a typical experiment, a compound labeled with tritium or carbon 14 is injected into an animal, sometimes under some specific experimen-tal conditions. Subsequently, the animal is killed and its pineal tissue is frozen and sectioned. The frozen sections are dried and apposed to photographic emulsion. The period of time of the exposure may be short (a few days) or long (many months). The films are developed and silver grain patterns show where the radioactivity localized. Relative amounts of radioactivity can be quantified by counting the silver grains or measuring their density.

2.4 Surgical Methods

Surgeries done in pineal studies include removal of pineal tissue as well as extirpation or lesion of other structures—photoreceptors, endocrine glands, brain regions, ganglia, and so forth. Most attempts at pineal ablation have so far utilized the surgical approach. However, an alternative has been to make antibodies to pineal constituents (e.g., melatonin) [12]. The antibodies have two advantages: (1) they should affect the molecule whether it is of nonpineal or pineal origin; and (2) the potential for chemically specific ablations exists.

2.4.1 Pinealectomy

Pinealectomy (PINx, pinx) is a common surgical method. Many small animals (rodents, birds) have pineal glands whose club-shaped tops

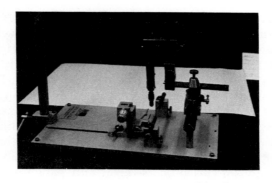

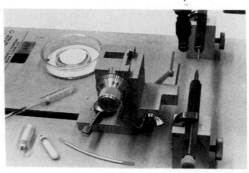

Figure 2.2 The photograph illustrates the Hoffman Reiter pinealectomy instrument in which the animal's head is held stationary with ear bars and a circle of skull is drilled with a trephine. The arrangement of the dental drill driving the trephine in the instrument makes it possible to do one animal after another with the same settings. On the base of the instrument rest (counter-clockwise) are: an organ culture dish used for in vitro pineal cultures, a glass microhomogenizer used to puree pineals, a programmed microinfusion capsule, a miniosmotic pump, and a Silastic® capsule.

are accessible at the meninges just below the skull. Practiced investigators pinealectomize animals rapidly (1–2 minutes) with no mortality (sparrows [3, 8], hamsters [9], rats [10]).

In the procedures the animal is first anesthetized. The head of the animal is immobilized in a holder fixed with ear bars and a method of trapping the teeth or beaks (Fig. 2.2). The immobilization is necessary for drilling through the skull. An incision is made along the midline in the skin over the top of the skull (scalp) running about 0.5 in. from anterior (level of the eyes) to posterior (base of the skull). The skin over the skull is loose in most animals and the skull can be exposed by pulling the skin laterally.

The location for drilling is based on landmarks provided by the sutures on top of the skull. Pineals are located in the midline beneath the point where the sutures converge. In some species muscle masses must be scraped back from the region to permit drilling. For mammals with skulls that have relatively even thickness in the pineal region, the hole is drilled with a trephine (a disk drill or small circular saw) with a collar to control the depth of penetration. The trephine does not work well in birds, however, because the skull in the pineal region has uneven thickness and the bone has a spongy structure. In birds, a circular piece of skull can be drilled freehand. In small animals, jewelers' loupes or a boom-type dissecting microscope are useful for the drilling and pinealectomy. It is best in either case to remove the bone disk before completely drilling through it, exposing the meninges above the brain over the pineal region. The operation is virtually bloodless to this point.

The pineal gland is usually not visible (it is only 0.3–0.5 mm in diameter in a sparrow or hamster) because of the surrounding venous sinuses. Hamster pineal glands can be removed by "inserting an open pair of watchmaker's forceps into the junction of the two sinuses, grasping the stalk and removing gland and stalk in one motion" [9]. To get the sparrow pineal, three tears are made with microscissors or sharp forceps over the brain in the meninges surrounding the pineal region. In making these tears, the venous sinuses are avoided so that bleeding does not occur. The pineal gland and the piece of overlying meninges are grasped with fine mouse tooth forceps (at this point bleeding begins, so the grasp must be maintained), and the remaining meninges are cut with microscissors. The meninges and pineal gland are removed by pulling gently (so as not to break the stalk, which can usually be seen as it emerges). Bleeding is prevented (in either hamsters or sparrows) by quick replacement of the bone disk and the application of moderate pressure. The skin flaps are sutured or stapled. Postoperative treatments have generally not been required.

Sham operations include removing a bone disk and tearing meninges, but leaving the blood vessels and pineal gland undisturbed. As will be explained in later chapters, the pineal is not the only source of melatonin, so that pinealectomy should not be assumed to remove all melatonin.

2.4.2 Pineal transplants

Transplanting pineals (between animals) was successful when the pineal glands were transplanted to the anterior chamber of the eye [27], although other loci have been used. In the procedure, the recipient is anesthetized. A slit is made near the edge of the cornea of the eye. The pineal gland from the donor is inserted through the slit with fine forceps and placed at the edge of the iris. The implant is thus visible and its postoperative progress can be followed by subsequent examination of the eye. Revascularization and reinnervation occur.

The donor pineal (obtained from a freshly killed animal or removed surgically) is prepared by removing meninges and blood. Some investigators feel that success is enhanced if the pineal gland is snipped a few times with fine scissors before implantation. The procedure has several advantages in addition to simplicity and the implant visualization: (1) the transplanted pineal is in a position where it can be exposed to light-dark treatments; (2) more than one pineal can be implanted; (3) the implant can be removed by enucleation (surgical removal of the eye); and (4) the recipient may be unoperated or pinealectomized. Sham operations are similar without actual implantation of pineal tissue.

2.4.3 Superior cervical ganglionectomy

Superior cervical ganglionectomy (SCGx) is used with species, such as rats, whose pineals are controlled by the superior cervical ganglia. Ganglionectomized rats can be obtained commercially or the ganglia can be removed quickly (in less than 5 minutes) from adult or neonatal rats in the following manner [5]: The rats are anesthetized. The ventral neck is opened with a 2–3 cm incision. Salivary glands and muscles are separated with a blunt probe. The omohyoid muscle is cut, revealing the carotid artery and associated structures including the superior cervical ganglion. The carotid artery is grasped with a forceps and the ganglion is dissected free with watchmaker's forceps, being careful to get the entire ganglion. The operation is repeated on the other side. Jewelers' loupes are used to magnify the surgical site. The incision is closed with surgical staples. With practice, there was no mortality for adult rats; survival rate for pups was 70% with mortality due to surgical trauma and/or maternal cannibalism.

Successful ganglionectomy can be assessed immediately following recovery from anesthesia. Ptosis (drooping of the eyelid) means that a ganglion was removed. Sham operations are the same except for grasping the carotid artery and removing the ganglion.

2.4.4 Suprachiasmatic lesions

Suprachiasmatic lesions (SCNx) are effective in species in which the suprachiasmatic nuclei of the hypothalamus direct pineal melatonin synthesis. These bilateral structures at the base of the brain (Fig. 2.3) can be manipulated with electrical lesion or knife cuts. An anesthetized animal is placed in a stereotaxic instrument and bilateral electrolytic lesions are placed using coordinates from brain atlases. Alternatively, cuts can be made with a Halasz knife. A bent wire is placed within a tube and the end of the tube is implanted stereotaxically. The wire is extruded from the tube in the desired location and rotated in an arc to make a cut. Location of the lesion is determined by histological examination of the brain upon completion of the experi-

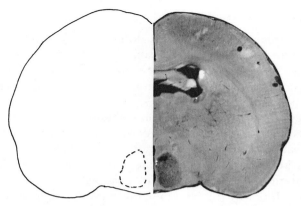

Figure 2.3 Half of a section through a brain with the other half sketched in to show the location of the suprachiasmatic nuclei (*dashed line*), in a rodent.

ment. Sham operations are lesions deliberately placed outside the nuclei and/or the "misses" found in the histological examination.

2.4.5 Laparotomy and vaginal smears

The pineal has a role in reproduction. In assessing this role the size and conditions of the gonads are often measured. Gonad size can be determined by (1) wet weights of gonads of freshly killed animals, (2) weights of gonads preserved in formalin, or (3) caliper measurements of length and diameter. In some experimental protocols, progress of gonad size changes can be followed by laparotomy. In this procedure, a small incision is made and the gonads are inspected and even measured (length and/or diameter) in situ. Estimates of testis weight can be made from standard series of similar measurements of dimensions and weights made on testes from killed animals. Further assessment of gonad function (e.g., whether or not sperm are being made) is possible from histological examination. An assessment of female reproductive function can also be made (usually in small rodents) by examining vaginal smears. The cytology of the smears reflects the stage of the female reproductive cycle and is an indicator of the presence of estrogen (which causes cornified cells to appear in the smears).

2.5 Pharmacological Methods

Original efforts to replace pineal function focussed on pineal extracts, but most of the recent replacement studies have utilized pure hormones, such as melatonin. A myriad of other chemicals have been used to study the pineal.

2.5.1 Melatonin replacement

Melatonin replacement has been done a number of ways to solve problems with solubility and the timed nature of its function.

Melatonin has compensated for some deficiencies resulting from pinealectomy. However, melatonin is relatively insoluble in water. It is soluble in ethanol, oil, and waxes. Low concentrations of melatonin can be gotten into aqueous solution if the melatonin is first dissolved in a small quantity of ethanol. In experiments with melatonin, then, controls treated with vehicle (ethanol, ethanol water, oil, wax, etc.) are necessary. Melatonin has been effective when administered orally (pills or solutions), injected, and in capsules.

Experimenters who injected melatonin produced negative or equivocal results for years. Melatonin is more effective at some times of day than others, so that the timing of the injections must be taken into consideration for more meaningful results. Repetition of injections (at the same time every day) may be required.

Long-term continuous melatonin administration has been achieved with pellets and capsules. In one method of making pellets, melatonin can be dissolved in beeswax. The warm solution is sucked into a piece of tubing. The cooled tubing is cut into sections that constitute the pellets. Controls are similar pellets without melatonin. In a second method previously developed for reproductive steroids [24] silicon Silastic® capsules are prepared. Silicon tubing is plugged at one end with liquid silicon, which is allowed to cure. The tube is then packed with crystalline melatonin and the other end is plugged with liquid silicon. The dose is controlled by varying the length of the capsule. Investigators have estimated that a 50-mm capsule delivers 26 μg of melatonin per day. Controls are empty capsules.

Timed programs of melatonin can be administered automatically by programmed microinfusion. In this ingenious technique, a program of melatonin is loaded into capillary tubing which has been preformed into a coil [15]. The microsyringes alternately force separate individual components of the desired infusate via a manifold placed so that they are linearly arranged in the tube. A solution of melatonin dissolved in phenolsulfonphthalein (PSP, an indicator) alternates with an inert solution with which it cannot mix (e.g., light mineral oil). The program can be examined because the melatonin solution is colored red. The coiled program tube is then placed around an osmotic minipump, which forces solution out at a given rate (e.g., 1 μl/hr) over 1–4 weeks. The pump with its coil is implanted subcutaneously. Controls are programmed pumps without the melatonin. Indicator in the animals' urine provides confirmation of the proper operation of the pump and program.

One common feature of melatonin replacement studies has been that large doses of melatonin have been required. As a result,

TABLE 2.1 N-acetyltransferase (NAT) response to isoproterenol in vivo

Species	NAT (pmol/pineal/hr)	
	Control	Isoproterenol
Sparrow	177 +/− 31	225 +/− 27
Chick	3094 +/− 191	2723 +/− 394
Hamster	294 +/− 66	438 +/− 55
Rat	185 +/− 16	2635 +/− 280
Rat (pump)	500 +/− 200	7900 +/− 190

Note: Isoproterenol injections (10 mg/kg) raised NAT in 3-4h in rats but not sparrows, hamsters, or chickens. Isoproterenol also raised NAT in rats when it was administered with miniosmotic pumps for 8-16h.

researchers worry that the effects are "pharmacological" and do not mimic normal physiology. However, melatonin is produced in large amounts and it has a high turnover rate so that the "effective" doses at the level of the target organ could be physiological.

2.5.2 Pineal stimulation and inhibition

Stimulation and inhibition of pineal glands can be obtained with a variety of compounds. In a typical experiment, a drug (or a combination of drugs or a sequence of drugs) is injected and the subsequent effect on the pineal (enzymes or hormones) is measured. Controls are similar injections of the diluents used for the drugs. In these studies, time of day and light-dark conditions are important parts of the protocols. Table 2.1 shows the results of an experiment of this type that measured the effect of injected isoproterenol on N-acetyltransferase (NAT) activity. Of the four species studied, rats responded most dramatically to the stimulus.

2.6 In Vitro Techniques

Experiments involving the living animal (in vivo experiments) have a drawback. An observed effect can be due to a secondary, unidentified process. That is, it is not possible to know whether an injected drug that stimulates the pineal gland to produce melatonin acts directly on the pineal or exerts its influence through a secondary structure that in turn causes the pineal response. This problem is obviated in studies where the living pineal or pineal cells are isolated and supported with nourishing medium and essential gases to mimic the normal blood supply. The disadvantage to culture techniques is that cultured tissues may produce responses that have no complement in the

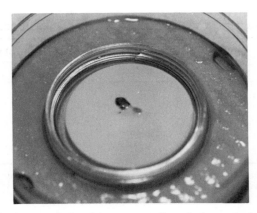

Figure 2.4 A chick pineal gland (*center*, stalk and choroid plexus usually not included extending to the right) resting on a millipore filter to illustrate culture and anatomy of the chick pineal gland. The millipore filter is 2.5 cm in diameter.

normal physiology of the animal. Responses in culture that have correlates in the normal physiology of the animal are sought for experimentation.

2.6.1 Organ culture

Intact pineal glands can be obtained from freshly killed animals, cleaned of adhering meninges and blood, and placed into culture. Organ cultures [11] work for the pineals of small animals because the small size of the gland permits gas and nutrient exchange for at least the outer layers of cells. In a typical technique (which has been used for chick, rat, hamster, and sparrow pineals), one to three pineals are placed on millipore filters that are 2.5 cm in diameter (Fig. 2.4). The filter rests atop a 1-ml well which has 1 ml of culture medium (containing amino acids, salts, antibiotics, and vitamins). Covered culture dishes are placed in a water-jacketed incubator to maintain temperature at 37°C. A gas (95% oxygen, 5% carbon dioxide) atmosphere interacting with the culture medium buffer provides a pH of 7.4 for the glands. The cultures last for several days or more. Histological examination of pineals subjected to culture revealed some necrosis (cell death) in the centers of the glands, which is probably due to insufficient gas or nutrient exchange.

Experimental treatments can be applied to the glands—light or dark, addition of stimulating or inhibiting drugs, or provision of radioactive substrates (e.g., tryptophan, a precursor of serotonin and melatonin). Measurements can be made on the pineals (uptake of radiolabeled compounds, melatonin, enzyme activities) or on the culture medium (melatonin, production of radiolabeled products).

TABLE 2.2 N-acetyltransferase (NAT) response to norepinephrine in vitro

Species	NAT (pmol/pineal/hr)	
	Control	Norepinephrine 10^{-3}M in culture medium
Sparrow	69 +/− 25	49 +/− 17
Chick	2258 +/− 403	1187 +/− 97
Hamster	86 +/− 36	137 +/− 57
Rat	100 +/− 17	1756 +/− 14

Table 2.2 shows the results of an organ culture experiment that measured the effects of norepinephrine on NAT activity in pineal cultures.

2.6.2 Superfusion culture

Using peristaltic pumps, it is possible to provide a constant supply of fresh culture medium to pineals and to collect fractions of effluent medium that have been exposed to a pineal [23]. This is called *superfusion*. Single pineals are placed in vessels designed to permit influx and outflow of medium. Some investigators recommend "mincing" the glands because small pieces might permit better gas and nutrient exchange. The superfused glands can be subjected to treatments (such as drugs or light-dark) and measurements (e.g., of melatonin) can be made on the fractions to obtain time profiles.

2.6.3 Cell culture

Pineal cells can be grown in layers [18] or in suspensions [6]. To grow pineal cells in a monolayer (Fig. 2.5), the pineal (e.g., from a freshly killed rat or chick) is cleaned of adherent meninges and vascular tissue. The gland is then teased into smaller pieces (explants) with fine forceps. The pieces from several glands are dispersed into tissue culture plates containing medium. The cultures are maintained at pH 7.0 and 37°C in a humidified incubator with 5% carbon dioxide in air. The cells migrate from the explants and, after a couple of weeks, can be dissociated into single-cell suspensions with a trypsin solution. The number of cells in the suspension can be counted with a hemacytometer. The suspensions can be replated to grow even monolayers of cells. The appearance of the cells is observable throughout the culturing process with an inverted microscope. The cells can be treated with drugs (e.g., isoproterenol), and cells harvested with a rubber policeman can be subjected to measurements (e.g., of enzyme activities).

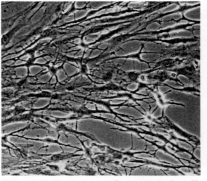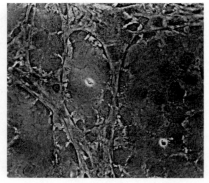

Figure 2.5 Views of rat pineal cells in monolayer cultures. (Photos courtesy of Nathanson, Hilfer, and Binkley.)

The advantage of the cell culture technology is that events can be attributed to particular kinds of cells. The disadvantage is that the proportions of cell types in the population of cells in culture may not reflect the composition of cells in the pineal in situ.

2.6.4 Homogenates

For enzyme assays and other measurements, pineals are homogenized (in glass homogenizers consisting of a tube with a fitted pestle) or sonicated in solutions (typically a 1 mg pineal in 30 or 50 µl of 6.8 phosphate buffer) to break open the cells. The homogenates may be centrifuged to pellet the debris. The properties of pineal enzymes can be studied in the homogenates or supernatants. Treatments include temperature (37°C or cold) inhibiting compounds, and substances that "protect" enzyme activity.

2.7 Indole Assays

Indoleamines in pineal extracts have been measured with bioassays [16, 21] and various chemical techniques [13, 14, 19, 20].

2.7.1 Tissue handling

For biochemical measurements, pineals must be specially handled. Some of the enzymes, especially N-acetyltransferase, are unstable at body temperature. Pineals for biochemistry are usually rapidly dissected (in a minute or less) and frozen. While many investigators have traditionally used dim red light for killing the animals, hoping to reduce inhibitory effects, red light should not be considered a "safelight" or a substitute for rapid killing. It is practicable to freeze small pineal glands in the 0.1-ml wells of plastic microtest plates precooled on dry ice. The glands stick by freezing to the wells. While it is preferable to make chemical assays within a week, pineals kept frozen at $-70°C$ retain most of their enzyme activity for years. Frost-free freezers are not recommended for pineal storage as the glands desiccate.

2.7.2 Indole separation

Pineal indoles can be separated with extraction and chromatography. Melatonin can be extracted from incubation medium or pineal homogenate by shaking the sample with 5–10 ml of chloroform saturated with borate buffer (pH 10.0). The chloroform is then washed (e.g., with borate buffer). Evaporation of the chloroform leaves melatonin in the residue, which can be redissolved in various solutions.

Thin-layer chromatography has been used to separate indoles. In one two-dimensional chromatographic technique used to separate N-acetylserotonin and melatonin from serotonin, methoxyindoles, and hydroxyindoles, the sample is spotted in the bottom left corner of a glass plate coated with silica gel. The plate is developed in chloroform, methanol and glacial acetic acid (90:10:1). The plate is then turned 90° and run in the second direction in ethyl acetate. Indole spots are visible under ultraviolet light.

High-performance liquid chromatography (HPLC) has also been used to separate indoles including melatonin. A liquid phase (e.g., citrate-acetate buffer) is forced at high pressure over a column containing a solid phase (e.g., cation exchange resin). The indoles separate and come off the column in fractions. Molecules can be detected electrochemically or spectrofluorometrically.

In gas chromatography (GC), a gas phase is forced through a column containing a stationary liquid phase and separated molecules are monitored in the effluent. Detection procedures include electron-capture (GC-EC) and mass spectrometric detection (GC-MS). The latter technique permits absolute identification of a molecule.

2.7.3 Melatonin assay

Melatonin bioassays are based on skin color lightening properties of lower vertebrates. For the most part, the bioassays have been replaced by radioimmunoassays.

McCord and Allen [16] fed pineals to tadpoles and found that, within 30 minutes, the color of their dark skin lightened so as to become translucent. This response is the basis for melatonin bioassays (Fig. 2.6). In one of these assays [21], *Rana pipiens* larvae are used on the 12th day after fertilization (developmental stage 25). The tadpoles are cultured in LD 15:9 (lights on at 6 A.M.) and are optimally sensitive from 1 to 4 P.M. Ten such light-adapted tadpoles are placed in 2-ml samples of melatonin solution (standards or unknowns) in disposable 15-ml beakers. The beakers are illuminated on a white background. After 30 minutes, 2 ml of formalin are added to kill and fix the tadpoles. The tadpoles are examined under a dissecting microscope; specifically the melanophores are examined in an area on the left side of the head between the eye and mouth. The degree of dispersion of pigment in the melanophores is compared visually to standard melanophore appearances ("indexes") in order to assign numerical values. Melatonin results in aggregation of the pigment (reduced amount of dispersion) and lightens the overall appearance of the tadpoles.

Quay [19, 20] used spectrofluorometric techniques to separate pineal indoles. First, he applied selective extraction techniques to isolate indoles (e.g., melatonin is extracted with p-cymeme and an alkaline solution). Next, he quantitated them with the fluorescence the molecules exhibit in strong mineral acid. To measure the fluorescence (which is emitted at 540–550 nm) the samples are activated with light at 295 nm. A fluorometer is used to make the measurement.

Radioimmunoassay (RIA), measurement of hormones with antibodies and radioactive materials using the method that was developed by Yalow and Berson [26], has been applied to the pineal gland [1, 22]. There are now a large number of melatonin RIAs similar in principle but different in detail and several are commercially available. In the assays, antisera containing antibodies to melatonin-protein molecules are reacted with samples and with radioactive melatonin tracers (triated or iodinated). If a sample contains melatonin, the native melatonin competes with the tracer for sites on the antibody. In a typical melatonin RIA, samples are extracted with chloroform and washed with sodium bicarbonate buffer to remove interfering molecules. The chloroform is evaporated under nitrogen and the purified samples (containing melatonin) are redissolved and washed with petroleum ether. Aliquots of the samples and standard melatonin solutions are then mixed with ^{125}I-labeled melatonin analog (tracer) and antisera containing antibodies that react with melatonin. After about 70 hours of incubation at 4°C, the antigen-antibody complex is precipitated with ethanol. The solution is centrifuged and the pellet is counted in a gamma counter. Melatonin is determined in "unknowns" by comparing the radioactivity with values obtained for known concentrations of melatonin. Sometimes it is necessary to dilute samples to get them in the range of detection of the assay. Validation of the melatonin RIA is required when a new type of tissue sample is to be assessed. Validation is accomplished by adding pure melatonin to tissue samples, then measuring "recovery" in a subsequent RIA. Melatonin is difficult to measure in blood of some species because of low levels and, possibly, because of interfering substances.

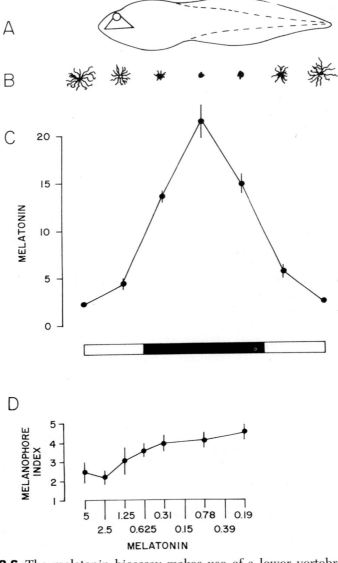

Figure 2.6 The melatonin bioassay makes use of a lower vertebrate (e.g., tadpoles of *Rana pipiens or Xenopus laevis*). The tadpoles (A) exhibit dark or light coloration due to changes in the distribution of pigment containing organelles (melanosomes) in skin cells (melanophores). The melanophores (B) are diagrammatically represented over a graph of chick pineal melatonin and correlate with the way they appear at the times indicated in the graph (C) that was measured with a bioassay. In the dark-time, homogenates of the chick pineals aggregated the pigment, producing dot-like melanophores (punctate), and in the light-time the chick pineal homogenates spread out (dispersed) the pigment in the melanophores. A dose-response curve for pure melatonin is graphed in D. The numbers on the ordinate represent the melanophore (Hogben) index for classifying melanophore dispersion. (Unpublished data collected by Binkley, MacBride, Klein, Ralph, Rubin, Mosher, and White).

2.8 Enzymes

Pineal enzymes, especially those that synthesize melatonin, have been studied and measured under a variety of environmental conditions. Tissue handling is similar to that discussed for indoles. A few examples of the assays are presented here to illustrate the principles for assay of pineal enzymes. The assays here all measure "activity" of an enzyme (i.e., how much product can be formed from a given substrate), not numbers of molecules of the enzyme. Units for the enzyme activities are given in product formed per pineal gland (or weight pineal or amount pineal protein) per unit of time.

2.8.1 Tryptophan hydroxylase

Tryptophan hydroxylase catalyzes the conversion of tryptophan to 5-hydroxytryptophan. In a typical assay [11], a whole pineal gland is incubated for 60 minutes at 37°C in 60 μl of Ringer's solution with ^{14}C-radiolabeled tryptophan and m-hydroxybenzylhydrazine (a decarboxylase inhibitor). Then 1 ml of acetone and hydrochloric acid with unlabeled 5-hydroxytryptophan are used to stop the reaction. The solution is homogenized and centrifuged. An aliquot of the supernatant is dried, redissolved, and chromatographed with thin-layer chromatography. Ninhydrin spray makes the spots visible and the 5-hydroxytryptophan spot can be scraped off and counted with a scintillation counter.

2.8.2 N-acetyltransferase

N-acetyltransferase (NAT, NATase, SNAT) catalyzes the acetylation of serotonin to N-acetylserotonin utilizing acetyl coenzyme A (acetyl CoA) as the acetyl donor. There are two assays for N-acetylserotonin. The first measures melatonin and N-acetylserotonin production from serotonin, the "natural" substrate of the enzyme. The second measures the production of N-acetyltryptamine from an "artificial" substrate, tryptamine. The two assays do not give identical quantitative results, which is a factor to consider when comparing data.

Serotonin substrate ^{14}C-radiolabeled serotonin and acetyl CoA are mixed with pineal homogenate [11]. It is important for this assay that the homogenate (in 6.8 phosphate buffer) be prepared at 4°C and that the pineals (stored frozen at −70°C) are minimally thawed only to permit their removal from the storage plates. The assay is a "micro" assay so that total volume of the reaction mixture is only 20 μl. The pineal samples and similar tubes with buffer but no pineal ("blanks") are incubated at 37°C block heaters for precisely 10 minutes. The reaction is stopped with alcohol-hydrochloric acid containing ascorbic acid and "carrier" indole molecules. A sufficient amount of the reactant (serotonin) and products (N-acetylserotonin, melatonin, hydroxyindoleacetic acid, hydroxytryptophol, methoxyindoleacetic acid, methoxytryptophol—the "carriers") must be added to the mixture to permit visualization of the spots in the chromatography. The reaction tubes are centrifuged. The reactant (serotonin) and the now radiolabeled products are separated with thin-layer chromatography. The spots representing N-acetylserotonin and melatonin (products of N-acetyltransferase) are scraped off and counted together as a measure of enzyme activity.

Tryptamine substrate Fifty microliters of pineal homogenate (cold, 6.8 phosphate buffer) are mixed in 1.5 ml plastic centrifuge tubes with tryptamine and ^{14}C-acetyl CoA [4, 7]. The mixture is incubated at 37°C for 20 minutes in block heaters and is stopped by addition of chloroform saturated with buffer. The 5-hydroxytryptamine (product) is extracted into chloroform by shaking for 5 minutes at room temperature, centrifuging at 3600 rpm for 1 minute, and removing the aqueous layer. The chloroform, washed with buffer, is evaporated to dryness in a counting vial and counted in a scintillation counter.

2.8.3 Hydroxyindole-O-methyltransferase

Hydroxyindole-O-methyltransferase (HIOMT) catalyzes the methylation of N-acetylserotonin to produce melatonin. S-adenosylmethionine is the methyl donor. The enzyme is assayed [2, 11] by mixing pineal homogenate with the substrates, N-acetylserotonin and ^{14}C-S-adenosylmethionine. After 60 minutes at 37°C, the reaction is stopped with borate buffer (pH 10.0). The radiolabeled melatonin is extracted into chloroform, which is washed, evaporated to dryness, and counted in a scintillation counter. The optimal concentration of the reactants is dependent upon species.

2.8.4 Enzyme isolation

Early attempts have been made to purify and characterize the enzymes found in pineals. Limitations include the small size of the gland, the fact that some of the enzyme activities vary with time of day, and the instability of the enzymes. However, progress has been made using protecting compounds to preserve the enzyme activity. In addition to telling us about the nature of the enzymes and how they work, successful enzyme isolation permits the generation of antibodies to that enzyme. These antibodies can be used to determine the locus of the enzyme and to study its function.

2.9 Environmental Lighting

Because pineal function is dependent upon light and dark, specification of the light sources used in experiments is necessary. There is no consensus as yet as to the "preferred" light source, but whatever light source is used should be described. A description includes as much information as possible: (1) the brand name, wattage, and bulb number; (2) the distance of the animals from the light source; and (3) the measured intensity in the region of the animals. Most investigators have used "white" or "full-spectrum" fluorescent lights (available commercially) and intensities in the range of 500–1500 lux for pineal experiments; a very few have used natural light.

The quality of the "dark" can be crucial to experimental results. The hamster gonad regression response is especially sensitive and even minor "light leaks" in the experimental room may block the response. Some investigators have used red light for the "dark" portion of a cycle (viewing red light as a "safe" light, especially in experiments with rats); however, animals such as chicks perceive red light. In addition to specification of the quality of light and dark, the timing of light and dark are programmed. For most studies, 24-hour timers are usually sufficient, but programmable timers and computers are also used to obtain more complex light and dark regimens.

In considering the effects of light and dark on pineal function of various species, some thought should be given to the organisms' natural environmental lighting conditions. The sun is the principal light source and it is much brighter than light sources used in the laboratory. Diurnal (day-active) birds are by necessity exposed to sun or shade throughout the day. Some nocturnal (night-active) animals retreat to burrows in the daytime where they may experience dark or very dim light. Burrowing animals may expose themselves to the sun only at dawn and/or dusk. Humans use artificial lighting to extend natural lighting and to shift the time of light, and they use watches and clocks for time cues.

REFERENCES

1. Arendt, J., L. Paunier, and P. Sizonenko. 1975. Melatonin radioimmunoassay. *J. Clin. Endocrinol. Metab.* 40:347–350.
2. Axelrod, J., and H. Weissbach. 1961. Purification and properties of hydroxyindole-O-methyltransferase. *J. Biol. Chem.* 236:211–213.
3. Binkley, S., E. Kluth, and M. Menaker. 1971. Pineal function in sparrow: Circadian rhythms and body temperature. *Science* 174:311–314.
4. Brammer, M., and S. Binkley. 1981. Pineal glands of immature rats: Rise and fall of N-acetyltransferase activity in vitro. *J. Neurobiol.* 12:167–173.

5. Brammer, M., S. Binkley, and K. Mosher. 1982. The rise and fall of pineal N-acetyltransferase in vitro: Neural regulation in the developing rat. *J. Neurobiol.* 13:487–494.

6. Buda, M., and D. Klein. 1978. A suspension culture of pinealocytes: Regulation of N-acetyltransferase activity. *Endocrinology* 103:1483–1493.

7. Deguchi, T. 1972. Sensitive assay for serotonin N-acetyltransferase activity in rat pineal. *Anal. Biochem.* 50:174–179.

8. Gaston, S. 1969. The effect of pinealectomy on the circadian activity rhythm of the house sparrow, *Passer domesticus.* Ph.D. diss., Univ. of Texas.

9. Hoffman, R., and R. Reiter. 1965. Rapid pinealectomy in hamsters and other small rodents. *Anat. Rec.* 153:19–22.

10. Kitay, J., and M. Altschule. 1954. *The pineal gland: A review of the physiologic literature.* Cambridge, Mass.: Harvard Univ. Press. Pp. 8–9.

11. Klein, D. 1972. Melatonin synthesis. In *The thyroid and biogenic amines,* ed., I. Rall and J. Kopin, pp. 550–568. Amsterdam: North-Holland.

12. Knigge, K., and M. Sheridan. 1976. Pineal function in hamsters bearing melatonin antibodies, *Life Sci.* 19:1235–1238.

13. Lynch, H. 1983. Assay methodology. In *The pineal gland,* ed. R. Relkin, pp. 129–149. New York: Elsevier.

14. Lynch, H., Y. Ozaki, and R. Wurtman. 1978. The measurement of melatonin in mammalian tissues and body fluids. *J. Neural Trans. Suppl.* 13:251–264.

15. Lynch, H., R. Rivest, and R. Wurtman. 1980. Artificial induction of melatonin rhythms by programmed microinfusion. *Neuroendocrinology* 31:106–111.

16. McCord,, C. P., and F. P. Allen. 1917. Evidences associating pineal gland function with alterations in pigmentation. *J. Exp. Zoo.* 23:207–224.

17. Møller, M., and Th. Van Veen. 1981. Fluorescence histochemistry of the pineal gland. In *The pineal gland I: Anatomy and biochemistry,* ed. R. Reiter, pp. 69–93. Boca Raton, Fla.: CRC Press.

18. Nathanson, M., S. Binkley, and R. Hilfer. 1977. Cultivation of mammalian pineal cells: Retention of organization and function in tissue culture. *In Vitro* 13:843–848.

19. Quay, W. 1963. Differential extraction for the spectrophotofluorometric measurement of diverse 5-hydroxy- and 5-methoxyindoles. *Anal. Biochem.* 5:51–59.

20. ———. 1964. Circadian and estrous rhythms in pineal melatonin and 5-hydroxyindole-3-acetic acid. *Proc. Soc. Exp. Biol. Med.* 115:710–713.

21. Ralph, C., and H. Lynch. 1970. A quantitative melatonin bioassay. *Gen. Comp. Endocrinol.* 15:334–338.

22. Rollag, M., and G. Niswender. 1976. Radioimmunoassay of serum concentrations of melatonin in sheep exposed to different lighting regimens. *Endocrinology* 98:482–489.

23. Takahashi, J., and M. Menaker. 1980. Circadian rhythms of melatonin release from individual superfused chicken pineal glands in vitro. *Proc. Nat. Acad. Sci. USA* 77:2319–2322.

24. Turek, F., C. Desjardins, and M. Menaker. 1976. Melatonin: Effects on circadian locomotor rhythm of sparrows. *Science* 194:1441–1443.

25. Vollrath, L. 1981. *The pineal organ.* Berlin: Springer-Verlag.

26. Yalow R., and S. Berson. 1960. Immunoassay of endogenous plasma insulin in man. *J. Clin. Invest.* 39:1157–1175.

27. Zimmerman, N., and M. Menaker. 1979. The pineal gland: A pacemaker within the circadian system of the house sparrow. *Proc. Natl. Acad. Sci. USA* 76:999–1003.

3

Pineal Anatomy

"From a phylogenetic aspect, few organs have undergone such change in form and cytological differentiation as the pineal organ. Consequently it is very difficult to present a short comparative review that gives a clear, general picture and still does not treat the important facts too briefly. Among the lower vertebrates the pineal organ is a sense organ containing receptor and nerve cells; in some forms it resembles an eye. In reptiles and birds and even in some lower forms a structural change to an endocrine gland is apparent. Comparative analysis is difficult because the roof of the vertebrate brain, from which the pineal organ is derived, gives rise, in the very same region, to still other organ-like differentiations. One of these is the parapineal organ, which is very closely associated with the pineal organ.

As shown by fossil skulls, both of these organs are phylogenetically very old having appeared first in certain Devonian (and Silurian) tetrapods, the ancestors of recent amphibians and lizards."

A. Oksche [13]

TABLE 3.1 Anatomical changes in the Gerbil Pineal over 24 hours

Time	Nadirs	Peaks
7 Light	Pinealocyte SER volume Pinealocyte lysozomes volume Pinealocyte microtubules volume Pinealocyte RER + ribosomes volume Pinealocyte mitochondria volume	
9 Light	Pinealocyte mean caliper diameter Pinealocyte nuclear volume Pinealocyte cytoplasmic volume	
11 Light	Pinealocyte cell volume Mean nuclear profile diameter Nucleoli Vv	
13 Light	Glial cell Vv Concretions and vacuoles Vv Other Vv Pinealocyte cytosol volume Pinealocyte secretory vesicles volume Pinealocyte Golgi apparatus volume	
15 Light	Pinealocyte nuclei Vv	Pinealocyte cytoplasm Vv
17 Light		Glial cell nuclei Vv
19 Light	Pinealocyte DCV	Pinealocyte mean nuclear profile diameter

Time	Nadirs	Peaks
	Pinealocyte synaptic ribbon volume	Pinealocyte mean caliper diameter
		Pinealocyte nuclear volume
		Pinealocyte DVC volume
		Pinealocyte secretory vesicle volume
		Pinealocyte microtubule volume
		Pinealocyte subsurface cisternae volume
		Pinealocyte synaptic ribbon volume
		Pinealocyte Golgi apparatus volume
21 Dark	Glial cell nuclei Vv	Pinealocyte nucleoli volume
		Pinealocyte SER volume
		Pinealocyte RER + ribosomes volume
		Pinealocyte synaptic ribbon volume
23 Dark		Glial cell cytoplasm Vv
1 Dark	Pinealocyte subsurface cisternae volume	Pinealocyte nuclei Vv
		Concretions and vacuoles Vv
		Other Vv
		Pinealocyte cytosol volume
		Pinealocyte mitochrondria volume
3 Dark		Pinealocyte cell volume
5 Dark	Pinealocyte cytoplasm Vv	Pinealocyte DCV volume
		Pinealocyte lysozome volume
		Pinealocyte synaptic ribbon volume

Source: Based on data from Welsh, Cameron, and Reiter [24].
Note: The table has been constructed from data provided in a morphometric analysis of the gerbil pineal over a period of 24 hours. On the left, the time and the light or dark condition (of LD 14:10) are arranged vertically in chronological order. Those anatomical parameters whose values were low are listed under "Nadirs," and the anatomical parameters that were high are listed under "Peaks." Thus, most parameters appear at least twice. A striking change (from nadirs to peaks) occurs in most of the parameters as dark approaches. The measurements noted "Vv" represent volume occupied by the structures in a known volume of tissue.

3.1 Variation

The principal characteristic of pineal anatomy is variation. There is diversity in both gross and microscopic anatomy. Pineal structure is peculiar to species, time of day, season, reproductive state (sex, pregnancy, ovarian cycle stage, puberty), and age. Table 3.1 shows how the microscopic anatomy of the gerbil pineal varies according to time of day and light-dark conditions.

3.2 Gross Anatomy

Pineal glands vary considerably in gross morphology in different species. The morphological differences may have functional significance. Classification schemes (which are beyond the scope of this book) are based on the pineal relationship to the corpus callosum, the pineal location with respect to the third ventricle, and the shape of the pineal [23]. In general, however, the pineal occurs as a single organ located in the fissures formed by the meeting of the cerebellum and cerebral hemispheres. A pine cone–shaped top may extend to the meninges just beneath the skull; an elongated stalk may reach inward to meet the choroid plexus. But, as stated above, each species has its own characteristic pineal gross anatomy. Differences between the pineal anatomy of a hamster and a lizard are diagrammed in Fig. 3.1.

First, the weight of the pineal gland is not necessarily proportional to the size of the animal. Voles, for example, have large pineal glands compared to mice and hamsters. According to Reiter [18], the largest pineal glands weigh in at 3500 mg (Weddell seals and walruses) and the smallest pineal glands, 0.2 mg, are found in *Mus musculus* (house mouse).

Second, the bulk of the pineal gland may be located just beneath the skull (as in sparrows or chicks) or it may be enfolded so that it lies underneath the cerebral hemispheres and cerebellum.

Third, the length, continuity, and/or thickness of the pineal stalk is not the same in all species—the stalk is long (about 0.5 cm) and thick in the rabbit; it is shorter (about 4 mm) and thinner in sparrows.

Fourth, in some species (e.g., hamsters) the pineal gland may be "segmented" or divided by a constriction into two parts: a "deep" pineal gland (dorsal posterior diencephalon) and a "superficial" pineal gland (beneath the surface of the skull and meninges at the juncture of the transverse and superior sagittal sinuses).

Fifth, the pineal gland may not exist as a structure discrete from brain (e.g., in crocodiles, alligators, anteaters, sloths, dugongs, and armadillos). In this last condition, however, there may be "pineal tissue" in the subcommissural region.

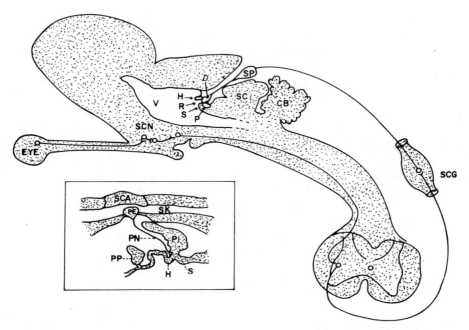

Figure 3.1 Diagrammatic representations of pineal anatomy showing deep and superficial structures as they might appear in animals such as a hamster, *above*, and a lizard, *below*. Structures are labeled as follows: *D*, deep pineal; *H*, habenular commissure or complex; *P*, posterior commissure; *PE*, parietal eye; *PN*, parietal nerve; *PP*, paraphysis; *R*, pineal recess; *S*, subcommissural organ; *SC*, superior colliculus; *SCG*, superior cervical ganglion; *SCN*, supra-chiasmatic nuclei; *V*, ventricle. Neural information is transmitted by a circuitous route beginning at the eye and ending at the pineal: eye → hypothalamus (SCN) → superior cervical ganglia → pineal. (Redrawn after diagrams by Reiter [18].)

Variation in gross anatomy of the pineal poses a problem for the surgical removal of the gland. While the superficial pineal may be accessible for extirpation, the deep pineal or functional equivalents of pineal cells may be capable of carrying on pineal function after superficial pinealectomy. In addition, other tissues (e.g., the retinas of some species) are capable of melatonin synthesis, which confounds experiments in which pinealectomy is used to remove the source of melatonin.

3.3 Histology

The light microscope (LM) has been a useful tool in following the development of the pineal, in comparing the anatomy of the pineal, and in verifying surgical success in pinealectomy with postmortem examination. For example, sparrow pineal tissue stains more darkly than surrounding brain with hematoxylin-eosin and this was used to verify pinealectomy in that species [3]. Under the light microscope, the pineal has an appearance that suggests glandular function; it does not look like brain, for example. Moreover, if care was taken in processing the pineal, so that its orientation is known, the pineal is not without structure—it has a top, bottom, left, right, front and back.

The light microscopist may note other organization that is characteristic of the pineal in addition to the arrangement of its stalk and body. For example, in the developing chick pineal (Fig. 3.2), cells line up in a layer (that appears to be one or two cells thick) along the length of the gland so as to form a cylinder in three dimensions (a so-called *primary follicle*). The same kinds of cells in a similar layer are organized in spheres in three dimensions (the spheres have been called secondary follicles, lobules, or rosettes). The layers that make up the follicles have a structure—there is an inner side (next to a space called the *lumen* or rudiment of a lumen) and an outer side. The tendency for pineal cells to organize into lobules has been noted in cell cultures as well as in sections of pineal.

3.4 Ultrastructure

Electron microscopy (TEM, transmission electron microscopy) has been employed to look closer at pineal cells. Cells of pineals are not identical (Fig. 3.3), and their peculiarities have been used to "typecast" them into categories. The organelles (e.g., mitochondria, Golgi bodies) and membranes that form the cells have also been examined.

3.4.1 Cell types

In examining the literature on cell types of the pineal gland (Figs. 3.3–3.8), the reader is reminded of the blind men trying to describe an elephant. In the case of the pineal, however, the men were not blind and there was more than one elephant. There is no single opinion of the cell types, and there is not a common nomenclature. One problem is the possibility that even when two cells look very different, they may in fact represent separate stages of the cell cycle or development of a single cell type. Another problem in sorting out pineal cells is that, in the gland, the cells are interdigitated.

Pévet [14] surveyed the literature on mammalian pineal glands and attempted a categorization. He divided the cells that make up the follicle layers by location. In his division, *first category cells* form the majority of pineal parenchymal cells and contain granular vesicles. *Second category cells*, found in fewer numbers alongside the first category cells, were near the perivascular or extracellular spaces.

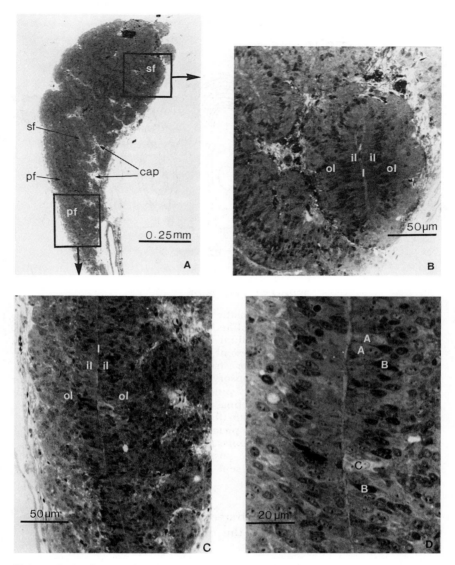

Figure 3.2 Photomicrograph of a chick (*Gallus domesticus*) pineal (LM, dark-time, CT 20). The sagittal section (part *A*) is through the entire gland, which is in its normal orientation with the anterior to the right. The posterior side of the lumen (or residual lumen) is lighter and the cells to the anterior side are darker. Successive magnifications of the primary follicle (*pf*) are shown in parts *C* (where *il* indicates inner layer; *ol*, outer layer; and *l*, lumen) and *D* (where three kinds of cells are shown: *A*, gray pinealocytes; *B*, dark glial cells; and *C*, cells that didn't stain). An estimate of the ratio of the three kinds of cells in the anterior primary follicle was *A*:*B*:*C*::27:9:1. Secondary follicles (*sf*) are present and an enlargement with the layers indicated is shown in part *B*. The orientation with respect to the primary follicle is a guide for the Figures 3.4–3.7. (Photos courtesy of Cioffi and Binkley.)

LUMEN

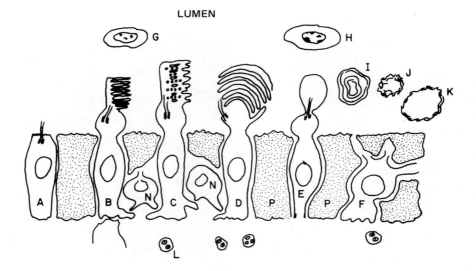

PERIVASCULAR SPACE

Figure 3.3 A generalized diagrammatic representation of pineal cells in the pineal "epithelium." Such a simplified epithelium does not exist in any species [2, 7, 11, 23]. The "epithelium" forms the walls of the primary and secondary follicles. Cells *A–F* represent the variety of pinealocytes found in different species. These and other structures are labeled as follows: *A*, pinealocyte with a cilia; *B*, a sensory pinealocyte with cone-like outer segment (e.g., in fish); *C*, a sensory pinealocyte with tubular and vesicular structures; *D*, a cell found in the "retina" of the pineal organ (brook lamprey); *E*, a pinealocyte with a bulbous cilium (9 + 0) (e.g., chicken); *F*, a "secretory" pinealocyte (mammals); *G, H*, macrophages and lymphocytes; *I, J, K*, lamellar whorl and degenerated outer segments; *L*, autonomic nerve fibers; *N*, pineal neurons with processes to indicate possible synaptic contacts with pinealocytes. The stippled areas represent supportive cells (glia, interstitial, ependymal).

Variation in pineal cells is illustrated in Fig. 3.3; examples of pineal cells drawn from one species, the developing chick, are shown in Figs. 3.4–3.7.

Pinealocytes Most of the cells referred to as *pinealocytes* fall into Pévet's first category (Fig. 3.5). They were subcategorized by some investigators as being "light," "dark," or "clear." In Pévet's first category are also cells called parenchymal cells, and light and dark chief cells, specific cells, glandular cells, fundamental cells, pineal cells, and light cells. Pévet suggested that all these cells may belong in a single functional group [14, 15, 16] and, moreover, that the cells may have the same phylogenetic derivation as the sensory cell line [2]. Cells belong to this group if they have cilia or ciliary derivatives with the 9 + 0 tubular pattern. Pineal cells have also been called

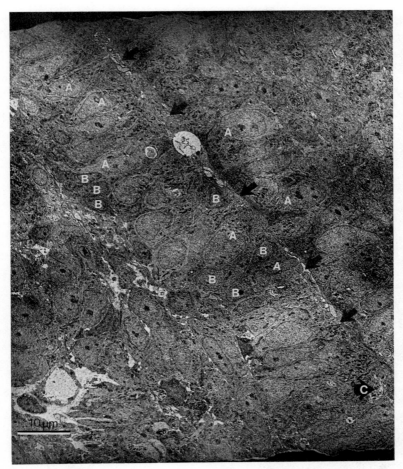

Figure 3.4 Low-power electron micrograph of the chick pineal (in dark-time, CT 20) showing the primary follicle. Again, the overall difference in darkness on the two sides of the lumen can be seen. Cell types A, B, and C are those shown in Fig. 3.2. (Photo courtesy of Cioffi and Binkley).

pineocytes and Reiter [18] characterizes them as having one to several processes that originate from the cell body or perikaryon and end in perivascular spaces. The cells may be modified photoreceptor cells. Some authors have subdivided the pinealocytes into two or more categories based on characteristics of the cell nuclei (large and variably shaped, or smaller and oval), nuclear to cytoplasm ratio, and nuclear or cytoplasmic inclusions.

A generalized description of a pinealocyte starting at the lumen and ending at the perivascular space would include (1) a residual lumen; (2) an outer segment; (3) a 9 + 0 cilium; (4) an inner segment with two centrioles, mitochondria, and microtubules; (5) the Golgi region; (6)

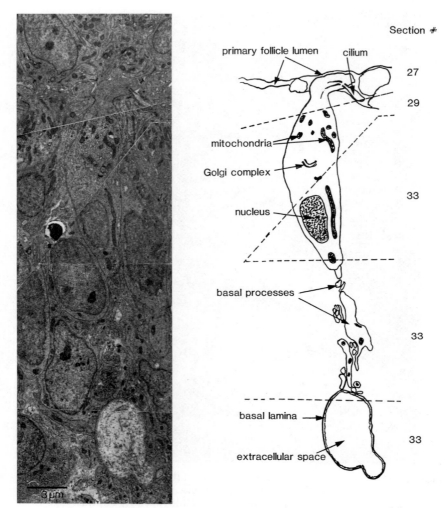

Figure 3.5 The photograph, *left*, is a reconstruction made from a series of chick pineal sections (TEM, light-time, CT 14) in order to visualize the convoluted pinealocyte (A of Figs. 3.2 and 3.4) from its cilium to the basal lamina. The cell has been traced, *right*, and its parts labeled. (Photo courtesy of Cioffi and Binkley.)

the nucleus; (7) a synaptic pedicle with vesicle-crowned rodlets; (8) processes extending from the cell soma to the synaptic pedicle; and (9) space with connective tissue. Variability in pinealocytes among species is found principally in the photoreceptor-like structures, the inner and outer segments.

Glial cells Most of the cells referred to as *glial cells* fall into Pévet's second category, (Fig. 3.6) which also includes the interstitial cells,

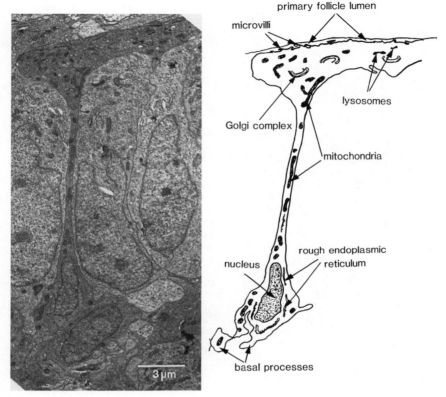

Figure 3.6 Photograph, of a chick pineal section (TEM, dark-time, CT 20) through the cell noted in Figs. 3.2 and 3.4 and **B**. Pinealocytes (**A** in Figs. 3.2 and 3.4) are on either side and the cell is in the same orientation with respect to the layers as in Fig. 3.4. The cell has been traced, *right*, and its parts labeled. (Photo courtesy of Cioffi and Binkley.)

dark cells, neuroblasts, stellate cells, and astrocytes. Many investigators do not consider the cells to be glial cells, but the use of this term to name the cells is widespread.

Other cells According to Quay [17], there may also be plasma cells, mast cells, melanocytes, and fibrocytes in the pineal gland. Lymphocytes, macrophages, contractile muscle cells, nerve cells, and nerve fibers have also been described in sections of pineals or in pineal cell cultures.

3.4.2 Cell parts and extracellular spaces

A variety of structures have been found in the pineal and in its cells. However, not all of the structures appear in all species.

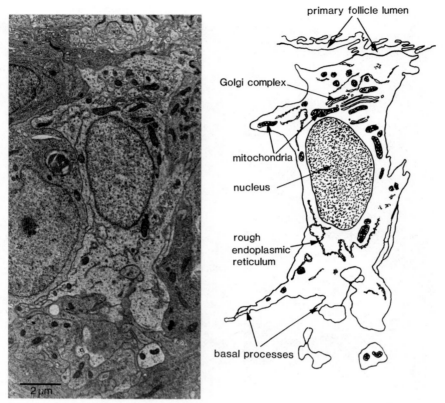

Figure 3.7 Photograph, *left*, of a chick pineal section (TEM, dark-time, CT 20) through the cell noted in Figs. 3.2 and 3.4 as **C**. These pale cells are prominent but less numerous (less than 1 per 1000 cells) in the inner layer of the follicle. The cell is in the same orientation as in Figs. 3.4 and 3.5. The cell has been traced, *right*, and its parts labeled. (Photo courtesy of Cioffi and Binkley.)

Concretions The pineal of humans is characterized by the presence of many calcareous inclusions [19, 20]. The concretions (also called *corpora acervuli*, *corpora arenacea*, *pineal acervuli*, *calcospherulites*, or *pineal sand*) have also been found in sheep, horses, donkeys, gerbils, oxen, pigs, goats, bats, gnus, mink, mules, geese, and herons. The concretions appear to increase in number with increasing age. The morphology of the concretions varies from amorphous to a more organized mulberry appearance. In section, concentric rings can be seen. They are supposed to be similar to enamel, composed of carbonate-containing hydroxyapatite. Pineals of human females may be heavier than those of males due to increased calcification. The incidence of concretions in human pineals is less in African than American blacks. Superior cervical ganglionectomy reduces the num-

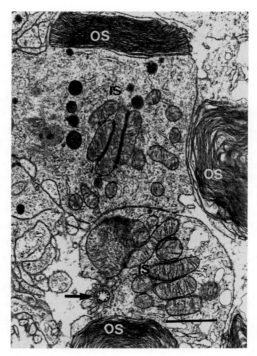

Figure 3.8 Pineal photoreceptor inner segments (*IS*) and outer segments (*OS*), which are interconnected by a 9 + 0 cilium (*arrow*) in goldfish. Mitochondria are typically concentrated in the inner segments. (Photo courtesy of J. McNulty.)

bers of concretions in gerbils, so it seems possible that their formation is a consequence of some aspect of pineal function.

Fibers Fibers, which may be collagen, occur between lobules and delimit their circumference. In developing vertebrates, separate fibers can be seen, but as the animal ages, dense connective tissue is found. Other fibers (so-called *oxytalan fibers*, which are also found in periodontal ligament, dermis, and cornea) occur in the connective tissue spaces [1].

Nerves According to Pévet [16], there are four categories of nerve fibers: sympathetic, parasymphathetic, commissural, and peptidergic. The ones most studied are those originating in the superior cervical ganglia. These last fibers disappear following ganglionectomy. Nerve fibers are found within the pineal gland. Both green fluorescence (characteristic of norepinephrine) and yellow fluorescence (characteristic of serotonin) associate with the fibers. However, not all the serotonin may originate in the cells from which the fibers emanate; it is possible that the serotonin is acquired by the fibers when they enter the pineal and may comprise 30% of pineal serotonin content.

Nerve terminals   Nerve endings are observed in most pineals. The terminals contain granular and/or nongranular vesicles. Some of the terminals are adrenergic and fluoresce. Terminals may form traditional morphological synapses with pinealocytes, but they are more commonly found in the vicinity of capillaries or pinealocyte processes.

Cell membrane and processes   Pinealocytes are distinguished by the variation of their processes. Some pinealocytes end in a club-shaped terminal (found in the lumen or rudimentary lumen of the primary follicle or the rosettes). The "neck" of the process, compared to inner segments, is characterized by intermediate or tight junctions. Other cell contact regions have been described (gap junctions, zonulae adhaerentes, zonulae occludentes, fenestrated communicating zonules) [21]. In some species, the pinealocyte possesses a ciliary (9 + 0) structure (Fig. 3.5). The cilia may end in a whorl of concentric lamellae or connect to an outer-segment-like structure (Fig. 3.8). In other species these cilia are not found. Glial cell processes end at the perivascular space, on other glial cells, or among pinealocytes.

Cytoplasm and contents   The cytoplasm of pinealocytes of various species includes numerous kinds of small bodies—lozenges, paracrystalline structures, proteinaceous accumulations, lysozomes, glycogen granules, dense bodies, laminar lipids or lipid inclusions, multivesicular bodies, glycogen-bound vacuoles and granular vesicles. Vacuoles often contain flocculent material which investigators speculate may represent secretory material.

Mitochondria in pinealocytes are large and numerous. Some of the mitochondria have been described as tigroid-like mitochondria, presumably for the distinct cristae in the horizontal axis, which give the mitochrondria a striped appearance. Other mitochondria have cristae arranged on the longitudinal axis. Usually the mitochondria are found in concentration in the inner-segment-like process. Intramitochondrial crystalloid inclusions (composed of a lattice of electron-dense lines) or microcylinders have been reported in pineal mitochondria [5, 9].

Smooth endoplasmic reticulum is found in pinealocytes. Some descriptions note a peculiarly shaped endoplasmic reticulum with flattened cisterns. Golgi apparatus, subsurface cisterns, ribosomes, and rough endoplasmic reticulum may be present. Often they are located in the region between the nucleus and the neck of the inner-segment-like process. Agranular reticulum has been found in

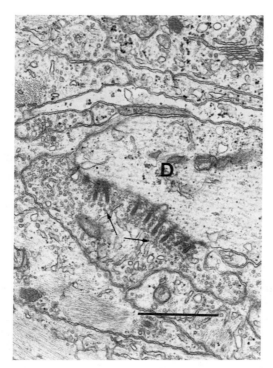

Figure 3.9 Pineal photoreceptor basal pedicle containing synaptic ribbons (*arrows*) lining the plasma membrane adjacent to a ganglion cell dendrite (*D*) in goldfish. (Photo courtesy of J. McNulty.)

strange hexagonal configurations of pores and fenestrations; Lin [10] referred to these as *canaliculate lamellar bodies.*

Vesicle-crowned rodlets (synaptic ribbons, Fig. 3.9) are composed of an electron-dense rod surrounded by a layer of small vesicles. These structures are found in most pineals and in retinas. Usually they are in the end of the pinealocyte opposite to the end that has the cilium. Much functional importance has been attached to their apparent daily cycles and changes in response to physiological alterations. These structures form part of synaptic junctions in retina and in the hypothetically parallel structures in the pineal.

Microtubules, microfilaments, and centrioles have been found. Parallel microfilaments in cell processes are characteristic of the glial cells.

Nuclei   The nuclei of pinealocytes may be oval or irregular in shape; in the latter case there are cytoplasmic invaginations or nuclear creasing (often a single such invagination is seen). The nuclei are rarely seen in mitoses, even in young animals. When dividing cells are observed, it is difficult to tell which kind of pineal cell is in the process of division. Pairs of sister cells, however, are often seen aligned as though just having divided. The nuclei are characterized by having dark inclusions (one to two nucleoli, sometimes large) and light inclusions. The nuclear membrane has channels leading into the cytoplasm. Curious spherules or nuclear pellets, called *Kernkugeln,* could be artifacts of fixation, trapped cytoplasmic vesicles, or enlarged nuclear masses [17].

Extracellular spaces   There are at least two kinds of extracellular spaces in the pineal gland. The first kind is the lumen or residual lumen of the primary and secondary follicles. This lumen contains the macrophages, lymphocytes, and outer-segment-like processes. The second kind of space, the perivascular space, is outside of the follicles and usually contains the connective tissue and nerve terminals.

3.5 Vascularization

As much as 4 ml/min/g of blood circulates through the pineal. This blood supply is second only to that of the kidney [4], which supports the idea that the pineal has functions in which the circulation plays some role. Reiter [18] described the pineal arterial supply and venous drainage; it is variable among species, but his description which is derived from many studies, provides the general picture:

> The major blood supply to the pineal gland is provided by (2–6) branches of the posterior choroidal arteries that derive from the posterior cerebrals as they course around the dorsolateral aspect of the mesencephalon. The arteries branch extensively in the capsule of the gland before they penetrate the parenchyma. In glands that are subdivided by connective tissue trabeculae, the arteries are most commonly found in this structure. In those glands in which the parenchyma is not divided into lobules by septae, the arteriolar character of the entering vessels is lost soon after they enter the gland. In most mammals, all areas of the gland are abundantly supplied with capillaries. . . . the venous drainage is via the distal end of the great cerebral vein. . . . the (6–12) superficial collecting veins of the pineal . . . enter the great cerebral vein that drains directly into the superior sagittal sinus (which is closely associated with the pineal).

The capillaries of the pineal may possess tight endothelial junctions or such junctions may be missing, depending on species [12]. When animals are injected with dyes, the pineal gland is stained. This has been accepted as evidence that the pineal gland is "outside" of the blood-brain barrier. This idea is buttressed by the fact that the pineal responds to drugs injected systemically (e.g., isoproterenol).

3.6 Innervation

Innervation of several types has been proposed: sympathetic, parasympathetic, commissural, and peptidergic. Sympathetic, cholinergic, and peptidergic nerve terminals in the pineal have been separated anatomically with consideration of the nature of vesicles that are present [8].

3.6.1 Sympathetic innervation

Sympathetic innervation of the superficial pineal gland [6, 18, 22] emanates from the superior cervical ganglia. The nerve cells are adrenergic (postganglionic sympathetic neurons) and have their cell bodies located in the ganglia. The pathway from the ganglia to the pineal follows the course of blood vessels (internal carotid plexus to tentorium cerebelli). According to Reiter [18], the deep pineal is innervated sympathetically by way of the superficial pineal so that superficial pinealectomy denervates the deep pineal. The fibers may penetrate the pineal capsule at its apex (distal end) via paired or fused nervi conarii. Alternatively, in some species, the fibers follow the vascularization—perivascular space or arterioles, venules, and capillaries [16, 18]. The superior cervical ganglia in turn receive light information from the eyes coordinated with rhythm information from the suprachiasmatic nuclei of the hypothalamus. It is noteworthy for consideration of pineal function that the ganglia also are the source of adrenergic fibers to the eyes, which in some species are like pineals in being able to synthesize melatonin at night.

The neurotransmitter within adrenergic nerve terminals is contained in vesicles, often dense core, about 50 nm in diameter.

3.6.2 Parasympathetic innervation

The parasympathetic innervation may consist of preganglionic (extrapineal) and postganglionic (intrapineal) nerve cells. In this less-studied pathway, the preganglionic cell bodies are located in the superior salivatory nuclei of the lower brain. The fibers of the preganglionic cells project together with the facial nerves, course with the greater petrosal nerve (some synapsing with postganglionic cells), and reach the pineal by the nervi conarii. Intramural pineal postganglionic parasympatheic nerve cells synapse with the preganglionic fibers. The cholinergic vesicles lack the dense core and are about 50 nm in size in the terminals.

3.6.3 Commissural fibers

The commissural fibers form interesting, but unexplained, hairpin loops. The loops occur within the pineal body, mostly in the stalk.

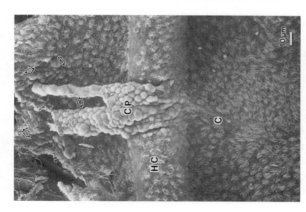

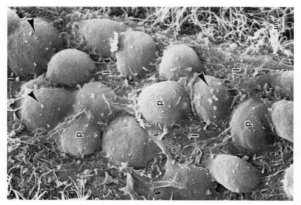

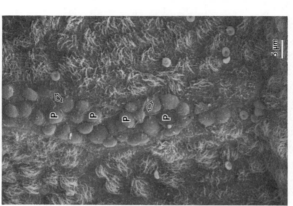

Figure 3.10. Scanning electron micrographs (SEMs) of pineal structures of the Mongolian gerbil. *A,* low magnification SEM of the pineal and suprapineal recesses in the gerbil shown below and above the habenular commissure (*hc*). The cells of the central zone (*c*) of the pineal recess appear relatively devoid of surface specializations. Numerous CSF-contacting pinealocytes (*arrows*) are present in the suprapineal recess. What is presumed to be part of the cells of the choroid plexus are present (*cp*). *B,* scanning electron micrograph of pinealocytes (*p*) of the deep pineal. These pinealocytes extend into the cerebrospinal fluid of the pineal recess. The CSF-contacting pinealocytes have occasional processes (*arrows*) that extend short distances on the ventricular surface of the deep pineal. *C,* scanning electron micrograph of CSF-contacting pinealocytes (*p*) of the deep pineal extending into the CSF of the pineal recess. The pinealocytes have numerous processes (*clear arrows*) and surface blebbing (*arrow heads*). The ventricular surface (*i*) between the CSF-contacting pinealocytes consists of processes from both the pinealocytes and from the underlying glial cells of the deep pineal. (Photo courtesy of M. Welsh.)

They are found in the pineals of most species studied and the loops connect the habenula to the posterior commissure.

3.6.4 Peptidergic fibers

Peptidergic fibers are found in the pineal stalks of some animals and a periventricular nuclear origin has been suggested. They have been dubbed *peptidergic* because the putative neurotransmitter is a peptide such as vasopressin, oxytocin, luteinizing hormone releasing hormone (LRH), vasoactive intestinal peptide, or arginine vasotocin (AVT). Pévet [16] suggests a hypothalamic link could explain the presence of these peptides in the pineals. The peptidergic terminals are dominated by 100-nm granular vesicles.

3.7 Pineal Recess

The pineal recess is the area of the third ventricle of the brain where the stalk of the pineal attaches. Depending on the species, few or many pinealocytes are thus in proximity to the cerebrospinal fluid (CSF) (Fig. 3.10). This close relationship has caused many investigators to suggest the possibilities of an intraventricular route of secretion of pineal products or of accumulation of CSF substances by the pineal. The cells of the pineal recess (ependymal cells, tanycytes) may be capable of bidirectional transport. The cells are described by Pévet [16]:

> These cells are generally characterized by a well-developed Golgi apparatus and granular endoplasmic reticulum and by the presence of a deeply invaginated nucleus. The apical cell surface is . . . packed with microvilli and cilia. Ependymal cells arranged in rosettes are also seen in the pineal parenchyma, but most often near the pineal recess.

REFERENCES

1. Calvo J., and J. Boya. 1983. Oxytalan fibres in the rat pineal gland. *J. Anat.* 136:363–366.
2. Collin, J., and A. Oksche. 1981. Structural and functional relationships in the nonmammalian pineal gland. In *The pineal gland I: Anatomy and biochemistry*, ed. R. Reiter, pp. 27–67. Boca Raton, Fla.: CRC Press.
3. Gaston, S. 1969. The effect of pinealectomy on the circadian activity rhythm of the house sparrow, *Passer domesticus*. Ph.D. diss., Univ. of Texas.
4. Goldman, H., and R. Wurtman. 1964. Flow of blood to the pineal body of the rat. *Nature* 203:27–88.
5. Heidbuchel, U. 1982. Intramitochondrial crystalloids in rat pinealocytes. *Cell Tiss. Res.* 221:693–696.

6. Kappers, J. 1960. The development, topographical relationships and innervation of the epiphysis cerebri in the albino rat. *Z. Zellforsch.* 52:163–215.

7. Karasek, M. 1983. Ultrastructure of the mammalian pineal gland: Its comparative and functional aspects. In *Pineal research reviews I*, ed. R. Reiter, pp. 1–48. New York: Alan R. Liss.

8. Korf, H., and M. Møller. 1984. The innervation of the mammalian pineal gland with special reference to central pinealopetal projections. In *Pineal research reviews II*, ed. R. Reiter, pp. 41–46. New York: Alan R. Liss.

9. Lin, H. 1965. Microcylinders within mitochondrial cristae in the rat pinealocyte. *J. Cell Biol.* 25:435–441.

10. ———. 1967. Peculiar configuration of agranular reticulum (canaliculate lamellar body) in the rat pinealocyte. *J. Cell Biol.* 33:15–25.

11. McNulty, J. 1985. Personal communication.

12. Matsushima, S., and R. Reiter. 1975. Ultrastructural observation of pineal gland capillaries in four rodent species. *Amer. J. Anat.* 143:265–282.

13. Oksche, A. 1965. Survey of the development and comparative morphology of the pineal organ. In *Structure and function of the epiphysis cerebri*, ed. J. Kappers and J. Schade. pp. 3–29. Progress in Brain Research 10. Amsterdam: Elsevier.

14. Pévet, P. 1977. On the presence of different populations of pinealocytes in the mammalian pineal gland. *J. Neural Trans.* 40:289–304.

15. ———. 1981. Ultrastructure of the mammalian pinealocyte. In *The pineal gland I: Anatomy and biochemistry*, ed. R. Reiter, pp. 121–154. Boca Raton, Fla.: CRC Press.

16. ———. 1983. Anatomy of the pineal gland of mammals. In *The pineal gland*, ed. R. Relkin, pp. 1–75. New York: Elsevier.

17. Quay, W. 1965. Histological structure and cytology of the pineal organ in birds and mammals. In *Structure and function of the epiphysis cerebri*, ed. J. Kappers and J. Schade, pp. 49–86. Progress in Brain Research 10. Amsterdam: Elsevier.

18. Reiter, R. 1981. The mammalian pineal gland: Structure and function. *Amer. J. Anat.* 162:287–313.

19. Relkin, R. 1983. The human pineal. In *The pineal gland*, ed. R. Relkin, pp. 273–274. New York: Elsevier.

20. Scharenberg, K., and L. Liss. 1965. The histologic structure of the human pineal body. In *Structure and function of the epiphysis cerebri*, ed. J. Kappers and J. Schade, pp. 193–217. Progress in Brain Research 10. Amsterdam: Elsevier.

21. Taugner, R., and A. Schiller. 1981. Gap junctions between pinealocytes. *Cell Tiss. Res.* 218:303–314.

22. Thiéblot, L., J. Naudascher, and H. Lebars. 1947. Modifications histologiques de l'épiphyse à la suite d'excitation électrique du ganglion cervical supérieur chez le chat. *Ann. Endocrinol.* 8: 468–469.

23. Vollrath, L. 1981. *The pineal organ.* Berlin: Springer-Verlag.

24. Welsh, M., I. Cameron, and R. Reiter. 1979. The pineal gland of the gerbil, *Meriones unguiculatus*, II: Morphometric analysis over a 24 h period. *Cell Tiss. Res.* 204:95–109.

4

Pineal Biochemistry

"The activity of *N*-acetyltransferase in the rat pineal gland is more than 15 times higher at night than during the day. This circadian rhythm persists in complete darkness, or in blinded animals, and is suppressed in constant lighting. The *N*-acetyltransferase rhythm is 180 degrees out of phase with the serotonin rhythm and is similar to the norepinephrine and melatonin rhythms. Experiments in vitro indicate that norepinephrine, not serotonin, regulates the activity of *N*-acetyltransferase through a highly specific receptor."

D. Klein and J. Weller [6]

4.1 Indoleamines

The principal biosynthetic pathway that has been studied in the pineal is that of the indoleamines [10, 11]. Indoleamine synthesis probably occurs in the cells designated as pinealocytes. The amino acid, tryptophan, is the precursor of the hydroxyindole, serotonin (5-hydroxytryptamine, 5-HT). Serotonin is the precursor of the pineal secretory product or hormone, melatonin (M, MEL, MT), and 6-hydroxymelatonin is a metabolite of melatonin.

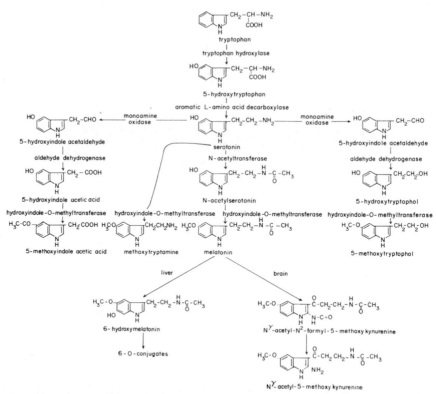

Figure 4.1 Biochemical pathway for serotonin and melatonin synthesis and metabolism.

4.1.1 Biosynthesis and metabolism

The biochemical pathway for the synthesis and metabolism of serotonin and melatonin is shown in Figure 4.1. Pineals produce melatonin from radiolabeled tryptophan in organ culture and therefore can make serotonin. They may also garner serotonin from other sources (blood, cerebrospinal fluid, or nerve terminal emissions). The concentrations of serotonin are higher in the pineal gland than in other tissues, and most serotonin is found in the pinealocyte cytoplasm. That tryptophan, the amino acid precursor of serotonin, is not found in quantity in the pineal could be due to uptake, then rapid conversion to other indoleamines.

Serotonin can have one of several fates. It can be converted to 5-hydroxyindole acetaldehyde by oxidative deamination with the enzyme monoamine (monamine) oxidase (MAO). The acetaldehyde is converted into four other indoleamines with aldehyde dehydrogenase and hydroxyindole-O-methyltransferase: 5-hydroxyindole acetic acid (5-HIAA), 5-methoxyindole acetic acid (5-MIAA), 5-hydroxytrypto-

TABLE 4.1 Tissue uptake of 3H-melatonin 1 hour after injection into cats

Tissue/organ	μg/100g
Pineal	26
Eye	6
Ovary	6
Pituitary	3
Sympathetic chain	3
Peripheral nerve	2
Testes	2
Thyroid	2
Adrenal	2
Kidney	1
Uterus	1
Liver	1
Other[a]	<1

Source: Based on data from Wurtman, Axelrod, and Potter [17].
[a] Pancreas, salivary glands, spleen, plasma, heart, skin, brain, diaphragm, and adipose tissue.

phol, and 5-methoxytryptophol. Alternatively, serotonin can be acety-lated by N-acetyltransferase (NAT) to produce N-acetylserotonin (NAS). Acetyl coenzyme A (acetyl CoA) is the acetyl group donor for the reaction; coenzyme A is the byproduct. NAS in turn is methylated with the enzyme, hydroxyindole-O-methyltransferase, in the presence of a methyl donor, S-adenosylmethionine.

Melatonin disappears from the blood quickly; and, according to Quay [10, 11], there may be a two-step process of elimination. In the first 10 minutes after an injection of radioactive melatonin in mice, there is a rapid decrease (half-life 2 minutes), but by 40 minutes the half-life is 35 minutes. There is hydroxylase in the liver that converts melatonin to 6-hydroxymelatonin. This step is then followed by conjugation with sulfate or glucuronic acid, the products being excreted in urine.

There are other proposed metabolic fates for indoles. Melatonin may be converted in the brain to N^γ-acetyl-N^2-formyl-5-methoxykyn-uramine, which in turn is a precursor of N^γ-acetyl-5-methoxykyn-urenine. Melatonin, serotonin, and 5-methoxytryptamine may undergo cyclohydrogenation in the pineal to form β-carboline derivatives: 6-hydroxytetrahydroharman, 6-methoxytetrahydrohar-man, and 6-methoxyharmalan. The compounds are interesting because they are psychoactive (producing tremors, convulsions, and hallucinations) and can inhibit enzymes (MAO, cholinesterase).

4.1.2 Loci

The enzymes and substrates necessary for the synthesis of melatonin are present in the pineal gland, but they are also distributed in other tissues (Table 4.1). The distribution of NAT shows that other tissues can acetylate serotonin, but the largest daily cycle was found in the pineal gland (Table 4.2). NAT and melatonin cycles have also been found in the eyes (Fig. 4.2); the ratio of pineal to ocular NAT varies from one species to the next (NAT is comparable in eyes and pineals of chickens and quail; there is less NAT in eyes than pineals of hamsters, sparrows, and rats). As would be predicted from the species and tissue distribution of the various components of the melatonin biosynthetic machinery, pinealectomy or pinealectomy-plus-blinding does not always remove all circulating melatonin (Table 4.3).

TABLE 4.2 Tissue Distribution of *N*-acetyltransferase (NAT) activity in the rat and chick

Tissue/organ	Rat	Chick
Pineal[a]	62.0	6.9
Thyroid	2.0	0.7
Cerebrum	1.5	0.6
Cerebellum	1.4	1.9
Olfactory lobe	1.3	—
Spleen	0.9	0.5
Pituitary	0.9	1.6
Optic lobe	—	0.5
Heart	1.1	1.9
Kidney	1.4	0.8
Intestine	1.0	1.3
Adrenal	1.0	0.9
Submaxillary gland	1.2	—
Liver	1.5	1.2
Hypothalamus	—	1.8
Thymus	—	1.6
Gonad	—	0.5
Breast muscle	—	0.5
Skin	—	1.0
Pancreas	—	2.2
Lung	—	1.3

Source: Based on data from Ellison, Weller, Klein [4] and Binkley [1].
Note: NAT activity is expressed as a ratio (dark-time/light-time) adjusted for the weight of the tissue.
[a] Dark-time pineal NAT was 2.7 nmol/mg/hr for the rat and 7.6 nmol/mg/hr for the chick.

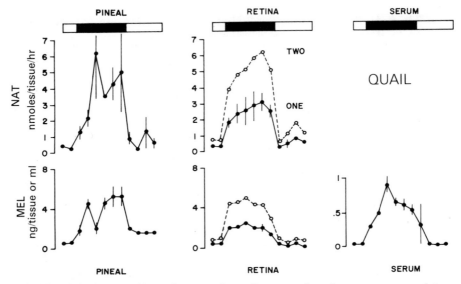

Figure 4.2 Time profiles of *N*-acetyltransferase and melatonin measured in quail pineal, retina, and serum over 24 hours. (Unpublished data of Underwood, Siopes, Binkley, and Mosher.)

4.1.3 Enzymes

The enzymes related to indoleamine biosynthesis in the pineal gland are important because the enzymes in any pathway may control the rates of production of a biochemical and, thus, the amount of the biochemical that is present or secreted. In the pineal, there are many aspects of the enzymology to consider: the reaction catalyzed, daily and seasonal rhythms, effects of light and dark, purification status, properties, activation, inhibition, and possible loci. Complete information is not available for all the enzymes for all these parameters. Enzyme activity—the amount of product produced by an enzyme under given substrate and chemical conditions—has most frequently been characterized for pineal enzymes; activity of the enzyme is physiologically relevant because, if substrate is available and other chemical conditions are favorable, the activity of the enzyme determines the amount of product that has been produced. Activity of an enzyme is usually represented as (1) amount of product produced per tissue (whole organ or per milligram) which indicates the physiological potential, or (2) amount of product produced per amount of protein present (specific activity). This latter measurement is most useful when purified preparations of the enzyme are being discussed. Once an enzyme has been isolated, its absolute amounts (concentration) can be designated.

TABLE 4.3 Melatonin in the blood (pg/plasma or serum) of animals subjected to pinealectomy and/or blinding

Species	Control	Pinx	Blind	Blind + Pinx
Rat	9, 47	9, 12	—	—
Chicken (a)	ND, 71	ND, ND	—	—
Chicken (b)	50, 300	50, 75	—	50, 40
Quail	10, 430	10, 200	10, 250	10, 100

Sources: Based on data from Ozaki and Lynch [8]; Pelham [9]; Reppert and Sagar [12]; and Underwood et al. [14].
Note: Melatonin was measured by RIA for the rats, chickens (b), and quail and by bioassay for chickens (a). The data are given in pairs of numbers—the first number is the light-time value; the second is the dark-time value. ND = not detectable.

Tryptophan hydroxylase Tryptophan hydroxylase catalyzes the hydroxylation of tryptophan to produce 5-hydroxytryptophan (5-HTP) and may be the rate-limiting step in serotonin formation. The enzyme is present in tissues other than the pineal gland, including the raphe nuclei of the brain. Tryptophan hydroxylase is probably localized in the mitochondria of pinealocytes. The reaction requires a pteridine cofactor; tetrahydrobiopterin (BH_4) is a possible cofactor and is found in the pineal. Attempts at purification have so far suggested a 30,000 MW enzyme which may be identical to phenylalanine hydroxylase. Klein et al. [5] demonstrated a possible activation mechanism involving reducing agents (e.g., borohydride) and suggested a possible means of physiological regulation of the enzyme through thiol reactions. The enzyme in pineal homogenates is inhibited by p-chlorophenylalanine (pCPA). Rhythms in the activity of the enzyme have been sought by various investigators, at most, a 1.5-fold increase in the enzyme at middark was found.

Aromatic-L-amino acid decarboxylase Aromatic-L-amino acid decarboxylase converts 4-HTP to serotonin using pyridoxal phosphate as a cofactor. The enzyme is generally present in tissues, and in the pineal it is found in the pinealocyte cytoplasm. Constant light may double the activity of the enzyme compared to constant dark but no daily rhythm has been discerned.

N-acetyltransferase NAT catalyzes the acetylation of serotonin with acetyl CoA as the acetylating agent. The product of the reaction is N-acetylserotonin. The enzyme is distinguished by its daily cycles in the pineal gland and the retina: 6 to 100 times the NAT activity is present in the night compared to the day. The enzyme is probably the rate-limiting enzyme for the nightly production of melatonin. Serotonin can be acetylated by enzymes in the homogenates of most other tissues (e.g., liver), but the other tissues do not have the enzyme activity rhythm, and the characteristics of their enzymes (stability, substrate specificity, etc.) differ from the characteristics of pineal NAT. Pineal NAT is located in the cytoplasm, probably of pinealocytes. The properties of NAT are similar when the enzyme is obtained from pineals of different species (e.g., rats, chicks), and the NAT in the retina may be an identical or very similar enzyme.

NAT is unstable at 37° C in pineal homogenates [2, 3, 5] (Fig. 4.3), and this fact has impeded attempts at its purification; early efforts point to a molecular weight of 39,000. The enzyme is protected from inactivation by cold temperature, by dilution, by its substrate, acetyl CoA, and by molecules that contain a subunit like cysteamine (as does acetyl CoA). Inactivation of NAT is accelerated by disulfide molecules such as insulin [3, 5, 7]. The protection-inactivation mechanism could have physiological importance to the regulation of NAT, because the time course of loss of activity in homogenates is similar to that in pineals in vivo.

NAT can be stimulated (e.g., in rats) or inhibited (e.g., in chicks) by

Figure 4.3 *N*-acetyltransferase loses activity rapidly in homogenates kept at 37°C. The rate of activity loss is less when the pineal extract is more dilute. (Data are for chick pineal glands from Binkley, Klein, and Weller [3].)

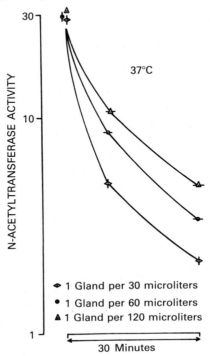

adrenergic agonists and cyclic adenosine monophosphate analogs. The stimulation is blocked by cycloheximide (a protein synthesis inhibitor) and, in some experiments, by actinomycin D (which inhibits RNA synthesis).

Klein et al. [6] considered the possibility that NAT may be the rate-limiting enzyme in melatonin synthesis in pineals of rats:

> It seems that N-acetyltransferase is the rate-limiting enzyme in melatonin synthesis during the day. At night, when N-acetyltransferase activity increases 10- to 30-fold, it seems probable that the rate of production of N-acetylserotonin exceeds the maximum possible rate of O-methylation. Although a small diurnal rhythm of hydroxyindole-O-methyltransferase has been observed, the highest activity reported does not exceed the activity of N-acetyltransferase at night. This situation might result in the accumulation of N-acetylserotonin followed by a gradual conversion to melatonin. HIOMT would regulate the rate of production of melatonin under these conditions. The amount of melatonin produced during one 24-hour period, however, would be limited by the amount of N-acetylserotonin synthesized by N-acetyltransferase.

However, it should be pointed out that HIOMT activities are much higher in some other species (e.g., chickens) than in the pineals of rats, and, furthermore, availability of the substrates (serotonin acetyl CoA, and S-adenosylmethionine) could influence the actual amount of melatonin synthesized.

Hydroxyindole-O-methyltransferase HIOMT produces melatonin by methylating its substrate, N-acetylserotonin. The methyl donor is S-adenosylmethionine. HIOMT also methylates other substrates (e.g., 5-HIAA, hydroxytryptamine, and hydroxytryptophol) producing products other than melatonin. HIOMT comprises 2–4% of the proteins in pineal cytoplasm. There may be more than one form of HIOMT, but one proposal is that it has a molecular weight of 78,000 with two 39,000 subunits. Oxaloacetate and bicarbonate are activators and pyridoxal phosphate is an inhibitor of the enzyme. Constant dark increases the number of HIOMT molecules produced over a period of days or weeks, while constant light decrease HIOMT activity. Small daily changes (e.g., 1.2-fold, peak in the dark-time) have been found.

Monoamine oxidase As pointed out, there is an alternate route for metabolism of serotonin. Monoamine oxidase produces 5-hydroxyindole acetaldehyde from serotonin, and aldehyde dehydrogenase and HIOMT further convert the acetaldehyde to other deaminated products. Monoamine oxidase is a mitochrondrial enzyme that is not specific to pineal tissue (where one form, B, is found in pinealocytes and a second form, A, is in the nerve endings). Monoamine oxidase also functions in catecholamine metabolism (e.g., epinephrine and norepinephrine are substrates), so its function is not limited to serotonin metabolism.

4.2 Nonindoles

Molecules in categories other than indoles and their related enzymes have been studied in the pineal. Some of these other molecules included ions, amino acids, catecholamines, nucleotides, lipids, carbohydrates, inorganics, nucleic acids, and enzymes (Fig. 4.4).

4.2.1 Amino acids

Pineal amino acid levels have been determined for a number of species (see Table 4.4 for bovine levels) and compared to amounts for other tissues [10, 11].

Tryptophan and methionine are very low in the pineal. This may be due to their depletion by use as substrates for serotonin and melatonin production, though it might be argued that one would expect higher values because of their role as substrates.

Glutamic acid (accounting for 21% of bovine pineal free amino acids) is in high concentration in pineal but not as high as in brain. The glutamic acid metabolite, GABA, which may function as an inhibitory neuron transmitter in brain, is in low concentration.

Sulfur-containing amino acids, taurine and cystathionine, are present in high concentrations in some pineals, but the pattern is variable from species to species. They may function as constituents of pineal peptides and proteins, in the methylation of N-acetylserotonin, and in the regulation of NAT activity. Taurine, for example, exhibits a rhythm that parallels that in norepinephrine (nadir at lights-out, peak at mid-light). Klein [5] postulates an extracellular messenger role for taurine where it would interact with presynaptic norepinephrine (NE) terminals to change the release of NE.

4.2.2 Catecholamines

Most of the work pertaining to pineal catecholamines is from rats. DOPA (3,4-dihydroxyphenylalanine), dopamine (DA), and norepinephrine (NE) are found in nonmyelinated pineal nerve fibers and terminals (in the granular center of dense core vesicles that are 300–600 Å in diameter). The nerve endings in the pineal gland have the enzymes (phenylalanine hydroxylase, tyrosine hydroxylase) and the precursors (phenylalanine, tyrosine) to synthesize the catecholamines. The pineal can also take up norepinephrine from blood and extracellular fluid in amounts that exceed those of other tissues by twofold or more. Quay [10] lists four possible fates for pineal norepinephrine:

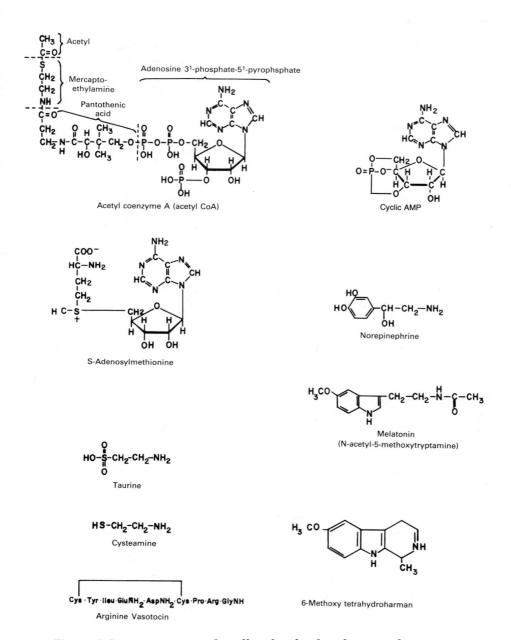

Figure 4.4 An assortment of small molecules found in pineals.

TABLE 4.4 Free amino acids in bovine pineals

Amino acid	Percent of total amino acids
Cystathionine	35.9
Glutamic acid	21.0
Taurine	18.2
Glycine	3.4
Glutamine	3.4
Alanine	2.2
Serine	1.6
Aspartic acid	1.5
Valine	1.5
Leucine	1.1
Threonine	0.9
Histidine	0.8
Lysine	0.7
Arginine	0.7
α-Aminobutyric acid	0.6
Isoleucine	0.6
Tyrosine	0.6
β-Aminobutyric acid	0.6
Proline	0.4
Phenylalanine	0.4
Citrulline	0.4
Methionine sulfoxide	0.4
Cystine	0.3
Ornithine	0.3
γ-Aminobutyric acid	0.3
3-Methyl histidine	0.1
Hydroxyproline	0.1
Methionine	0.0
Tryptophan	0.0

Source: Data are reorganized from a table presented by Quay [10].

1. Interaction with receptors in pinealocytes or smooth muscle of the blood vessels
2. Uptake or re-uptake and storage in dense core vesicles of the sympathetic nerve endings
3. Loss as free NE to the capillaries
4. Conversion to physiologically inactive metabolites by MAO in the terminals and by pineal catechol-O-methyltransferase (COMT)

4.2.3 Nucleotides and their derivatives

There are some facts known about pineal nucleotides and their derivatives: (1) adenosine injections dilate pineal blood vessels [10,

11]; (2) adenosine triphosphatase (ATPase) activity at the interface between glial cells and pinealocytes encouraged Quay [10] to suggest a "nurse" or nutritive function for the glial cells; and (3) ATP and ATPase are found in the several pineal cell types.

The second messenger, cyclic AMP (cyclic adenosine monophosphate, a cyclic nucleotide), is present in amounts in pineals. The cyclic nucleotide is synthesized from ATP by pineal adenyl cyclase (adenyl cyclase is an enzyme common to the plasma membrane of many cells that respond to hormones). Cyclic guanosine monophosphate (cGMP) rhythms matching the phase of NAT are found in chick pineals [15], but the diurnal changes were not accompanied by diurnal cycles in the accompanying enzymes (cGMP phosphodiesterase, guanylate cyclase, GTPase) [16].

S-adenosylmethionine (SAM, SAMe) is synthesized from ATP with methionine-activating enzyme. The levels of SAM in the pineal (38 μg/g) are considered high (matching the amounts in the liver and adrenal); the possible physiological significance of this is that the SAM distribution matches its use as a methylating agent in enzyme reactions (e.g., synthesis of catecholamines and melatonin).

4.2.4 Macromolecules

Total pineal RNA has been measured and found to be rhythmic (peak at early light-time in rats). Total pineal protein peaks in the late subjective day (rats). Other than that, most of our knowledge of pineal macromolecules has to do with the pineal enzymes and their activities. Quay [10, 11] lists a number of enzymes whose activity has been detected in the pineal gland, as well as some that have not (see Table 4.5). In addition to structural proteins and enzymes, the possibility exists that the pineal gland secretes a peptide product. The major candidate for such a peptide product is arginine vasotocin. Pigments that may be found in some pineals include rhodopsin, melanin, lipofuscin, and an iron-containing pigment.

4.2.5 Lipids

There does not appear to be anything particular to pineal lipids beyond the usual functions in membranes and metabolism. According to Quay [10, 11], 3–10% of pineal wet weight is lipid. Glycerides and cholesterol make up less than half of the lipid; the remainder is phosphatidyl choline, phosphatidyl ethanolamine, and sphingomyelin. Pineal lipids may be altered by light and reproductive state.

4.2.6 Carbohydrates

The pineal has no carbohydrates that are peculiar to it [10, 11] Ascorbic acid, neuraminic acid (a sialic acid), and glycogen have been

TABLE 4.5 Enzymes detected in pineal

Indoleamine pathways
      Tryptophan hydroxylase
      Aromatic-L-amino acid decarboxylase
      N-acetyltransferase
      Hydroxyindole-O-methyltransferase (HIOMT)
      Aldehyde dehydrogenase
      Monoamine oxidase (MAO), type B

Catecholamine pathways
      Phenylalanine hydroxylase
      Aromatic-L-amino acid decarboxylase
      Tyrosine hydroxylase
      Dopamine β-hydroxylase
      Monoamine oxidase (MAO), type A
      Catechol-O-methyltransferase (COMT)
      Phenylethanolamine-N-methyltransferase (PNMT)

Other enzymes
      Adenyl cyclase
      Phosphodiesterase
      ATPase
      Cyclic AMP-dependent protein kinase
      Acetyl CoA hydrolase
      Rhodopsin kinase
      Lactate dehydrogenase
      3-Hydroxybutyrate dehydrogenase
      Malic dehydrogenase
      Isocitrate dehydrogenase
      Glucose-6-phosphate dehydrogenase
      Glycerolphosphate dehydrogenase
      Succinate semialdehyde dehydrogenase
      Succinate dehydrogenase (SDH)
      Glutamate dehydrogenase
      Glutamate decarboxylase
      NADPH$_2$ diaphorase
      Diaphorase
      Cytochrome oxidase
      Histamine-N-methyltransferase (HNMT)
      Choline acetylase (ChAc)
      Acetylcholinesterase (AChE)
      Cholinesterase
      Thiolesterase
      Glycogen phosphorylase
      Glucose-6-phosphatase
      Aspartate aminotransferase
      Alanine aminotransferase
      Tyrosine aminotransferase
      Aminobutyrate aminotransferase
      Creatine kinase
      Lipase
      Alkaline phosphatase
      Acid phosphatase

TABLE 4.5 (Continued)

5'-Nucleotidase
Alpha amylase
Sucrase
Maltase
β-Glucuronidase
Leucine aminopeptidase
Glutaminase
Fructose diphosphate aldolase
Carbonic anhydrase (CA)
Fumarase
Aconitase
Glucose phosphate isomerase

Sources: Compiled from Quay [10] and Somers and Klein [13].
Note: Enzymes were detected with histochemistry or biochemistry in pineals of various species (mainly humans, rats, and lambs). Some enzymes are found in one species but not in others (e.g., PNMT is found in bird pineal but not rat pineal). Other enzymes are present at some but not all stages of development. A number of enzymes have daily cycles.

measured. Glycogen levels may exhibit a daily cycle and are depressed by constant light.

4.2.7 Inorganic constituents

Inorganic substances detected in the pineal gland include copper, manganese, zinc, iron, calcium, magnesium, and phosphorus. Pineals also take up radiolabeled rubidium, potassium, iodine, and inorganic phosphate. Phosphate uptake may be altered by light, age, stress, and reproductive state.

REFERENCES

1. Binkley, S. 1981. "Pineal biochemistry: Comparative aspects and circadian rhythms." In *The pineal gland I: Anatomy and Biochemistry*, ed. R. Reiter, pp. 155–172. Boca Raton, Fla.: CRC Press.

2. Binkley, S., D. Klein, and J. Weller. 1976. Pineal serotonin N-acetyltransferase activity: Protection of stimulated activity by acetyl-CoA and related compounds. *J. Neurochem.* 26:51–55.

3. Binkley, S., J. Riebman, and K. Reilly. 1979. Regulation of pineal rhythms in chickens: N-acetyltransferase activity in homogenates. *Comp. Biochem. Physiol.* 63C:291–296.

4. Ellison, N., Weller, J. and D. Klein. 1972. Development of a circadian rhythm in the activity of pineal serotonin N-acetyltransferase. *J. Neurochem.* 19:1335–1341.

5. Klein, D., D. Auerbach, M. Namboodiri, and G. Wheler. 1981. Indole metabolism in the mammalian pineal gland In *The pineal gland I: Anatomy and biochemistry*, ed. R. Reiter, pp. 199–228. Boca Raton, Fla.: CRC Press.

6. Klein, D., and J. Weller. 1970. Indole metabolism in the pineal gland: A circadian rhythm in *N*-acetyltransferase. *Science* 169:1093–1095.

7. Namboodiri, M., J. Favilla, and D. Klein. 1981. Pineal *N*-acetyltransferase is inactivated by disulfide-containing peptides: Insulin is the most potent. *Science* 213:571–573.

8. Ozaki, Y., and H. Lynch. 1976. Presence of melatonin in plasma and urine of pinealectomized rats. *Endocrinology* 99:641–644.

9. Pelham, R. 1975. A serum melatonin rhythm in chickens and its abolition by pinealectomy. *Endocrinology* 96:543–546.

10. Quay, W. 1974. Pineal chemistry. Springfield, Ill.: Charles C. Thomas.

11. ———. 1981. General biochemistry of the pineal gland of mammals In *The pineal gland I: Anatomy and biochemistry*, ed. R. Reiter, pp. 173–198. Boca Raton, Fla.: CRC Press.

12. Reppert, S., and S. Sagar. 1983. Characterization of the day-night variation of retinal melatonin content in the chick. *Invest. Opthalmol. Vis. Sci.* 24:294–300.

13. Somers, R., and D. Klein. 1984. Rhodopsin kinase activity in the mammalian pineal gland and other tissues. *Science* 226:182–184.

14. Underwood, H., S. Binkley, T. Siopes, and K. Mosher. 1984. Melatonin rhythms in the eyes, pineal bodies, and blood of Japanese quail. *Gen. Comp. Endocrinol.* 56:70–81.

15. Wainwright, S. 1980. Diurnal cycles in serotonin acetyltransferase activity and cyclic GMP content of cultured chick pineal glands. *Nature* 285:478–480.

16. Wainwright, S., and L. Wainwright. 1983. Enzymes of guanine nucleotide metabolism and the diurnal cycle in cGMP content of the chick pineal gland. *Can. J. Biochem. Cell Biol.* 61:137–143.

17. Wurtman, J., J. Axelrod, and L. Potter. 1964. The uptake of 3H-melatonin in endocrine and nervous tissues and the effects of constant light exposure. *J. Pharmacol. Exp. Ther.* 143:314–318.

References · **69**

5

Pineal Regulation
by Light and Dark

"Pineal 5-hydroxy- and 5-methoxyindoles of domestic pigeons were measured by differential extractions and spectrofluorometry. . . . Experimental changes in the timing of light and darkness showed that:

1. precocious morning rise in 5-HT could be caused by early onset of light, and possibly as well by early start of darkness during the previous evening;
2. delayed start of light did not inhibit the early morning rise;
3. continuation of light through the evening inhibited the usual nocturnal decline in 5-HT.

Thus primary phases in the daily rhythm in pineal 5-HT can be triggered in part by light and darkness."

W. B. Quay [16]

5.1 Interaction of Light and Circadian Clocks

In order to appreciate the function and biochemistry of the pineal, an understanding of the principles of circadian rhythms and their regulation is crucial. A circadian rhythm is a repetitive cycle that has a period length close to 24 hours that persists (free-runs) under constant conditions. Circadian rhythms are ubiquitous and are even found in single-celled organisms. The rhythms are probably a consequence of evolution under the influence of the earth's 24-hour rotation. The cycles that persist in constant conditions (e.g., in the laboratory with the lights on or off all the time and with invariant temperature) are not exactly 24 hours, however. They are brought into synchrony by time cues from the environment, a process called *entrainment.*

Understanding entrainment is not a simple matter. There must be a rhythm (that can be observed in constant conditions) for entrainment to occur. When one rhythm (e.g., the light-dark cycle of the external environment) synchronizes another (e.g., the locomoter activity rhythm of a sparrow), entrainment is said to occur. Synchronization may also be observed between two rhythms within an organism (e.g., the locomotor activity rhythm and the body temperature rhythm). Internal synchronization can be attained in two ways: (1) both rhythms synchronize to a third rhythm, or (2) one rhythm synchronizes the other (i.e., acts as a driver).

A number of environmental signals can act as entraining agents. Temperature, humidity, social interactions, and barometric pressure changes may act as time cues (*Zeitgebers*) for rhythms. But the most pervasive and widespread time-setting agent is light and dark. Light and dark have certain advantages: the timing of their occurrence is precise; they provide a "clock" in the form of two daily cues (dawn and dusk); and they give a calendar in the form of seasonally changing photoperiods (length of light) and scotoperiods (length of dark).

When organisms travel in an east-west direction, their circadian clocks must adjust to the new time by resetting. Such resetting becomes obvious when we travel and is partly responsible for the ill feelings called "jet lag." Resetting, however, recurs on a daily basis when an organism remains in one location. Most organisms have internal clocks that are not exactly 24.0 hours long and so must be reset each day in order for their owners to be in step with the timing of the environment. The resetting of circadian clocks has been extensively studied. In one type of protocol, resetting is studied following an advance or delay in time of the environmental cycle. The position of the ensuing rhythm (its new phase) is measured as it adapts to the new cycle. In another kind of protocol, light or dark pulses are provided to the organisms and the subsequent phase of their rhythm is assessed. A plot of such phases versus pulses administered at a sequence of times over 24 hours is called a phase response curve (PRC). Typically, rhythms are delayed by light pulses in the early subjective night and advanced by light pulses in the late subjective night, and there are relatively insensitive times in the day and mid–subjective night. The responses to dark pulses are out of phase with those for light pulses by 6–8 hours.

Single cells have circadian rhythms but in higher organisms the rhythms of various organs and tissues must be synchronized or provoked. Specialized areas (e.g., the optic lobes of roaches and the eyes of sea slugs) may act as pacemakers and provide the internal time cues. In some species the pineal may be a pacemaker; in other species the pineal is driven by a pacemaker believed to reside in the hypothalamus. Neuroendocrine hierarchies have been proposed to explain how a pacemaker can synchronize and drive the physiology of vertebrates.

Most of the pineal's operation and its role in the body involve daily and seasonal cycles. Associating the cycles with the gland led to an understanding of its function and sparked general interest in endocrine rhythms. Pineal rhythms follow most of the "rules" for circadian rhythms in general.

5.2 Daily Cycles

Daily cycles in pineal biochemical events are illustrated by time series or time profiles—a sequence of points obtained over 24 or more hours. Such profiles are usually obtained sequentially in LD 12:12 or LD 14:10, but an alternative method is to sample populations of organisms kept for 2 weeks or more in light-dark cycles whose dawn and dusk times are different. In either case, the time profiles are characterized by their shape—that is, by their amplitude and the timing of the maximum value (peak) and minimum value (nadir).

Quay [18] observed an interesting change in rat pineal indoleamine metabolism (Fig. 5.1): serotonin (5-HT) is high in the light and low in the dark. During the day, 5-hydroxyindole acetic acid (5-HIAA), the product of the conversion of serotonin by monoamine oxidase, is also high. But at night, 5-HIAA is low; instead, melatonin has its peak.

Profiles of pineal enzyme activities provide an explanation for melatonin production in the dark (Fig. 5.2). The activity of N-acetyltransferase (NAT) exhibits a pronounced daily cycle with a peak in the dark-time. Hydroxyindole-O-methyltransferase (HIOMT) has daily changes, but the day-night difference is small, usually less than twofold. Thus the shift in the fate of serotonin from 5-HIAA in the day to N-acetylserotonin at night is caused by the nightly activity of NAT. HIOMT, present day or night, produces methoxyindoles from whatever precursors are available. At night, when N-acetylserotonin is made by NAT, melatonin is formed by HIOMT. The time profiles of melatonin and NAT measured for all species so far have common features: peak NAT and melatonin occur in the dark-time irrespective of whether the organism has nocturnal or diurnal behavior. The serotonin profile, since it is affected by both synthesis and metabolism in the pineal, has a variable pattern—unimodal in the rat, bimodal in the chicken.

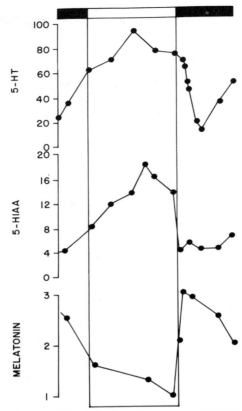

Figure 5.1 Daily time profiles for pineal serotonin (5-HT), 5-hydroxyindole acetic acid (5-HIAA), and melatonin in a nocturnal animal (rat). The figure shows the shift in the fate of serotonin from 5-HIAA in the light-time to melatonin in the dark-time. The horizontal bar over the profiles illustrates the LD 12:12 cycle that was used. All measurements are in ng/pineal. (Redrawn from Quay [18].)

Daily cycles are also found in other parameters of pineal biochemistry and anatomy (Fig. 5.3) and should not be considered to be limited to indoleamine biochemical events. However, the rhythms in melatonin and NAT are remarkable for their large amplitude, precise timing, regulation by light and dark, and dark-time peak.

5.3 Photoperiod

At most latitudes, the ratio of light to dark in the environment fluctuates with season of the year. Pineal measurements (e.g., enzyme activities and indole levels) have been made using photoperiods that are extremes or near the changes experienced normally by the

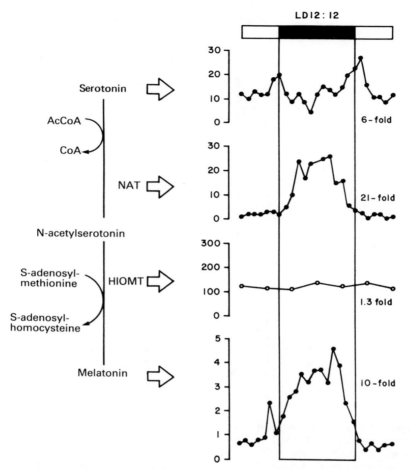

Figure 5.2 Daily time profiles for pineal serotonin, NAT, HIOMT, and melatonin in a diurnal animal (chick). Serotonin and melatonin are given as ng/pineal; NAT and HIOMT are given as nmol/pineal/hr. The horizontal bar illustrates the LD 12:12 cycle that was used. (From Binkley [3].)

organisms being studied. The changes in indoles are consistent with, and can be explained by, the consequence of the changes in the enzymes. Two types of changes have been obtained.

First, the shapes of the daily profiles change (Fig. 5.4). For example, NAT and melatonin exhibit longer periods of high levels when the dark period is lengthened (e.g., up to 12 hours in LD 8:16) and shorter periods of high levels (e.g., 4 hours) when the dark period is shortened. The amplitude of the NAT and melatonin is also affected, increasing in short dark and decreasing in long dark.

Second, long-term changes in enzyme activities and indole levels may occur. The most pronounced data for such long-term changes

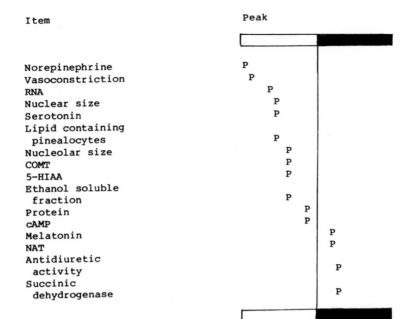

Item	Peak

Item		
Norepinephrine	P	
Vasoconstriction	P	
RNA	P	
Nuclear size	P	
Serotonin	P	
Lipid containing pinealocytes	P	
Nucleolar size	P	
COMT	P	
5-HIAA	P	
Ethanol soluble fraction	P	
Protein		P
cAMP		P
Melatonin		P
NAT		P
Antidiuretic activity		P
Succinic dehydrogenase		P

Figure 5.3 Peak times (*P*) of rhythmic events in the rat pineal gland. Abbreviations are as follows: *RNA*, ribonucleic acid; *COMT*, catechol-O-methyltransferase activity; *5-HIAA*, 5-hydroxyindole acetic acid; *cAMP*, cyclic adenosine 3′, 5′, monophosphate; *NAT*, N-acetyltransferase activity. (Redrawn from Quay [18].)

were obtained in sparrows under natural lighting where HIOMT varied markedly with season (Fig. 5.5). The data point out why caution should be used in denoting the rate-limiting enzyme for melatonin synthesis: in sparrows, the rate-limiting enzyme could be HIOMT in the season when the activity of the enzyme is low and it could be NAT in the season when HIOMT is not the limiting factor. A consequence of this might be alteration in the profile of indoles produced at different seasons. In other animals, the effect of photoperiod on HIOMT has been less dramatic than in sparrows. For example, in the laboratory, rat HIOMT after 6–12 weeks of long days is half the value it is after short days [17].

5.4 Constant Light and Constant Dark

The extremes of long and short photoperiods are constant light or constant dark. Here again, two types of effects are seen on pineal enzymes and indoles: (1) acute effects on the daily rhythms and (2) long-term effects. When constant dark is imposed, pineal N-acetyl-

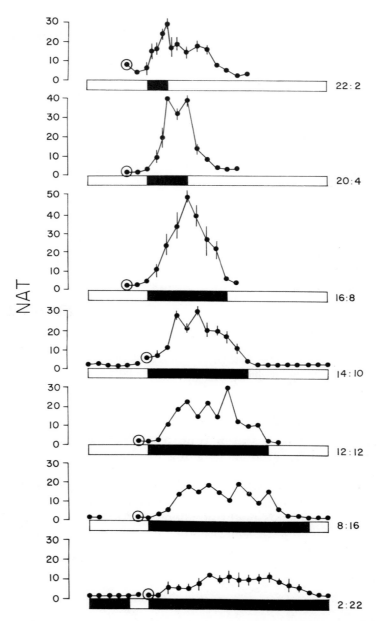

Figure 5.4 NAT profiles in chicks raised for 3 weeks in light-dark cycles with dark durations of 8–22 hours. The figure shows the effect of photoperiod on the pineal gland. The horizontal bar below each profile illustrates the 24-hour light-dark cycle that was used to obtain that profile. (From Binkley [3].)

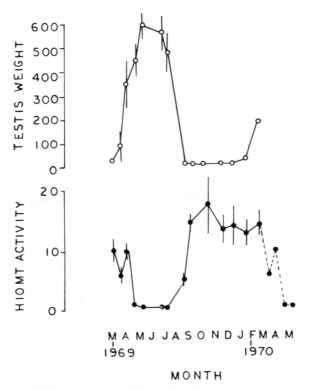

Figure 5.5 Pineal HIOMT (levels) measured in sparrows over the course of a year with concomitant testis weight. (Redrawn from Barfuss and Ellis [1].)

transferase and melatonin rhythms persist with periods close to 24 hours. The persistence of the rhythms is evidence that they are truly circadian in nature and not simply driven by the environmental lighting. In constant dark, the rhythms of some species exhibit damped amplitude compared to the amplitude achieved in LD (Fig. 5.6)

When constant light is imposed, pineal N-acetyltransferase and melatonin rhythms may persist with periods close to 24 hours. Usually, however, the rhythm is damped (reduced in amplitude) compared to the rhythm in either constant dark or LD. Sometimes, in constant light, the rhythms appear to be lost altogether (arrhythmia). Constant light and dark have effects on HIOMT similar to those of long and short photoperiods—that is, constant light reduces HIOMT to half the activity it has in constant dark.

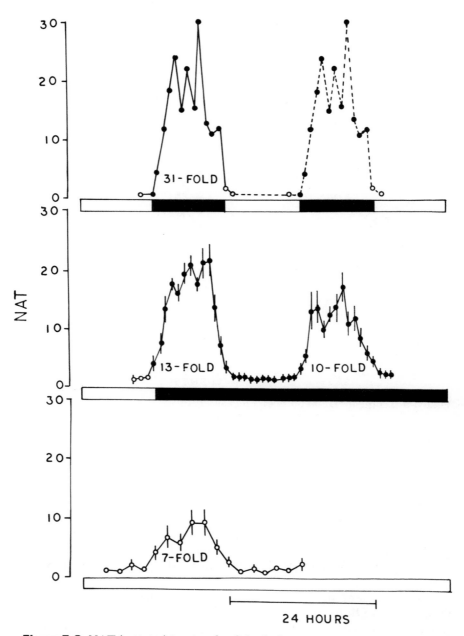

Figure 5.6 NAT (activity) in pineals of chicks kept in LD 12:12, constant dark (DD) or constant light (LL). The figure shows persistence of the rhythm in constant conditions and effects of constant dark and light on amplitude. The horizontal bar below the profiles illustrates the light or dark conditions. All the chicks were previously in the LD 12:12 cycle. Data for the first and second days of DD are shown. (From Binkley [3].)

5.5 Refractory Period and Rapid Plummet

The free-running rhythm in constant dark points up the fact that dark cannot continuously stimulate NAT and melatonin. NAT and melatonin production appear to occur cyclically under the influence of a clock providing a timed program. The pineal, then, is "refractory" to stimulation during part of the day, much as the heart is refractory to electrical stimuli during part of its cycle. The existence of a refractory period has been verified with other experiments. If animals (e.g., rats or chickens) are exposed to dark at various times over 24 hours, NAT activity increases only when the time of expected lights-out approaches or during the time of expected lights-out. In other words, dark will not provoke NAT in the early morning. The refractory period recurs on the next day, even if the animal was not exposed to dark but instead was kept in the light throughout a night. Thus, the timing of the rise in NAT appears to be controlled by a clock that provides a gate: if dark occurs in the gated periods, NAT increases.

On the other hand, extending light into the dark-time delays the rise in NAT and the decline in serotonin levels. Thus, the pineal has a means for designating the time of lights-out with respect to an internal standard provided by the circadian clock.

As we have said, light suppresses the amplitude of the daily cycle of NAT and the long-term level of HIOMT. Light has yet another suppressive effect on NAT. If animals are exposed to light unexpectedly, in the dark, when NAT is high, NAT falls rapidly with a halving time of 3–5 minutes and serotonin levels rise. The fall in NAT has been called the *rapid plummet*. The plummet occurs any time NAT is high, though it may be greater in the early than the late subjective night. The rapid plummet permits the pineal to denote the end of the scotoperiod. It has been pointed out that the rapid plummet may involve the sulfur-related instability of NAT because the time course for the rapid plummet in vivo is similar to the time course for loss of NAT in homogenates at 37° C or loss of NAT when an inhibitor is added to pineal cultures [6] (Fig. 5.7). If the light pulse falls in the early subjective night, NAT can rise again and appears to "complete" its programmed duration; but, if the light pulse falls in the late subjective night, NAT does not rise again as though the refractory period had begun and the pulse was considered a new dawn (Fig. 5.8).

Therefore, the pineal can keep track of light and dark. It can measure the length of the dark period. It can compare the length of an imposed dark period with that experienced on the previous day. Much as a yardstick is used to measure length, the interaction of light with the duration of NAT activity can be used as a "timestick" to measure scotoperiod. By secreting melatonin, the pineal can convey the time information to other cells.

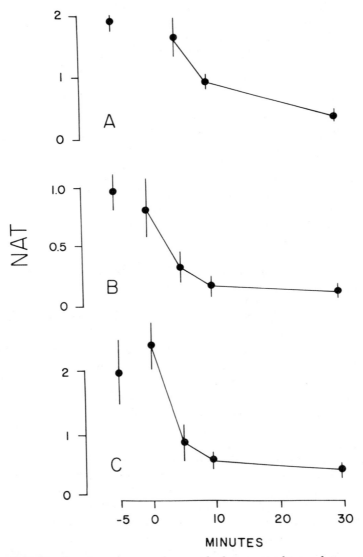

Figure 5.7 Similar time courses for rapid plummets obtained in rat pineal NAT (activity) with three different treatments. *A,* plummet observed in homogenates of dark-time rat pineals kept at 37°C. *B,* plummet observed in organ cultures of pineals stimulated with norepinephrine (NE), 10^{-4} M, and then inhibited with *N*-ethylmaleimide (NEM), 10^{-3} M. *C,* plummet obtained in rats exposed to light in the dark-time. (From Binkley [3].)

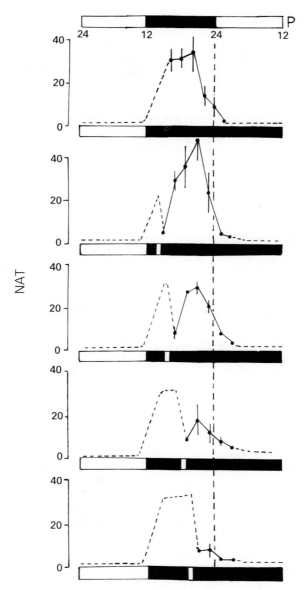

Figure 5.8 Rapid plummets and reinitiations of pineal NAT (activity) in chicks exposed to 1-hour-long light pulses. The NAT reinitiated and completed the subjective night with high activity if the pulse was imposed in the early subjective night. The NAT did not reinitiate if the pulse was imposed in the late subjective night when the chicks were refractory. The top horizontal bar illustrates the LD 12:12 in which the chicks were raised; the horizontal bars below each profile illustrate the actual light-dark treatments under which the profiles were measured. (From Binkley [4, 5].)

5.6 Resetting

Light and dark pulses not only delimit the duration of NAT, they can reset the clock for the next cycle. A light pulse in the early subjective night delays the next NAT cycle but a light pulse in the late subjective night advances the next NAT cycle (Fig. 5.9). Dark pulses have roughly opposite effects. Phase response curves for light and dark pulses for NAT are about 6 hours out of phase with one another (Fig. 5.10). The resetting responses of NAT are typical for circadian rhythms. As little as 1 minute of light shifts the phase of the rat NAT rhythm [12].

5.7 Light Quality

Most of the investigators who studied the pineal used experimental light sources that were cool white fluorescent tubes and had the animals in 300–1500 lux light intensities. More rarely, natural light was used or attention was paid to definition of the light source.

The effects of cool white fluorescent light intensity and light spectra on melatonin synthesis have been studied using the rapid plummet response. Results showed that 0.5 $\mu W/cm^2$ suppressed rat NAT by 50%; 15 $\mu W/cm^2$ produced full NAT inhibition [15]. Pigmented rats were more sensitive than albino rats [13]. The threshold for suppression of pineal melatonin and NAT in Syrian hamsters was 0.06 $\mu W/cm^2$ or 1.08 lux [8, 10]. The order of effectiveness for colors of light in suppressing pineal melatonin in Syrian hamsters was blue (most), green, yellow, near UV, and red (least) [9]. Isolated chick pineal glands had peak NAT suppression at 500 nm [11].

In another investigation, three different light intensities were used to make up two cycles, bright-dim and dim-dark. In these cycles, urinary melatonin peaked in the dim (of bright-dim) and the dark (of dim-dark) even though the dim light was the same. The experiment showed that peak melatonin occurs in the darker of two conditions and is not simply driven by the light intensity [14].

5.8 Photoreceptors

Photoreceptors for the mammalian pineal events and pineal-mediated events are the eyes. Bilateral orbital enucleation (blinding) eliminates the responses to light but not the rhythms. In mammals and birds, the expectation is that the traditional photoreceptors and photopigment (rhodopsin) are responsible for receiving and relaying the light-dark information to the pineal gland.

In the birds and lower vertebrates, however, blinding does not eliminate all pineal responses to light and dark. Pineals of some

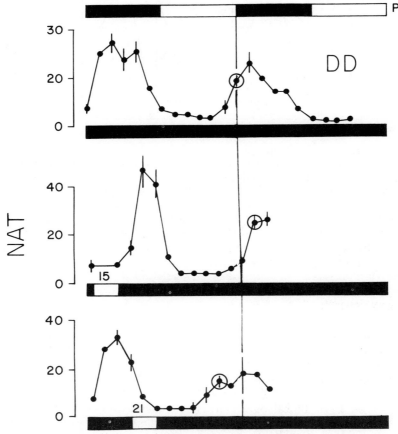

Figure 5.9 Subsequent NAT cycles were phase-shifted (*right*) if chicks were exposed to 4-hour-long light pulses (*left*). Constant dark controls and experimentals that delayed and advanced are shown. The top horizontal bar (*P*) illustrates the LD 12:12 in which the chicks were raised; the horizontal bars below each profile illustrate the actual one-time light treatments under which the profiles were measured. Experiments such as this produced data for the phase response curves plotted in Figure 5.10. (From Binkley [3].)

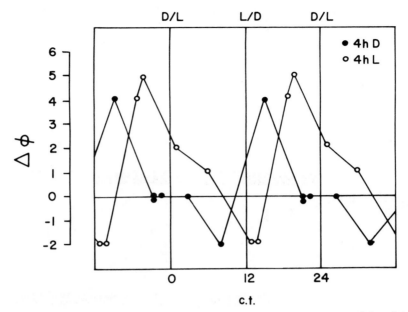

Figure 5.10 Light and dark pulse phase response curves measured for chick pineal NAT using 4-hour-long light or dark pulses. The phase shift ($\Delta\phi$) is in hours and the data have been duplicated horizontally in order to visualize the full peak and nadir. (From Binkley, White, and Mosher [7].)

species perceive light directly, though there is evidence that these pineals receive light and dark information from the lateral eyes as well. The rapid plummet, constant light suppression, and entrainment can all be obtained in blind birds.

REFERENCES

1. Barfuss, D., and L. Ellis. 1971. Seasonal cycles in melatonin synthesis by the pineal gland as related to testicular function in the house sparrow, *Passer domesticus. Gen. Comp. Endocrinol.* 17:183–193.

2. Binkley, S. 1976a. Pineal gland biorhythms: *N*-acetyltransferase in chickens and rats. *FASEB* 35:2347–2352.

3. ———. 1981. Pineal biochemistry: Comparative aspects and circadian rhythms. In *The pineal gland I: Anatomy and biochemistry*, ed. R. Reiter, pp. 155–172. Boca Raton, Fla.: CRC Press.

4. ———. 1983a. Rhythms in ocular and pineal *N*-acetyltransferase: A portrait of an enzyme clock. *Comp. Biochem. Physiol.* 75A:123–129.

5. ———. 1983b. Circadian rhythm in pineal *N*-acetyltransferase activity: Phase shifting by light pulses II. *J. Neurochem.* 41:173–276.

6. Binkley, S., D. Klein, and J. Weller. 1976. Pineal serotonin *N*-acetyltransferase activity: Protection of stimulated activity by acetyl-CoA and related compounds. *J. Neurochem.* 26:51–55.

7. Binkley, S., B. White, and K. Mosher. 1985. Circadian phase of sparrows: Control by light and dark. *Photochem. Photobiol.* 41:453–457.
8. Brainard, G., B. Richardson, T. King, S. Matthews, and R. Reiter. 1983. The suppression of pineal melatonin content and N-acetyltransferase activity by different light irradiances in the Syrian hamster: A dose-response relationship. *Endocrinology* 113:293–296.
9. Brainard, G., B. Richardson, T. King, and R. Reiter. 1984. The influence of different light spectra on the suppression of pineal melatonin content in the Syrian hamster. *Brain Res.* 294:333–339.
10. Brainard, G., B. Richardson, L. Petterborg, and R. Reiter. 1982. The effect of different light intensities on pineal melatonin content. *Brain Res.* 233:75–81.
11. Deguchi, T. 1981. Rhodopsin-like photosensitivity of isolated chicken pineal gland. *Nature* 290:706–707.
12. Illnerová, H., and J. Vaněček. 1984. Circadian rhythm in inducibility of rat pineal N-acetyltransferase after brief light pulses at night. Control by a morning oscillator. *J. Comp. Physiol.* 154:739–744.
13. Lynch, H., M. Deng, and R. Wurtman. 1984. Light intensities required to suppress nocturnal melatonin secretion in albino and pigmented rats. *Life Sci.* 35:841–847.
14. Lynch, H., R. Rivest, P. Ronsheim, and R. Wurtman. 1981. Light intensity and the control of melatonin secretion in rats. *Neuroendocrinology* 33:181–185.
15. Minneman, K., H. Lynch, and R. Wurtman. 1984. Relationship between environmental light intensity and retina-mediated suppression of rat pineal serotonin-N-acetyltransferase. *Life Sci.* 15:1791–1796.
16. Quay, W. 1966. Rhythmic and light-induced changes in levels of pineal 5-hydroxyindoles in the pigeon (*Columba livia*). *Gen. Comp. Endo.* 6:371–377.
17. ———. 1968. Relation of pineal acetylserotonin methyltransferase activity to daily photoperiod and light intensity. *Archives d'Anatomie, Histologie et d'Embryologie Normales et Experimentales* 51:567–571.
18. ———. 1974. *Pineal chemistry.* Springfield, Ill.: Charles C Thomas.

6

Neural and Endogenous Control of Pineal Function

"Pineal function in mammals is regulated by a system with four major neural components. The first is a retinohypothalamic projection from the ganglion cells of the retina to the suprachiasmatic nucleus of the hypothalamus. The suprachiasmatic nucleus appears to function as a circadian oscillating system projecting into the hypothalamus and this represents the second component. The third component is constituted of a brainstem pathway from the lateral hypothalamus to the intermediolateral cell column of the upper thoracic spinal cord. The fourth component is the preganglionic and postganglionic sympathetic system arising from the upper thoracic cord to innervate the superior cervical ganglion which, in turn, innervates the pineal gland."

R. Y. Moore [12]

6.1 Variation in Regulation

One scheme does not suffice to explain regulation of the pineal because of species variation. However, a reasonable tactic for understanding pineal regulation is to use the scheme that has been established for the adult laboratory rat [1] as a reference standard for the variations that are present in other species (Fig 6.1). In the rat, the

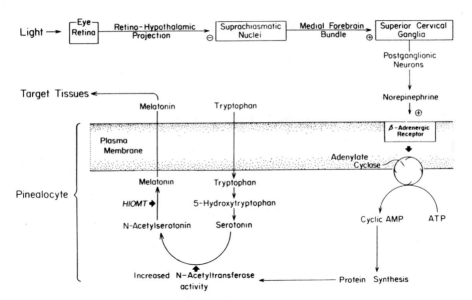

Figure 6.1 The pathway by which light perceived by the eyes regulates the production of melatonin in the pineal gland of the rat. (With permission of M. Hadley [8] and Prentice Hall.)

eyes are the only photoreceptor for acquiring light and dark information (Fig. 6.1). There is a neural route from the eyes to the pineal. The pineal cannot maintain repeated oscillations without neural input from the suprachiasmatic nucleus. The pineal is stimulated by adrenergic agents and is the major site of rhythmic melatonin synthesis. These facts are not applicable to all species.

The chicken is an example of a species in which regulation of the pineal is quite different [2, 3]. The pineal as well as the eyes can acquire light and dark information. While there is evidence for a neural route from the eyes to the pineal as in rats, the chick pineal can maintain repeated daily oscillations of melatonin synthesis isolated in organ culture. The pineal is inhibited rather than stimulated by adrenergic agents. The eyes as well as the pineal are capable of rhythmic melatonin synthesis. Thus, whereas the rat appears to have a single neural route for regulation of melatonin synthesis, the chicken pineal has two routes of control: (1) a neural route like that in the rat, and (2) the ability within the pineal to detect light and generate oscillation.

Regulation of the pineal, then, must be unraveled on a species-by-species basis. While this may at first glance be unsatisfying, from another point of view it is to be expected. The case that is developing for pineal function is based on the premise that the pineal is a gland involved in detection and use of environmental information, especially light, for temporal organization of an animal's physiology. Since different species have specialized environmental adaptations (e.g., they are nocturnal or diurnal in their behavior), their systems for temporal physiological organization must be themselves specialized.

6.2 Neural Pathway and Consequences

The principal neural pathway by which the pineal is controlled is that studied in rats [1]: the eyes act as photoreceptors; the light and dark information they detect is coordinated with time information from the suprachiasmatic nuclei acting as a circadian clock; rhythmic signals (integrating lighting with rhythm information) are then transmitted to the pineal via a neural route in which a component is the superior cervical ganglia.

6.2.1 Eyes

In mammals, the eyes are photoreceptors for regulation of the pineal. Blinding rats eliminates the pineal responses to light (e.g., attenuation by constant light, rapid plummet), but it does not eliminate pineal rhythms (e.g., N-acetyltransferase, NAT). The cells within the eyes that are responsible for receiving information that will affect the pineal melatonin synthesis have yet to be identified. Presently, rods and cones are the candidates and the proposed photopigment is rhodopsin.

Light information from the retina is conveyed to the hypothalamus by a special tract of nerve fibers called the *retinohypothalamic tract*. The fibers of this pathway (which proceed to the hypothalamus) are distinct from the fibers in the optic nerves (which proceed to the lateral geniculate nucleus and visual cortex).

6.2.2 Suprachiasmatic nuclei

Circadian clock information for the pineal gland (of some species, such as the rat) comes from two small areas of the hypothalamus, the suprachiasmatic nuclei (SCN). In adult rats, lesions of the nuclei abolish (1) the rhythm in NAT that is present in DD, and (2) responses of pineal NAT to light. The integration of the light information (as in entrainment) with the endogenous clock information may occur at the level of the SCN [12, 13]. Evidence that the SCN has rhythms comes from studies with 2-deoxyglucose [15]. Radioactive 2-deoxyglucose (2-DG) is a substance which some believe is taken up by nerve cells that are active; the 2-DG is not metabolized as is glucose; autoradiographic examination of sections of brain from animals treated with 2-DG may show which cells are active. Rat SCN take up more 2-DG

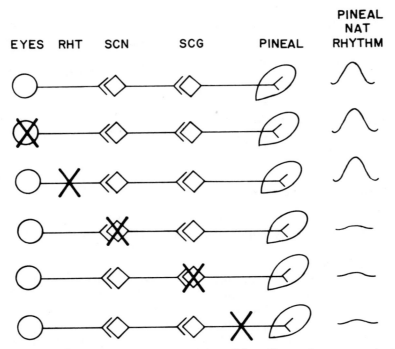

Figure 6.2 A diagrammatic representation of the effects of surgery or lesions of various structures upon the rat pineal NAT rhythm. the rhythm was abolished by lesions of the suprachiasmatic nuclei (SCN) and by denervation of the pineal.

in the light (3–4 hours after lights-on) than in the dark (3–4 hours after lights-off) of LD-12:12. Nerve tracts that eventually connect with the path to the pineal leave the posterior of the SCN because prechiasmatic cuts do not abolish the rhythm in pineal NAT but postchiasmatic cuts do abolish the cycles (Fig. 6.2).

The hypothesis that has been proposed is that the circadian rhythm originates in cells of the SCN and it is in the SCN that the information from the "clock" is integrated with the information from the eyes about the prevailing light conditions. The pathway from the point where the integrated neural information leaves the posterior SCN to the preganglionic neurons is still to be defined. The medial forebrain bundle may be in the pathway since its destruction abolishes the pineal NAT rhythm in rats.

6.2.3 Superior cervical ganglia

Preganglionic neurons in the intermediolateral cell column of the spinal cord have unmyelinated fibers that synapse with postganglionic cell bodies in the superior cervical ganglia (SCG) of the sympathetic chains [1]. Cells of the SCG that innervate the pineal are adrenergic neurons (producing norepinephrine). Removal of the SCG from adult rats (by surgery, by chemical sympathectomy with 6-OH dopamine, or by immunosympathectomy) eliminates the pineal NAT rhythm and light responses. Thus, the SCG regulate the pineal by providing neural signals to the pineal in response to signals that the SCG receive from the SCN. The role proposed for the SCG so far is only one of transmitting or conveying the signals from SCN; modification of the SCN information or integration of the signals with other information has not been proposed.

6.3 Pineal β-Receptors

The suggestion has been made for rats that stimulation of pineal melatonin synthesis by catecholamines is mediated by β-receptors [1, 4, 7]. The receptors are visualized as sites on pinealocyte membranes that chemically recognize catecholamines; because of this recognition, the receptors do something that activates the cells to produce melatonin. The hypothesis, then, is that the postganglionic fibers from the SCG release norepinephrine in the pineal and that the norepinephrine interacts with β-receptors which may be on pinealocyte cell membranes; in response to the stimulation, pineal cells produce produce melatonin.

6.3.1 Pharmacology

The evidence for receptors and how they act is mostly pharmacological. For in vivo experiments, animals are injected with drugs followed by measurement of pineal parameter, such as NAT in rat pineals. The effect of a drug in such a protocol can always be indirect; therefore, in order to verify that a compound acts on the pineal, in vitro pharmacological techniques have been used to isolate the pineal responses. Pineals are removed from animals and placed in organ or cell culture; drugs are added to the cultures followed by measurement of a pineal parameter, again such as NAT in rat pineals. Receptor types are assigned on the basis of which drugs stimulate a response (agonists) and which other drugs prevent a response (blockers). (See Table 6.1.) Adrenergic agonists, which should mimic norepinephrine, stimulate rat pineal NAT. Norepinephrine stimulates rat pineal NAT in vitro (See Table 2.2), but is less effective when injected, possibly because the norepinephrine is metabolized too rapidly. However, isoproterenol, an agonist that has a structure similar to norepinephrine, stimulates NAT both when it is injected into rats (Table 2.1) and when it is added to rat pineal cultures (Fig. 6.3).

Based on relative potencies of agonists and blockers, rat pineal melatonin synthesis has been classified as a β-adrenergic response

TABLE 6.1 Compounds that affect NAT in rat pineals in vivo and/or in vitro.

NAT stimulators	NAT blockers
L-norepinephrine	Propranolol
L-isoproterenol	Cycloheximide
L-DOPA	2-fluorohistidine
Epinephrine	Actinomycin D
Phenylephrine	Cordycepin
Terbutaline	α-Amanitin
Dobutamine	Serotonin
Desmethylimipramine	N-ethylmaleimide
Tyramine	Cystamine
Cocaine	Reserpine
Procaine	Indomethacin
Veratridine	Nialamide
0 KCl (Zero potassium chloride)	Tetrodotoxin
Chlorpromazine	Mecamylamine
Catron, pheniprazine	Nicotine
Pargyline	Methoxamine
Harmine	Anesthetic barbiturates
Theophylline	Morphine
Isobutylmethylxanthine	Lidocaine
Choleragen	Dibucaine
Dibutyryl cAMP	Potassium
Prostaglandin E_2	Carbachol
Vasoactive intestinal peptide	Atropine
Taurine	

Sources: Binkley [1] and Kaneko et al. [9].

[1]. A case has sometimes been made for a role of α-receptors in pineal regulation as well [17].

6.3.2 Supersensitivity

Pineal glands of rats that have been ganglionectomized exhibit larger-than-normal responses to adrenergic stimulation. For example, injected L-DOPA caused a 100-fold increase in rat pineal NAT in ganglionectomized rats but only a 30-fold increase in rat pineal NAT in unoperated rats [6, 7]. This phenomenon has been called *superinduction* or *supersensitivity*. The increased response could be explained if adrenergic receptor sensitivity or numbers were increased by deprivation of normal stimulation. Superinduction of pineals from ganglionectomized rats also occurs in vitro, implying that the cause of supersensitivity resides in the pineal gland.

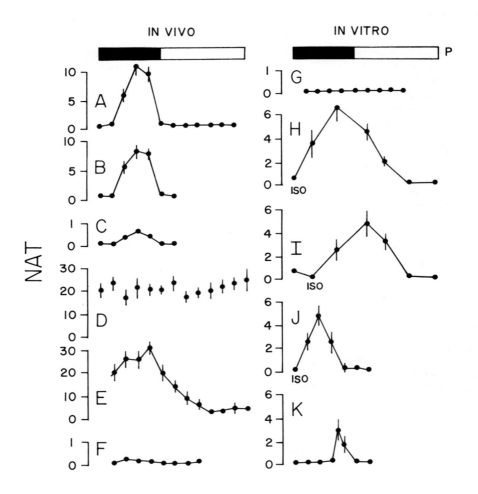

Figure 6.3 NAT activity in pineal glands of rats studied in vivo (*left*) and in vitro (*right*). The data show the effects of denervation and isoproterenol (*ISO*), regulation by light, and occurrence of a spontaneous NAT cycle in neonatal rat pineals. Rats in *A–I* were 3–4 weeks old; those in *J–K* were 10–14 days old. Conditions were as follows: *A*, NAT rhythm in LD 14:10; *B*, NAT rhythm in DD; *C*, NAT rhythm in LL; *D*, stimulation by single injections of isoproterenol in LL 4 hours prior to the time of each point; for this reason the points have not been connected; *E*, exhaustion by repeated injections of isoproterenol; *F*, superior cervical ganglionectomy; *G*, superior cervical ganglionectomy or control or 6-hydroxydopamine injected; *H, I*, isoproterenol added to culture medium at two different times; *J*, isoproterenol added to pineals from 10- to 14-day-old rats; *K*, cycle in pineals from 10- to 14-day-old rats. (Data from Binkley [1] and White, Mosher and Binkley [18].)

6.3.3 Subsensitivity or exhaustion

Rat pineals cannot be stimulated to continuous high NAT levels either in vivo (e.g., with repeated injections of L-isoproterenol) or in vitro (by continuous presence or additions of L-isoproterenol to culture medium). The terms *subsensitivity* or *exhaustion* have been used to denote this phenomenon [6, 7] and three explanations for subsensitivity can be suggested. The first, like that for supersensitivity, is based on receptors: the presence of a stimulating agent (e.g., L-isoproterenol) causes a reduction in receptor numbers. The second alternative is that the decrease in responsiveness occurs inside the pinealocyte due to exhaustion of something required for melatonin production (the RNA for NAT, NAT, a substrate, etc.) [18]. A third possibility is that decreased response is more complicated, to wit, that several phenomena—both receptor sensitivity and exhaustion of some required substance—are involved.

6.3.4 Sensitivity and the NAT rhythm

It is possible that the sensitivity/subsensitivity phenomena have roles in generation of the NAT rhythm. In reinitiation experiments, pineals (e.g., of rats and chicks), as noted in Chapter 5, exhibit a rapid plummet in response to light. When animals treated with light to produce the plummet were replaced in the dark, one of two events happened. After a light pulse in the early subjective night, NAT reinitiated and appeared to complete its normal time course. The pineals were still "sensitive" to stimulation by dark. The subsequent descent in NAT which occurred in the dark was only 1–2 hours later than in controls that experienced no plummet. After a light pulse in the late subjective night, NAT failed to reinitiate; the pineals were refractory—they were no longer sensitive to stimulation by dark.

Sensitivity status provides a possible explanation for circadian rhythm phase shifting and resetting, because sensitivity status when a light pulse occurs affects the timing of the subsequent cycle as well as the cycle in which it is imposed. If NAT is suppressed in the early subjective night—when the system is still sensitive to dark—the NAT reinitiates, the cycle is completed but ends slightly late; and the next cycle is slightly delayed. Delay phase shifts are thus produced by light pulses in the early subjective night. If NAT is suppressed by light in the late subjective night—when the system has become insensitive to dark stimulation—the NAT does not reinitiate, the cycle has ended early, and the next day's cycle is advanced. Light pulses in the late subjective night thus cause phase advances.

6.4 Second Messengers

The second-messenger hypothesis, as applied to the rat pineal, holds that once a neural signal has been perceived by β-receptors on a pinealocyte, the signal is conveyed to control intracellular processes by a second messenger, cAMP [1]. Dibutyryl cyclic AMP (a cell-penetrating analog of cAMP) provokes NAT and melatonin synthesis in the rat pineal; because of this, cAMP is probably the principal second messenger. We apply second-messenger tenets to propose a sequence of events in a pineal cell: (1) the interaction between the norepinephrine and the β-receptor is transduced to activate an enzyme, adenyl cyclase, in the pineal cell membrane; (2) the adenyl cyclase catalyzes the production of cAMP inside the cell; (3) the cAMP activates a protein kinase; and (4) a cascade of reactions result in NAT initiation by activation.

There is other evidence for a cAMP second messenger in the pineal. Inhibitors of phosphodiesterase (such as theophylline), which should raise cAMP levels, stimulate rat pineal NAT. Agents that increase pineal NAT also increase cAMP production and adenyl cyclase activity.

Some puzzles remain, however. First, supersensitivity and subsensitivity are seen for responses to dibutyryl cyclic AMP (which should bypass the receptors); this implies that super- and subsensitivity involve intracellular events, not β-receptors. Second, NAT initiation and maintenance requires new protein synthesis, not protein activation. The evidence for this is that cycloheximide, a poison that blocks protein synthesis, prevents stimulation of pineal NAT. Moreover, if cycloheximide is injected in the dark even after NAT has increased, NAT declines [6, 7]. These results with cycloheximide imply continuous new synthesis of NAT must occur throughout the night in order to keep NAT at high levels.

A role has been suggested for cAMP in the decrease in NAT as well as in its increase. A decline in cAMP was accompanied by a decline in NAT [10]. However, NAT declines even in the continued presence of high levels of dibutyryl cAMP. It is possible that cAMP decreases, signaling a rapid plummet (as in response to unexpected light); but it is also possible that there are other factors that can cause the cessation of NAT (as occurs without a light signal, in DD).

6.5 Intrapineal Control

The pineal is not a simple slave of neural signals in some species. There is evidence that the pineal can function by itself as clock or photoreceptor, but these capabilities are not found in the rat pineal.

6.5.1 Intrapineal clock

Pineals or pineal cells of some species (chickens, sparrows, quail, and lizards) are capable of initiating NAT or producing melatonin in vitro without β-adrenergic agents (as required by rats). They are capable not only of a complete cycle, but of repetitive cycles, or a rhythm. The cycles can be studied by assaying NAT in glands that have been cultured [3] or by measuring melatonin in effluent medium from single pineals in superfusion culture [16]. Pineals placed in culture do not simply begin the cycle as though rezeroed; rather, they commence from the time at which the pineals were removed from the animal and placed into culture (Fig. 6.4). This phenomenon has been called *timekeeping* [2]. The rhythm in vitro remains longer in the presence of a light-dark cycle than in DD. (Deguchi [5] claims 17 cycles for chick pineal cells in culture in LD). In constant dark, the rhythm damps in chick pineals but there are at least three to four cycles.

Generally, the amplitude of the first cycle in vitro is much larger than those of subsequent cycles (an observation that also applies to the NAT cycle measured in vivo in chicks in constant dark). Two explanations come to mind. The first is that some structure(s) present in the pineal responsible for the large rhythm deteriorates in the first day of culture. Pineals in vitro do show necrosis. The second is that the amplitude of pineal NAT is programmed by light and dark of the previous cycle and that this programming requires input from extra-pineal structures.

There is reason to believe that there are extrapineal influences (e.g., neural regulation) on pineals of animals, such as chickens, whose pineals are capable of rhythmic melatonin synthesis in vitro. First, the glands have terminals. Additions of NAT-stimulating agents (isopro-terenol, pargyline, dibutyryl cyclic AMP) to cultures of chicken pineals or injection of the compounds into chickens alters NAT but does not produce the maximal stimulation response obtained with rat pineals. Second, ablation of SCG abolishes the NAT rhythm in the chick pineal in constant dark, but removing the ganglia does not alter the NAT cycle in LD 12:12 [14]. Third, blinding chicks, as mentioned, reduces the magnitude of (but does not eliminate) the responses to light and dark in vivo.

The duration of high NAT or melatonin production is limited in the pineals of chicks—just as in rats—so the duration program may result from the same cause even though the mechanisms for initiation of the NAT may differ.

6.5.2 Pineal light perception

Pineals of some species (e.g., chickens) detect light in vitro [3] (Fig. 6.5). Constant light attenuates the amplitude of the NAT cycle [3].

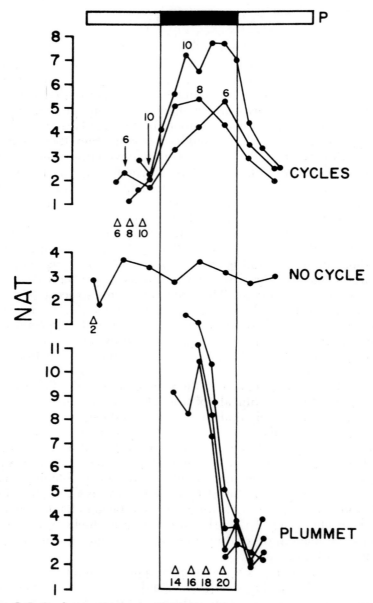

Figure 6.4 Cycles in chick pineal NAT in DD in vitro as a function of time. The Cultures were begun after lights-on in the previous (*P*) LD 12:12 regimen. The data show that the pineal exhibits a well-defined cycle when the culture was begun in the late subjective day, (6, 8, and 10 hr after lights-on) but not in the early subjective day (2 hr after lights-on). When the cultures were begun at several times in the dark-time (14, 16, 18, 20, hr after lights-on) NAT plummeted at one time. (After Binkley, Riebman, and Reilly [3].)

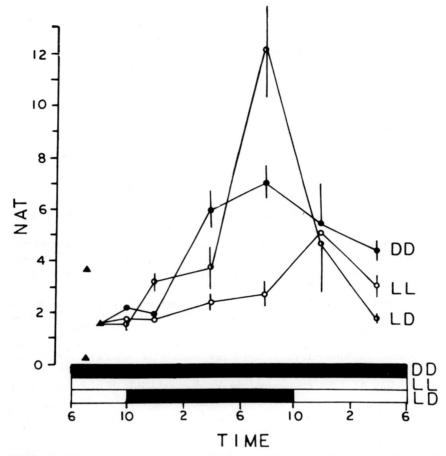

Figure 6.5 NAT measurements in chick pineals in vitro that were subjected to an LD cycle, DD, or LL while in culture prove that light directly affects chick pineal NAT. (After Binkley, Riebman, and Reilly [3].)

The rapid plummet response to light can also be obtained in vitro [5]. Presumably, the light is detected by pinealocytes (using photoreceptor-like structures denoted as inner and outer segments, the cilia and whorls) and the photopigment is rhodopsin-like.

6.6 Systemic Catecholamines

Because of the high degree of pineal vascularization, it would be surprising if the gland did not exhibit some responses to circulating substances. For example, it should be possible to elicit pineal adrenergic responses with stress via catecholamines from the adrenal. In fact, rats subjected to extreme stress (several hours of immobilization or swimming in the light-time) increase pineal NAT and melatonin more than six-fold [11]. Roles for circulating catecholamines in the normal function of the pineal have not been established.

REFERENCES

1. Binkley, S. 1983. Circadian rhythms of pineal function in rats. *Endocrine Rev.* 4:255–270.

2. Binkley, S., J. Riebman, and K. Reilly. 1977. Timekeeping by the pineal gland. *Science* 197:1181–1183.

3. ———. 1978. The pineal gland: A biological clock in vitro. *Science* 202:1198–1201.

4. Deguchi, T. 1978. Circadian rhythm of serotonin *N*-acetyltransferase activity in organ culture of chicken pineal gland. *Science* 203:1245–1247.

5. ———. 1979. A circadian oscillator in cultured cells of chicken pineal gland. *Nature* 282:1–3.

6. Deguchi, T., and J. Axelrod. 1972a. Control of circadian change of serotonin *N*-acetyltransferase activity in the pineal organ by the β-adrenergic receptor. *Proc. Nat. Acad. Sci. USA* 69:2547–2550.

7. ———. 1972b. Induction and superinduction of serotonin *N*-acetyltransferase by adrenergic drugs and denervation in rat pineal organ. *Proc. Nat. Acad. Sci. USA* 69:2208–2211.

8. Hadley, M. 1984. *Endocrinology.* Englewood Cliffs, N.J.: Prentice Hall.

9. Kaneko, T., P. Cheng, H. Oka, T. Oda, N. Yanaihara, and C. Yanaihara. 1980. Vasoactive intestinal polypeptide stimulates adenylate cyclase and serotonin *N*-acetyltransferase activities in rat pineal in vitro. *Biomed. Res.* 1:84–87.

10. Klein, D., M. Buda, C. Kapoor, and G. Krishna. 1978. Pineal serotonin *N*-acetyltransferase activity: Abrupt decrease in adenosine 3′, 5′-monophosphate may be signal for "turnoff". *Science* 199:309–311.

11. Lynch, H., J. Eng., and R. Wurtman. 1973. Control of pineal indole biosynthesis by changes in tone caused by factors other than environmental lighting. *Proc. Natl. Acad. Sci. USA* 70:1704–1707.

12. Moore, R. 1978. Neural control of pineal function in mammals and birds. *J. Neural Trans. Suppl.* 13:47–58.

13. Moore, R., and D. Klein. 1974. Visual pathways and the central neural control of a circadian rhythm in pineal serotonin *N*-acetyltranferase. *Brain Res.* 71:17–33.

14. Ralph, D., S. Binkley, S. MacBride, and D. Klein. 1975. Regulation of pineal rhythms in chickens: Effects of blinding, constant light, constant dark, and superior cervical ganglionectomy. *Endocrinology* 97:1373–1378.

15. Schwarz, W., and H. Gainer. 1977. Suprachiasmatic nucleus: Use of ^{14}C-labeled deoxyglucose uptake as a functional marker. *Science* 197:1089–1091.

16. Takahashi, J., H. Hamm, and M. Menaker. 1980. Circadian rhythms of melatonin release from individual superfused chicken pineal glands in vitro. *Proc. Natl. Acad. Sci. USA* 77:2319–2322.

17. Vaněcěk, J., D. Sugden, J. Weller, and D. Klein. 1985. Atypical synergistic α-1- and β-adrenergic regulation of adenosine 3′, 5′-monophosphate and guanosine 3′,5′-monophosphate in rat pinealocytes. *Endocrinology* 116:2167–2173.

18. White, B., K. Mosher, and S. Binkley. 1985. Rat pineal *N*-acetyltransferase (NAT): Stimulation, exhaustion, and recovery. *Endocrinology* 117: 1050–1056.

7

Mammalian Photoperiodism

"Exposure of male hamsters to cycles of 1 hour of light and 23 hours of darkness causes atrophy of the gonads. Pinealectomy prevents this atrophy, but has no effect on animals exposed to light-dark cycles of 16:8. Likewise, removal of both eyes induces gonad atrophy which is prevented by pinealectomy. These data emphasize the importance of the pineal gland in the regulation of photoperiodic influences on the gonads."

R. Hoffman and R. Reiter [7]

7.1 Introduction

The pineal has been studied with respect to a number of possible roles in reproduction of both males and females. Appreciation of these functions requires an understanding of the interaction of light and circadian rhythms in seasonal reproductive phenomena. Most attention has been directed toward the part played by the pineal in seasonal reproduction in hamsters. In addition to its role in seasonal breeding, the pineal may act in reproduction in puberty, in compensatory hypertrophy, and in the menstrual cycle.

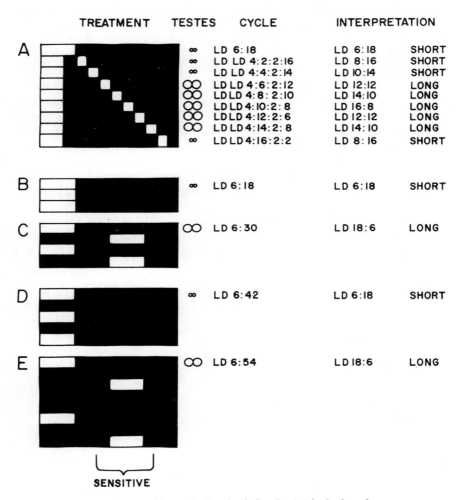

Figure 7.1 Illustration of light-dark schedules for (A) light-break experiments and (B–E) resonance experiments. Each horizontal bar represents 24 hours. Data in columns is as follows: *Testes*, the relative size (large or small) of the testis obtained with the cycle; *Cycle*, the LD ratios; *Interpretation*, the apparent way the cycle was interpreted based on testis size. In the light-break schedule, the bottom bar denotes a cycle that was interpreted as short—the animal chose the 2-hour pulse as dawn for this cycle. In all the cycles there was a reasonable way in which the animal could interpret the cycle as long or short. Examples of work with these protocols can be found in Menaker [8] and in Elliott, Stetson, and Menaker [5].

7.2 The Role of Circadian Rhythms

The timing of seasonal biological phenomena is influenced by environmental cues (e.g., changes in temperature and light) provided by the rotation of the earth and its annual orbital motion. Light is a major factor. At most latitudes, a precise calendar is provided by the length of the day (photoperiod), the length of the night (scotoperiod), and the direction of change (e.g., in northern latitudes, whether the photoperiod is shortening from the summer to the winter solstice or lengthening from the winter to the summer solstice).

The rationale for seasonal breeding appears to be the advantage in birth and rearing of young under the most propitious conditions (i.e., during periods of warm temperatures and abundant food). Seasonal breeders are classified by whether they breed in long days or short days. Gestation period may be a factor determining whether breeding occurs in the spring (short gestation) or fall (long gestation). Elaborate reproductive strategies, such as delayed implantation, have evolved which match the time from fertilization to birth to fall and spring seasons.

Daily light and dark synchronize the circadian clock, resetting it each day to maintain entrainment to 24.0 hours. Meanwhile, however, the photoperiod is lengthening or shortening. Many organisms adjust

Figure 7.2 Seasonal reproductive cycle in the male hamster and the times of refractoriness and spontaneous recrudescence (With permission from Stetson, M. and M. Watson-Whitmyre. Redrawn from Physiology of the pineal and its hormone, melatonin, in annual reproduction in rodents, in ed. R. Reiter, The pineal gland, 1984, Raven Press, New York).

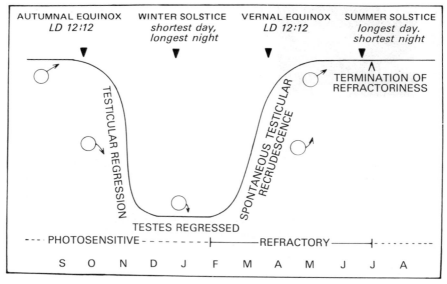

to the changes in day- and nightlength by altering their periods of activity and rest. In any case, a "memory" of the prior daylength to which the organism entrained makes it possible to use daylength as a calendar. The organisms could use the direction of change, the timing of light and dark with respect to their established circadian rhythms, the light-dark ratio, the absolute length of light, the absolute length of dark, or some combination of these for calendar information. The light-time duration at which an organism distinguishes a "long" day from a "short" day is called the *critical photoperiod*.

The question of how photoperiod is measured has been addressed in two types of ingenious, but complicated, experimental paradigms (Fig. 7.1). First, in a light-break experiment, the organisms are exposed to light-dark cycles consisting of a short photoperiod plus a brief light exposure (e.g., LDLD 4:6:2:12). A photoperiodic parameter (e.g., testis size) is then measured. The placement of the brief (e.g., 2-hour) light pulse is varied in different experimental groups, but the total duration of light exposure (e.g., 6 hours) is constant. Using this protocol, long-day responses can be obtained with total light durations that are less than the critical photoperiod. Second, in a resonance experiment, the organisms are exposed to light-dark cycles whose overall length adds to 24 hours or multiples of 24 hours (e.g., LD 6:18 and LD 6:42) and the results are compared with light-dark cycles whose overall length does not add to 24 hours (e.g., LD 6:30 and LD 6:54). Both of these experiments give the same result: photoperiod is

Figure 7.3 Effect of pinealectomy in the hamster (A), representation of the reproductive organs of normal hamsters in long photoperiod. (B), representation of the same organs from pinealectomized hamsters; the photoperiod was short. (C), representation of reproductive organs from hamsters deprived of light by blinding or by short photoperiod. (Based on data from Moore [10]; Reiter [14]; Reiter and Hester [16]; Silver and Bittman [17]; and Stetson and Watson-Whitmyre[18].)

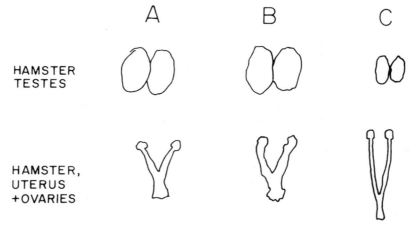

measured by when the light strikes the organism relative to its subjective time. The circadian clock is thought to be the timing device. The idea that photoperiodism is controlled by the time relationship of light with an internal rhythm of light sensitivity, is called the *Bünning hypothesis.*

An extension of the idea is the notion that there could be two kinds of coincidence [12]. In *external coincidence* models, a photoperiod is interpreted by the time light occurs relative to the timing of an internal oscillation. In *internal coincidence* models, the phase relationship of two oscillators (e.g., one that is synchronized with dawn and another that is synchronized with dusk) would be altered as photoperiod changed.

Regressed gonads (nonspermatogenic, paired weight about 300 mg) typify the male hamster in the nonbreeding, quiescent state. Cessation of estrous cycles (anovulation), which is accompanied by daily rhythms of luteinizing hormone (LH) and follicle stimulating hormone (FSH) surges, characterize the quiescent reproductive state seen in the nonbreeding season in female hamsters. The ovaries lack folliculogenesis. Recrudescence in the female (resumption of ovulation and 4-day estrous cycles) takes about 7 weeks following exposure to long days. In the male, the testes take about 10 weeks to grow full size (spermatogenic, paired weight about 3500 mg).

7.3 Seasonal Reproduction in Hamsters: The Role of Light

Hamsters are probably the most studied animals with respect to the role of the pineal in photoperiodic control of reproduction [1, 7, 14, 15, 17, 18, 19]. Although several species of hamster have been subjects of investigation, the discussion here refers to the golden hamster unless otherwise specified. Typically, testis size is the measurement made in male hamsters (large when breeding) and periodic appearance of cornified cells in vaginal smears (estrous cycles) is the measurement made in female hamsters.

Hamsters are long-day breeders. The critical photoperiod is 12.5 hours in males. Thus, long days cause hamster gonads to grow (recrudescence) and short days result in involution of the gonads (regression). Regression takes about 10 weeks in male hamsters and about 6–8 weeks in female hamsters. There is a complication to add to the simple effects of photoperiod. In hamsters exposed to short days for prolonged periods of time, however, the gonads enlarge (spontaneous recrudescence). That is, the hamsters become refractory to short days (Fig. 7.2). They can be caused to respond to short days again by exposing them to long days.

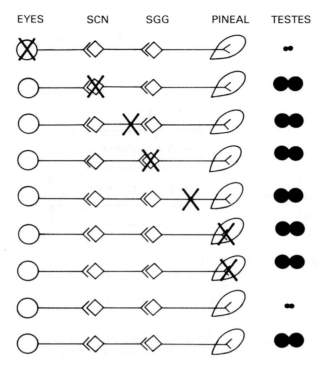

Figure 7.4 The response of hamster testes to ablations and cuts at different levels of a hypothetical pathway from the eye to the pineal gland. Conditions were *top line,* blind; *middle lines,* short photoperiod; *bottom line,* long photoperiod. (Based on information provided in Moore [10]; Reiter [14, 15]; and Stetson and Watson-Whitmyre [18].)

7.4 Seasonal Reproduction in Hamsters: The Role of the Pineal

Involution of the gonads and accompanying regression of the reproductive system does not occur in pinealectomized hamsters that are deprived of light (with short days, constant dark, or blinding) [7] (Fig. 7.3). Pinealectomized hamsters are aphotoperiodic and can reproduce. This finding was the basis for the hypothesis that the pineal gland is the source of an antigonadotropic agent.

The neural pathway by which photoperiod information is relayed to the hamster pineal was discovered in a series of ablation experiments (Fig. 7.4, 7.5). The eyes perceive light (there is no evidence for pineal and/or nonretinal light reception in hamster photoperiodism as there is for nonmammalian species, e.g., birds). The suprachiasmatic nuclei of hamsters has been identified as the site of the clock regulating estrous cycles and wheel-running rhythms. It is the probable site where light information transmitted from the eyes entrains the circa-

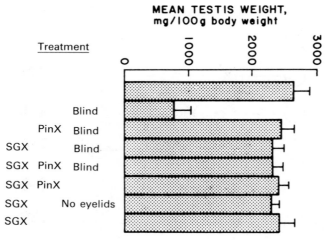

MEAN TESTIS WEIGHT,
mg/100g body weight

Treatment

Figure 7.5 The response of the hamster testes to combinations of blinding, pinealectomy (*Pinx*), and removal of the superior cervical ganglia (*SCGx*). The testes weights were reduced by light deprivation but the effect was reversed by either pinealectomy or blinding. (Redrawn from Reiter and Hester [16].)

dian clock. A retinohypothalamic tract (retino-SCN or receptor-clock pathway) has been identified in hamsters. The SCG receives information from the SCN via the paraventricular nuclei and relays it to the pineal. The proposed neural pathway for transmission of photic information from the eyes to the pineal of the hamster is the same as that suggested for the regulation of melatonin synthesis.

7.5 Melatonin Replacement

The hamster reproductive system responds to melatonin administered in oral doses, in beeswax pellets, in Silastic capsules, or by timed injections.

7.5.1 Antigonadal actions

Prolonged melatonin administration has been imposed on hamsters with oral doses, pellets, or capsules [11, 14, 18, 20, 23]. In the experiments, other treatments were given: (1) long photoperiod, (2) short photoperiod, (3) pinealectomy, and (4) superior cervical ganglionectomy. The essence of most of these studies is that melatonin treatment can sometimes cause the gonads of hamsters kept in long photoperiods to regress or can prevent recrudescence when hamsters are moved from short to long photoperiods. That is, the pineal antigonadotrophic effect can be mimicked with melatonin.

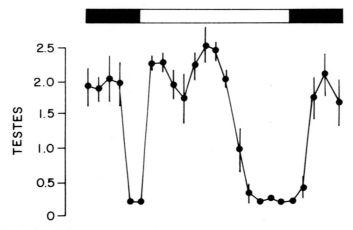

Figure 7.6 The daily response profile of golden hamster testes from hamsters subjected to single injections of melatonin (15 μg). (Redrawn from Stetson and Watson-Whitmyre [18].)

Experiments with single injections of melatonin produced results that were dependent upon time of injection (Fig. 7.6) [18, 19]. Melatonin had no effect at many times (in the morning, in the night) but did produce regression when it was administered in the intervals encompassing lights-on and lights-off (the transitions, dawn and dusk). A consequence of such injections would be to lengthen the duration of melatonin (as though a longer night were imposed). Experiments with single injections have led investigators to the conclusions that, in addition to a rhythm in melatonin secretion, there may also be a rhythm of sensitivity to melatonin. The rhythm of sensitivity may not reside in the pineal. When pinealectomized hamsters (which normally have large testes) are kept in short days they exhibit a rhythm of sensitivity to timed melatonin injections (daily for 10 weeks; sensitive CT 12 to CT 19) [25] (Fig. 7.7).

Melatonin treatment does not alter pineal melatonin production, and melatonin is effective in pinealectomized animals, so exogenous melatonin effects do not depend on product feedback inhibition of the pineal. The target of melatonin must be elsewhere. The sum of the experiments supports the hypothesis that melatonin is the antigonadotrophic factor from the pineal gland that makes the hamster reproductive system regress.

7.5.2 Progonadal actions

Paradoxically, in some experiments, melatonin implants or melatonin administered in the drinking water also block regression that should be obtained with short days or blinding [4, 23]. Reiter [14] called this the *counterantigonadotrophic* action of melatonin.

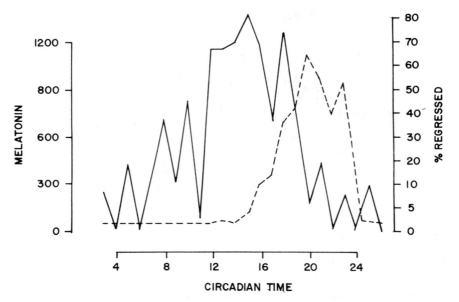

Figure 7.7 Rhythm of sensitivity *(solid line)* to melatonin injections in pinealectomized hamsters *(Pinx)* in LD 12:12. The data are plotted together with the rhythm of pineal melatonin content *(dashed line)* in unoperated hamsters *(Normal)* kept in LD 12:12 peaks later than the sensitivity rhythm. The horizontal bar over the co-plotted graphs represents the timing of darkness. (After Watson-Whitmyre [25].)

7.6 The Melatonin Hypothesis

The melatonin hypothesis (for reproduction) is the suggestion that melatonin mediates the reproductive response to seasonal changes in photoperiod. There are a number of ways this could be accomplished. A given species may have elaborated one or a combination of the possible strategies.

7.6.1 Duration

Pineal NAT and melatonin profiles in some species (quail, chickens, rats, and some species of hamster) are altered by photoperiod [1]. The duration of high NAT is shortened in long photoperiods (possibly with a lower limit of 6 hours) and is lengthened in short photoperiods (possibly with an upper limit of 12 hours). It seems reasonable to suggest that the duration of melatonin reaching targets, a consequence of melatonin production, as controlled by the photoperiod and scotoperiod acting on NAT, affects reproductive function. In short days (long nights) more melatonin is produced than in long days (short nights). However, even in species where duration is clearly altered by

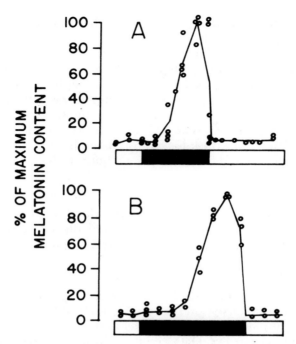

Figure 7.8 Daily cycles in golden hamster melatonin in (A) a long photoperiod (LD 14:10) and (B) a short photoperiod (LD 8:16). (Redrawn from Stetson and Watson-Whitmyre [18].)

photoperiod, the increase in synthesis is not necessarily proportional to the length of the dark-time. For example, total dark-time NAT was only 17% greater in chicks kept in LD 8:16 than in chicks kept in LD 16:8. The total quantity of enzyme activity was not doubled because the amplitude was less in LD 8:16 than in LD 16:8.

Golden hamsters are an exception; they have only small changes in the duration of melatonin production per day in response to altered photoperiod. It is possible, of course, that golden hamsters are exquisitely sensitive to small changes in melatonin duration, just as their reproductive systems are remarkably precise in their responses to small changes in photoperiod [4].

7.6.2 Phase

In golden hamsters, the fall in NAT and melatonin is locked to the time of lights-on. That means that lengthening the dark-time by 6 hours produces up to a 6-hour difference in the phase of the decrease in melatonin or a phase shift of at least 5 hours of the peak in melatonin (Fig. 7.8). The effectiveness of single melatonin injections at only certain times of day supports a phase model for melatonin mediation of photoperiod.

In an internal coincidence model, if there were a physiological rhythm locked to the time of lights-on (as melatonin is in the golden hamster) and a second physiological rhythm with its phase locked to the time of lights-out, the phase relationship between the two rhythms would be a function the difference between the times of lights-on and lights-off (or off and on). The existence of two oscillators, a dawn-locked oscillator and a dusk-locked oscillator, has been postulated for golden hamsters based on locomotor activity studies [12].

7.6.3 Phase and duration

The phase explanation encompasses the duration results. An alteration in phase relationships is an unavoidable consequence when duration of melatonin production is altered by photoperiod.

7.6.4 HIOMT

Some pineal parameters, HIOMT for one, have been shown to change when photoperiod or season is altered. Rat HIOMT is halved by 6–12 weeks of long days, and HIOMT has a reciprocal relationship with testis weight of sparrows. Data for hamsters are shown in Fig. 7.9. The HIOMT changes could modulate the amount of melatonin produced. An attractive hypothesis is that HIOMT would be responsible for seasonal modulation of the amplitude of melatonin produced on a daily basis, the daily cycle being due to rhythms in NAT. Clearly, in the golden hamster, the amplitude of the melatonin peak in the pineal was not altered by photoperiod (though blood levels and total production could be affected).

7.6.5 Interval timing

Silver and Bittman [17] coined the term *interval timer* to refer to "a mechanism that times behavioral or physiological events of durations shorter than 24 h and that does not oscillate or automatically reset . . . (such timers) can be quickly stopped and restarted and . . . can measure duration at any time of day." The pineal does not qualify for the interval timer (even though it may measure duration) since it cannot be started at any time of day (there is a refractory period). However, it is possible that a secondary event (the postulated other oscillation in the coincidence model) runs as an interval timer that interacts with the circadian melatonin signal.

7.7 Other Considerations

There are additional problems for understanding pineal function (or lack of it) in photoperiodic control of reproduction.

7.7.1 Species without a pineal role

There are photoperiodic species that lack a distinct pineal organ though the pineal is found in most vertebrates. Even when the gland is missing, however, melatonin has been found in blood [6]. The eye could be an alternate site for melatonin synthesis. More puzzling are photoperiodic species that have a pineal gland and whose reproduction is photoperiodic, but is not affected by pinealectomy [13]. A possible explanation comes from the fact that some of these species can also synthesize melatonin rhythmically in their eyes. However, blind pinealectomized sparrows respond to photoperiod [9].

7.7.2 Nonmelatonin hormones

The possibility exists that melatonin is not the pineal antigonadal hormone or not the only antigonadal pineal hormone. We know it is not the only pineal molecule affected by photoperiod since the daily profiles of other indoles (serotonin, N-acetylserotonin, etc.) are modified by photoperiod.

Peptides are present in pineals [2] and may have rhythms that are modulated by photoperiod. The most studied peptide is arginine vasotocin (AVT) which has a rhythm (peak at noon) in the pineal and may be altered by LL and DD [21]. There may be an interaction with

Figure 7.9 HIOMT in pineals of hamsters showing the higher activity correlates with conditions that reduce testis size. (Redrawn after Eichler and Moore [3].)

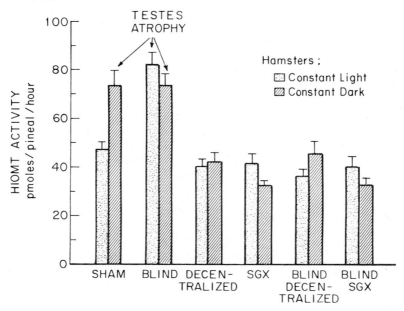

indoles; for example, melatonin may release AVT. AVT has been shown to affect reproductive parameters in a number of species. AVT treatment may impair the responses of mouse and rat reproductive systems to gonadotrophins. Daily AVT injections lengthen the mouse estrous cycle by prolonging diestrous. Rat LH surges can be delayed with an injection of AVT. Other candidates for a pineal antigonadotrophic peptide include arginine vasopressin, oxytocin, threonylseryllysine (TSL, thr-ser-lys), PAG (pineal antigonadotrophin), and E_5 peptide (14 amino acids, similar to AVT). There are also nonpeptides besides melatonin that have been mentioned (e.g., pteridines). These and other substances will be discussed in more detail in Chapter 11.

7.8 Nonseasonal Reproduction

There have been numerous attempts to associate the pineal with aspects of reproduction that are not a function of season.

7.8.1 Puberty

The possibility of a pineal role in puberty was recognized as early as 1896 [27]. It would make some sense that a gland that can function to turn the reproductive system on and off with season would also be involved in the reproductive life cycle—puberty and the climacteric. Pineal tumors were linked with early (precocious puberty) or late reproductive development. Attempts have been made to advance or delay puberty with experimental pinealectomy in mammals or birds with mixed success. Puberty may be assessed by the time of vaginal opening in rodents, the size of the gonads, onset of reproductive hormone secretion, and so forth.

Prepubertal effects aside from the timing of puberty onset (growth of the gonads, responses of gonads to hormones in vitro) have produced some positive indication for pineal and/or melatonin involvement in the regulation of the reproductive system before puberty. Serum melatonin was measured relative to stage of puberty (at 11 P.M.–1 A.M.) and found to have an inverse relationship with serum LH. Melatonin was high in children and declined at puberty, remaining low in adults [24].

7.8.2 Compensatory hypertrophy

When a testis or ovary is removed, the remaining gonad increases its function (size, hormone production, gamete production) and compensates for the lost organ [22]. The phenomenon is called *compensatory ovarian hypertrophy* (COH) in the female and *compensatory testicular hypertrophy* in the male. The COH response of mice has been used in conjunction with pineal studies of putative pineal hormones. Some of the pineal substances that inhibit COH are N-acetylserotonin, melatonin, 5-hydroxytryptophol, 5-methoxytryptophol, and vasopressin [21].

7.8.3 Menstrual cycle

Melatonin has been measured in humans throughout the menstrual cycle. Melatonin had a three- to sixfold change in morning values in November and December at different times of the menstrual cycle. Peak melatonin was measured at the time of menstruation and the nadir value occurred at the time of ovulation [26].

7.9 Nonreproduction

The focus of pineal involvement in photoperiodism has been on reproduction. There are, however, many other facets of physiology that are responsive to season. For example, body weight increases in the fall; fur and feathers turn white in some species in winter; and hibernation is a fall and winter event. These and other phenomena in which the pineal may be involved are discussed in more detail in Chapter 9.

REFERENCES

1. Binkley, S. 1976. Pineal gland biorhythms: N-acetyltransferase in chickens and rats. *Fed. Proc.* 35:2347–2352.
2. Blask, D., M. Vaughan, and R. Reiter. 1983. Pineal peptides and reproduction. In *The pineal gland,* ed. R. Relkin, pp. 201–223. New York: Elsevier.
3. Eichler, V., and R. Moore. 1971. Pineal hydroxyindole-O-methyltransferase and gonadal responses to blinding or continuous darkness blocked by pineal denervation in the male hamster. *Neuroendocrinology* 8:81–85.
4. Elliott, J. 1976. Circadian rhythms and photoperiodic time measurement in mammals. *Fed. Proc.* 35:2339–2346.
5. Elliott, J., M. Stetson, and M. Menaker. 1972. Regulation of testis function in golden hamsters: A circadian clock measures photoperiodic time. *Science* 178:771–773.
6. Harlow, H., J. Phillips, and C. Ralph. 1981. Day-night rhythm in plasma melatonin in a mammal lacking a distinct pineal gland, the nine-banded armadillo. *Gen. Comp. Endocrinol.* 45:212–218.
7. Hoffman, R., and R. Reiter. 1966. Pineal gland: Influence on gonads of male hamsters. *Science* 148:1609–1611.
8. Menaker, M. 1965. Circadian rhythms and photoperiodism in *Passer domesticus.* In *Circadian clocks,* ed. J. Aschoff, pp. 385–395. Amsterdam: North-Holland.

9. Menaker, M., R. Roberts, J. Elliott, and H. Underwood. 1970. Extraretinal light perception in the sparrow III: The eyes do not participate in photoperiodic photoreception. *Proc. Nat. Acad. Sci. USA* 67:320–325.

10. Moore, R. 1973. Retinohypothalamic projection in mammals: A comparative study. *Brain Res.* 49:403–409.

11. Pévet, P., and C. Haldar-Misra. 1982. Effect of orally administered melatonin on reproductive function of the golden hamster. *Experientia* 38:1493–1494.

12. Pittendrigh, C. 1972. Circadian surfaces and the diversity of possible roles of circadian organization in photoperiodic induction. *Proc. Nat. Acad. Sci. USA* 69:2734–2737.

13. Ralph, C. 1981. The pineal and reproduction in birds. In *The pineal gland II: Reproductive effects*, ed. R. Reiter, pp. 31–43. Boca Raton, Fla.: CRC Press.

14. Reiter, R. 1980. The pineal and its hormones in the control of reproduction in mammals. *Endocrine Rev.* 2:109–131.

15. ———. 1983. The pineal gland and its indole products: Their importance in the control of reproduction in mammals. In *The pineal gland*, ed. R. Relkin, pp. 151–199. New York: Elsevier.

16. Reiter, R., and R. Hester. 1966. Interrelationships of the pineal gland, the superior cervical ganglia and the photoperiod in the regulation of the endocrine systems of hamsters. *Endocrinology* 79:1168–1170.

17. Silver, R., and E. Bittman. 1983. Reproductive mechanisms: Interaction of circadian and interval timing. *Ann. N.Y. Acad. Sci.* 423:488–514.

18. Stetson, M., and M. Watson-Whitmyre. 1984. Physiology of the pineal and its hormone melatonin in annual reproduction in rodents. In *The pineal gland*, ed. R. Reiter, pp. 109–153. New York: Raven Press.

19. Tamarkin, L., C. Baird, and O. Almeida. 1985. Melatonin: A coordinating signal for mammalian reproduction. *Science* 227:714–720.

20. Turek, F. 1977. Antigonadal effect of melatonin in pinealectomized male hamsters. *Proc. Soc. Exp. Biol. Med.* 155:31–34.

21. Vaughan, M. 1981. Arginine vasotocin and vertebrate reproduction. In *The pineal gland II: Reproductive effects*, ed. R. Reiter, pp. 125–163. Boca Raton, Fla.: CRC Press.

22. Vaughan, M., R. Reiter, G. Vaughan, L. Bigelow, and M. Altschule. 1972. Inhibition of compensatory ovarian hypertrophy in the mouse and vole: A comparison of Altschule's pineal extract, pineal indoles, vasopressin, and oxytocin. *Gen. Comp. Endocrinol.* 18:372–377.

23. Vriend, J., and F. Gibbs. 1984. Coincidence of counter-antigonadal and counter-antithyroid action of melatonin administration via the drinking water in male golden hamsters. *Life Sci.* 34:617–623.

24. Waldhauser, F., H. Frisch, M. Waldhauser, G. Weisenbacher, U. Zeithuber, and R. Wurtman. 1984. Fall in nocturnal serum melatonin during prepuberty and pubescence. *Lancet*, February 18, pp. 362–365.

25. Watson-Whitmyre, M. 1985. Photoperiodism in the golden hamster: Dependence on rhythmic sensitivity to melatonin. Ph.D. diss., Univ. of Delaware.

26. Wetterberg, L., J. Arendt, L. Paunier, P. Sizonenko, W. van Donselaar, and T. Heyden. 1976. Human serum melatonin changes during the menstrual cycle. *J. Clin. Endocrinol. Metab.* 42:185–188.

27. Zrenner, C. 1985. Theories of pineal function from classical antiquity to 1900: A history. In *Pineal research reviews III*, ed. R. Reiter, pp. 1–40. New York: Alan R. Liss.

8

Circadian Rhythms

"The pineal organ of the house sparrow, *Passer domesticus*, is essential for persistence of the circadian locomotor rhythm in constant conditions. Upon removal of the pineal body, activity becomes arrhythmic. However, pinealectomy does not abolish the rhythm of locomotor activity in birds exposed to light-dark cycles."

S. Gaston and M. Menaker [16]

8.1 Introduction

In some species, the pineal controls circadian rhythms of locomotor activity and body temperature. In these species, pinealectomy abolishes the circadian rhythms that persist in constant conditions. The effects of pinealectomy on locomotor and temperature rhythms were initially discovered using house sparrows [16]. It was at first disappointing that some other avian and mammalian species were not as dramatically affected by pinealectomy, but the more recent discovery of the existence of melatonin synthesis rhythms in the eye and the presence of deep pineals in some species makes it necessary to reconsider a wider role for melatonin in circadian rhythms.

8.2 Surgery

Surgery has been used to study the pineal regulation of circadian rhythms of locomotor activity and body temperature (Figs. 8.1–8.3).

8.2.1 Rhythm abolition

House sparrows kept in constant dark exhibit free-running circadian perch-hopping (locomotor) activity (Fig. 8.1*B*). The circadian rhythm is classic in its responses to environmental lighting: (1) it is entrained by light-dark cycles; (2) the duration of activity is dependent upon photoperiod and light intensity; (3) constant light shortens the period length and/or abolishes the rhythm; and (4) light and dark pulses shift the phase of the rhythm. When sparrows were pinealectomized, however, the circadian rhythm was lost and the sparrows' perch hopping became aperiodic in DD [15, 16]. Surgical removal of the pineal was verified by histological examination of sparrows' brains following the experiment. Moreover, sparrows' body temperature rhythms were also abolished by pinealectomy [5]. The findings meant that the pineal could function as a circadian biological clock or as a means by which circadian clock information was transmitted to the rest of the body (by direct stimulation of rhythms or by acting as a coupling device between pacemaker and driven oscillations). Interestingly, blinding did not abolish normal or pinealectomized sparrows' responses to light; the birds have extraretinal light perception (Fig. 8.2) [24].

Abolition of rhythms by pinealectomy was subsequently found in some other species (some lizards, white-crowned sparrows, white-throated sparrows, and house finches) [33] but could not be obtained in still others (rats, hamsters, and chickens).

8.2.2 Abnormal entrainment

Pinealectomized sparrows placed in light-dark regimens entrain to the cycles. In entraining, they show anticipatory activity of the time of lights-on (Fig. 8.3) [16]. That means that removing the pineal does not remove all clock function—the pineal may be a clock but not the only clock. The entrainment patterns of pinealectomized sparrows were studied further [16, 23, 34]. When a circadian rhythm is entrained to a light-dark cycle, the relationship of the rhythm and the cycle is dependent upon the photoperiod. For example, in LD 2:22, sparrows begin hopping 6 hours or so before lights-on, while in LD 18:6 the sparrows begin hopping within seconds of lights-on. The sparrows' phase angle with respect to lights-on is different in the two cycles. Pinealectomized sparrows increase the time between starting to hop and lights-on by about 100 minutes.

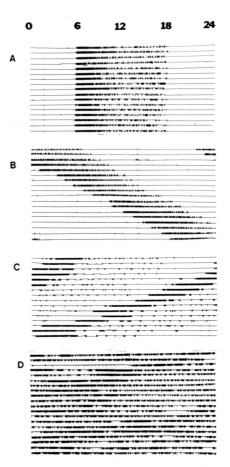

Figure 8.1 Examples of representative sparrow perch-hopping activity records. Each line is 24 hours long with midnight on the left. The lines are arranged vertically in chronological order.

Record *A* is from a sparrow entrained to LD 12:12, lights on from 6 A.M. to 6 P.M. (noted as *6* and *18*). In this regimen, activity occurs when the lights are on. The record illustrates entrainment and would be characteristic of normal or pinealectomized sparrows in LD 12:12. In shorter cycles, activity onset precedes lights-on and pinealectomy increases the anticipation [7, 15, 23, 36].

Record *B* shows a sparrow free-running with a period length longer than 24 hours. Such records are typical of sparrows kept in constant dark (DD).

Record *C* is from a sparrow free-running with a period length shorter than 24 hours. This record is typical for a sparrow kept in dim constant light (LL) [7] or in DD supplied continuously with melatonin (capsule) [6, 37].

Record *D* is from a sparrow that was arrhythmic in constant light (LL). Arrhythmia can be obtained in sparrows with bright LL [7]. Arrhythmia can also be obtained in sparrows in DD with pinealectomy [15, 16], melatonin implants [37], melatonin water [6], or lesions of the suprachiasmatic nucleus [35]. Similar arrhythmia can be obtained in DD in some chickens, quail, or pigeons with blinding or blinding plus pinealectomy [13, 26, 38].

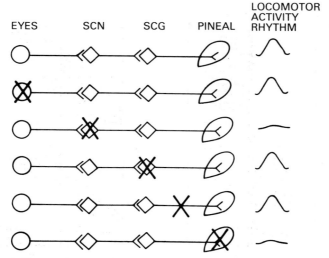

Figure 8.2 Effects of surgical procedures on avian locomotor rhythms [24, 43]. The connections and surgical procedures are based on the neural pathway proposed for mammals.

Skeleton photoperiods consist of two short light pulses (e.g., 1 hour each) every 24 hours to mimic dawn and dusk. Sparrows entrain to skeleton photoperiods in precise ways. They always choose dawn so that they entrain to the shorter of the two possible "photoperiods" [7, 31]. Pinealectomized sparrows were able to entrain to most skeleton photoperiods [34]. However, if the pinealectomized sparrows were first permitted to become arrhythmic in constant dark, then they exhibited abnormal patterns to LD 1:11 (skeleton of LD 13:11) showing bursts of activity during the light pulses and additional activity distributed throughout 24 hours (as opposed to the normal birds, which concentrated their activity between the two light pulses). The pinealectomized sparrows entrained to LD 1:11 if they were not first permitted to become arrhythmic.

8.2.3 Rate of reentrainment

Pinealectomy did not abolish the wheel-running (locomotor) activity of rats [11, 27, 30]. Rats entrain to light-dark cycles. When the phase of the light-dark cycle is shifted, the rats reentrain to the new cycle. Pinealectomy increases the rate at which reentrainment is achieved [22, 28].

8.2.4 Transplants

Transplanting pineal glands from donor house sparrows into the anterior chamber of an eye of pinealectomized recipient sparrows

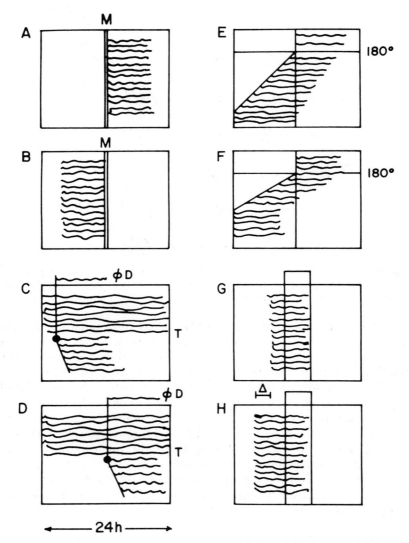

← 24h →

Figure 8.3 Diagrammatic representation of some effects of pineal surgeries on locomotor activity. The records are arranged in blocks with the horizontal axis equal to 24 hours. The wavy lines represent successive locomotor activity from one day to the next.

Record A represents the pattern of entrainment in a rat given daily melatonin injections at time M. The nocturnal rat synchronizes its activity onset with the injection. Record B represents the pattern of entrainment of a starling or lizard given daily melatonin injections at time M. the diurnal animals synchronized activity offset close to the time of the injection [17, 29, 40].

Records C and D represent the patterns of perching of arrhythmic pinealectomized recipient sparrows in DD that received pineal transplants (in the anterior chamber of the eye) at T [44]. The pineal glands came from donor restored the locomotor rhythm (which was absent after pinealectomy) in constant dark [44]. Moreover, the phase of the rhythm of locomotor activity after the transplant was determined by the phase of the donor bird's prior light-dark treatment.

8.2.5 Sympathetic regulation

The possibility that pineal effects on sparrow locomotor rhythms were a consequence of rhythmic signals from the superior cervical ganglia was investigated. Cutting and deflection of the pineal stalk (which should disrupt the sympathetic innervation) did not produce arrhythmia (Figs. 8.2–8.3). Chemical sympathectomy is possible with 6-hydroxydopamine. Injections of 6-hydroxydopamine abolished sparrow pineal norepinephrine fluorescence in 24 hours but did not cause arrhythmia [43, 44].

8.2.6 Suprachiasmatic nuclei

The suprachiasmatic nuclei have been lesioned in sparrows [12, 35]. In house sparrows, the lesions produced results similar to those obtained with pinealectomy: the sparrows became arrhythmic in constant dark but still entrained to light-dark cycles. Not all species have the 2-deoxyglucose uptake rhythm seen in rats and hamsters; the rhythm was absent in a diurnal species, the ground squirrel [14].

8.3 Melatonin Replacement

Melatonin replacement studies have been made with several modes of melatonin administration—continuous, cyclic, and single.

---

sparrows whose perching (wavy line over the record, ϕ D) began at the time marked with the vertical line. The recipient sparrow resumed rhythmic behavior and the onset of the perching corresponded with the onset of the donor.

Record E represents the wheel-running pattern of a rat whose light-dark cycle was reversed (shifted by 12 hours) on the day marked 180°. The rat's rhythm drifts to the new cycle. Record F represents the pattern from a pinealectomized rat showing that it drifted more rapidly to the new cycle [22, 28].

Record G represents entrainment of a sparrow to a short photoperiod light-dark cycle where activity anticipates lights-on. Record H represents entrainment of a pinealectomized sparrow exposed to the same cycle showing its greater anticipation of lights-on. Delta (Δ) represents the change in onset for the pinealectomized versus the normal sparrow [6, 15, 23, 34].

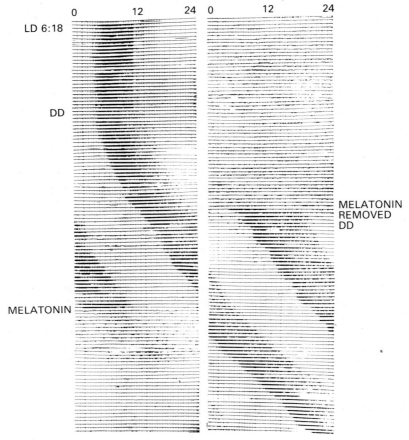

Figure 8.4 Record of a sparrow given continuous access to melatonin in its drinking water [6]. The sparrow entrained to LD 12:12, then free-ran in DD. It continued to free-run with increased period length when ethanol was added to the water. When melatonin (and ethanol) were added to the water, the sparrow became arrhythmic.

8.3.1 Continuous administration

When melatonin was implanted intraperitoneally (Silastic® capsules) in sparrows, two alternate results were obtained. First, in birds in which the rhythm persisted, the period length was shortened by about 1 hour [37]. Second, melatonin made some birds arrhythmic. More of the birds became arrhythmic at higher doses. The effects appeared immediately upon implantation of melatonin capsules and normal longer-period rhythms resumed as soon as the capsules were removed. A similar result was obtained when melatonin was placed in the drinking water and given to sparrows ad libitum [6] (Fig. 8.4).

Sparrows kept in LD 3:21 or LD 8:16 exhibited dose-dependent reductions in locomotor activity in response to melatonin capsule implants [20]. Thus, in the presence of the pineal gland exogenous melatonin administration is physiologically effective, and its actions cease when administration is halted.

8.3.2 Cyclic application

Daily melatonin injections have been administered to starlings, lizards, and rats to examine possible synchronization of rhythms and the phase of the rhythms. Daily melatonin injections (50 μg in 0.1 ml of sesame oil) into pinealectomized starlings synchronized the circadian perching rhythms of 21 of 22 birds to 24.0 hours [17] even though they were in dim constant light where their normal free-running period is less than 24 hours. The diurnal starlings ended their activity at or just before the melatonin injection. Diurnal lizards synchronized to melatonin injections choose a phase that would place the injections near the normal nocturnal rise [40]. Rats injected daily with melatonin [29] synchronized their circadian wheel-running rhythms to daily melatonin injections. The nocturnal rats synchronized the beginning of their activity with the melatonin injections. Thus, most of the animals of the three species studied synchronized with the timed melatonin so that the artificial melatonin increase from the injection occurred at a phase when melatonin would rise in the animal.

8.3.3 Single doses

Single melatonin injections have so far produced some results that are expected based on ablation studies. Pinealectomized sparrows lose their body temperature rhythms which are normally 4.4° C lower at night. Single melatonin injections (1.2–2.5 mg) lowered body temperatures in sparrows 4.7° C [2]. Melatonin may potentiate barbiturate-induced sleep, cause roosting posture in birds, and produce EEGs characteristic of sleep.

8.4 Eyes

The failure of pinealectomy to abolish circadian locomotor rhythms in some species has been partially ameliorated by the finding that the eyes may have pineal-like functions. Pinealectomized chickens did not lose their circadian rhythms, however; 50% of blinded chickens were arrhythmic in DD [26]. The combination of blinding with pinealectomy renders quail and pigeons arrhythmic where either operation alone leaves the animal rhythmic [12, 39].

Removing the eyes and pineal from chicks or quail lowers serum melatonin more than removal of either alone [39]. Moreover, when

N-acetyltransferase (NAT) and melatonin rhythms were measured in chicks and quail, both the eyes and pineal were found to have substantive NAT and melatonin rhythms [4, 18, 39]. The ocular NAT responds to lighting as does the pineal: rhythms persist in constant dark; NAT is suppressed by extending light into the dark-time; rhythms are abolished by constant light; NAT is refractory to stimulation by dark in the early subjective day; and there is a rapid plummet in response to light in the dark-time [4, 19, 39].

Possible interactions of the eyes and pineal of chicks were investigated using black eye or head patches (to reduce light reaching the eyes and pineal) and extension of light into the dark-time (which suppressed NAT, a test for light detection) [8]. As expected from studies where blind chicks exhibit less rapid plummet than intact ones, patching the eyes partially prevents suppression of NAT. Capping the pineal region did not affect NAT in the eyes, but light suppression of NAT was prevented in an intact eye if that eye was covered. Patching one eye did not affect the other. Thus, the eyes influence the pineal gland but the eyes are independent of the pineal and of each other [4, 9].

Eyes and pineal respond differently to isoproterenol depending on where it is injected. Intraocular isoproterenol suppresses NAT in the eye but not in the pineal; subcutaneous isoproterenol suppresses NAT in the pineal but not in the eye. Cycloheximide injections lowered pineal and retinal NAT when the injection was intraocular, but subcutaneous cycloheximide injections only affected the pineal. Thus, the ocular NAT response may be protected from molecules circulating in the blood (a blood-eye barrier) whereas the molecules can affect pineal NAT (the absence of a blood-pineal barrier) [4, 9].

8.5 Pineal and Ocular Cycles

Pineal glands of young chickens (1–3 weeks old) continued to exhibit circadian cycles when they were removed from the birds and maintained in organ cultures in DD. The pineals, as assessed by NAT responses, are sensitive to light in the cultures: LD enhances the amplitude of the rhythm; LL suppresses the rhythm; lights-on causes a rapid plummet; and light pulses shift the rhythm [5, 21, 32, 41, 42]. When chick, sparrow, pigeon, quail, or lizard pineals are placed in superfusion culture, rhythmic melatonin profiles can be assessed in sequential aliquots of effluent medium [3, 25, 32]. When *Xenopus* (frog) eyecups (sclera, choroid, and retina) are studied in vitro, they exhibit an NAT cycle [1].

Thus, both pineals and eyes have the ability to synthesize melatonin in a circadian fashion. They make melatonin in the subjective night. The relative abilities of the eyes and pineal are consistent with the ablation and melatonin replacement studies in a given species. Melatonin rhythms may be responsible for circadian behavioral rhythms, at least in some species.

REFERENCES

1. Besharse, J., and P. Iuvone. 1983. Circadian clock in *Xenopus* eye controlling retinal serotonin *N*-acetyltransferase. *Nature* 305:133–135.
2. Binkley, S. 1974. Pineal and melatonin: Circadian rhythms and body temperature. In *Chronobiology*, ed. L. Scheving, F. Halberg, and J. Pauly, pp. 582–585. Tokyo: Igaku Shoin.
3. ———. 1980. Functions of the pineal gland. In *Avian endocrinology*, ed. A. Epple and M. Stetson, pp. 53–74. New York: Academic Press.
4. Binkley, S., M. Hryshchyshyn, and K. Reilly. 1979. NAT responds to environmental lighting in the eye as well as in the pineal gland. *Nature* 281:279–281.
5. Binkley, S., E. Kluth, and M. Menaker. 1971. Pineal function in sparrows: Circadian rhythms and body temperature. *Science* 174:311–314.
6. Binkley, S., and K. Mosher. 1985. Oral melatonin produces arrhythmia in sparrows. *Experientia*. 41:1615–1617.
7. Binkley, S., K. Mosher, and K. Reilly. 1983. Circadian rhythms in house sparrows: Lighting ad lib. *Physiol. Behav.* 31:829–837.
8. Binkley, S., K. Reilly, and T. Hernandez. 1980. *N*-acetyltransferase in the chick retina II: Interactions of the eyes and pineal gland in response to light. *J. Comp. Physiol.* 140:181–183.
9. Binkley, S., K. Reilly, and M. Hryshchyshyn. 1980. *N*-acetyltransferase in the chick retina I: Circadian rhythms controlled by environmental lighting are similar to those in the pineal gland. *J. Comp. Physiol.* 139:103–108.
10. Binkley, S., J. Riebman, and K. Reilly. 1978. The pineal gland: A biological clock in vitro. *Science* 202:1198–1201.
11. Cheung, P., and P. McCormack. 1982. Failure of pinealectomy or melatonin to alter circadian rhythm of the rat. *Amer. J. Physiol.* 242: R261–R264.
12. Ebihara, S., and H. Kawamura. 1981. The role of the pineal organ and the suprachiasmatic nucleus in the control of circadian locomotor rhythms in the Java sparrow, *Padda oryzivora*. *J. Comp. Physiol.* 141:207–214.
13. ———. 1984. Circadian organization in the pigeon, *Columba livia*: The role of the pineal organ and the eye. *J. Comp. Physiol.* 154:59–69.
14. Flood, D., and F. Gibbs. 1982. Species difference in circadian (^{14}C)-2-deoxyglucose uptake by suprachiasmatic nuclei. *Brain Res.* 232:200–205.
15. Gaston, S. 1971. The influence of the pineal organ on the circadian activity rhythm in birds. In *Biochronometry*, ed. M. Menaker, pp. 541–548. Washington D.C.: National Academy of Sciences.
16. Gaston, S., and M. Menaker. 1968. Pineal function: The biological clock in the sparrow? *Science* 160:541–548.

17. Gwinner, E., and I. Benzinger. 1978. Synchronization of a circadian rhythm in pinealectomized European starlings by daily injections of melatonin. *J. Comp. Physiol.* 127:209–213.

18. Hamm, H., and M. Menaker. 1980. Retinal rhythms in chicks: Circadian variation in melatonin and serotonin *N*-acetyltransferase. *Proc. Natl. Acad. Sci. USA* 77:4998–5002.

19. Hamm, H., J. Takahashi, and M. Menaker. 1983. Light-induced decrease of serotonin *N*-acetyltransferase activity and melatonin in the chicken pineal gland and retina. *Brain Res.* 266:287–293.

20. Hendel, R., and F. Turek. 1978. Suppression of locomotor activity in sparrows by treatment with melatonin. *Physiol. Behavior* 21:275–278.

21. Kasal, C., M. Menaker, and R. Perez-Polo. 1979. Circadian clock in culture: *N*-acetyltransferase activity of chick pineal glands oscillates in vitro. *Science* 203:656–658.

22. Kincl, F., C. Change, and V. Zbuzkova. 1970. Observation on the influence of changing photoperiod on spontaneous wheel-running activity of neonatally pinealectomized rats. *Endocrinology* 87:38–42.

23. Laitman, R., and F. Turek. 1979. The effect of pinealectomy on entrainment of the locomotor activity rhythm in sparrows maintained on various short days. *J. Comp. Physiol.* 134:339–343.

24. Menaker, M. 1968. Light perception by extra-retinal receptors in the brain of the sparrow. *Proc. APA.*, pp. 299–300.

25. Menaker, M., and S. Wisner. 1983. Temperature-compensated circadian clock in the pineal of *Anolis. Proc. Natl. Acad. Sci. USA* 80:6119–6121.

26. Nyce, J., and S. Binkley. 1977. Extraretinal photoreception in chickens: Entrainment of the circadian locomotor activity rhythm. *Photochem. Photobiol.* 25:529–531.

27. Quay, W. 1968. Individuation and lack of pineal effect in the rat's circadian locomotor rhythm. *Physiol. Behav.* 3:109–118.

28. ———. 1970. Physiological significance of the pineal during adaptation to shifts in photoperiod. *Physiol. Behav.* 5:353–360.

29. Redman, J., S. Armstrong, and K. T. Ng. 1983. Freerunning activity rhythms in the rat: Entrainment by melatonin. *Science* 219:1089–1091.

30. Richter, C. 1965. *Biological clocks in medicine and psychiatry.* Springfield, Ill.: Charles Thomas.

31. Takahashi, J. 1981. Neural and endocrine regulation of avian circadian systems. Ph.D. diss., Univ. of Oregon.

32. Takahashi, J., H. Hamm, and M. Menaker. 1980. Circadian rhythms of melatonin release from individual superfused chicken pineal glands in vitro. *Proc. Natl. Acad. Sci. USA* 77:2319–2322.

33. Takahashi, J., and M. Menaker. 1979. Physiology of avian circadian pacemakers. *Fed. Proc.* 38:2583–2588.

34. ———. 1982a. Entrainment of the circadian system of the house sparrow: A population of oscillators in pinealectomized birds. *J. Comp. Physiol.* 146:245–253.

35. ———. 1982b. Role of the suprachiasmatic nuclei in the circadian system of the house sparrow, *Passer domesticus. J. Neurosci.* 2:815–828.

36. ———. 1984. Multiple redundant circadian oscillators within the isolated avian pineal gland. *J. Comp. Physiol.* 154:435–440.

37. Turek, F., J. McMillan, M. Menaker. 1976. Melatonin: Effects on the circadian locomotor rhythm of sparrows. *Science* 194:1441–1443.

38. Underwood, H. 1984. Circadian organization in Japanese quail. *J. Exp. Zool.* 232:557–566.

39. Underwood, H., S. Binkley, T. Siopes, and K. Mosher. 1984. Melatonin rhythms in the eyes, pineal, and blood of Japanese quail. *Gen. Comp. Endocrinol.* 56:70–81.

40. Underwood, H., and M. Harliss. 1985. Entrainment of the circadian activity rhythm of a lizard to melatonin injections. *Physiol. Behav.* 35:267–270.

41. Wainwright, S., and L. Wainwright. 1978. Regulation of the diurnal cycle in activity of serotonin acetyltransferase in the chick pineal gland. *Can. J. Biochem.* 56:685–690.

42. ———. 1980. Regulation of the cycle in chick pineal serotonin *N*-acetyltransferase activity in vitro by light. *J. Neurochem.* 35:451–457.

43. Zimmerman, N., and M. Menaker. 1975. Neural connections of sparrow pineal: Role in circadian control of activity. *Science* 190:477–479.

44. ———. 1979. The pineal gland: A pacemaker within the circadian system of the house sparrow. *Proc. Natl. Acad. Sci. USA* 76:999–1003.

9

Other Functions of the Pineal and Melatonin

"Body pallor due to contraction of both deep and integumental mela-nophores occurs when either blinded or normal *Xenopus laevis* and other amphibian larvae are placed in the dark. The reaction is abolished by pinealectomy, but is induced by administration of pineal hormones. It is suggested that the normal body lightening reaction is mediated by the pineal gland."

J. T. Bagnara [1]

"The tadpoles employed were hatched in the laboratory and immediately placed upon a diet of pineal gland. On the tenth day of larval life it was readily observable that in the pineal-fed groups the coloration was uniformly lighter than in the control, muscle-fed groups. . . . Thirty minutes after feeding pineal tissue, the tadpoles which prior to the feeding had been uniformly dark, became so translucent that all the larger viscera were plainly visible through the dorsal body wall."

C. P. McCord and F. P. Allen [48]

9.1 Introduction

Other possible roles of the pineal that have been studied have attributes in common with pineal function in locomotion and reproduction. These include associations with (1) environmental lighting, (2) circadian rhythms, (3) the brain, and (4) the endocrine system.

9.2 Color Change

Integumental color change was one of the earliest functions to be associated with the pineal. Skin color change responds to environmental lighting, has circadian rhythms, and involves the endocrine system.

9.2.1 Lower vertebrates

Color changes in the lower vertebrates—reptiles, amphibians, and fish—may involve the pineal and melatonin as well as the pituitary and melanophore stimulating hormone (MSH, intermedin) [1, 2, 3, 31, 63, 68]. Some of the changes are slow, taking many weeks, but others are rapid, taking place in a few minutes. The rapid skin color changes may be used for camouflage, thermoregulation, protection of body tissues, and behavioral signaling (e.g., of sexual readiness or aggression). There are two types of rapid color change. First, there is rhythmic color change (dark-time pallor, blanching in dark) that is probably dependent upon the pineal gland and melatonin; this color change is considered to be more primitive, and may only be present early in development (e.g., primary stage tadpoles). Second, there is background adaptation, which is dependent upon the interaction of the lateral eyes with the hypothalamus-pituitary and the release of MSH. The ability to background-adapt arises after the rhythm in development (e.g., in secondary stage tadpoles) [25].

For both blanching and darkening, the rapid skin color changes are achieved by redistribution of pigment in specialized cells called *chromatophores* (Fig. 9.1). The dispersion of melanin (a brown or black pigment) in chromatophores called *melanophores* results in skin darkening. Skin darkening is enhanced by reduction of skin reflectance by altering distribution of reflecting platelets in other chromatophores called *iridophores*. Melanophore dispersion and reduction of reflectance are responses to MSH.

There is variation in the color responses from one species to the next, probably depending on the use made of color change by the animal and the distribution and type of chromatophores in the skin. A full understanding of any one species must thus be on a case-by-case basis for that species. Some generalizations appear to hold, however, for those species that exhibit color changes.

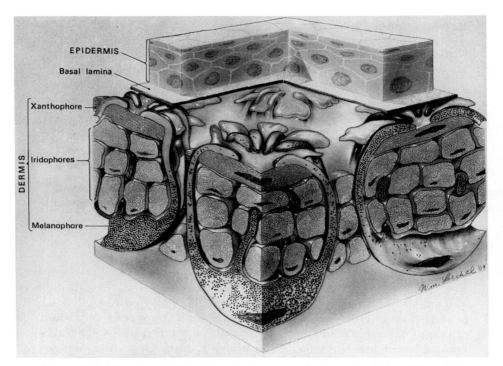

EPIDERMIS

Basal lamina

Xanthophore

DERMIS

Iridophores

Melanophore

Figure 9.1 Diagram of the dermal chromatophore unit of the skin of the lizard, *Anolis carolinensis*. Dark skin is attained by dispersion of melanosomes (organelles containing melatonin) through the basket-like processes of the melanophores (as in the cell at the right). Light skin is achieved by concentrating the melanosomes away from the epidermis (as in the cell at the left). (With permission from M. Hadley [25] and Prentice Hall.)

Species that become pale at night represent all groups of lower vertebrates, including lampreys, fish, tadpoles, frogs, and reptiles. During the daytime they may be light or dark, depending upon background. The rhythmic responses are typified by a lizard, *Anolis carolinensis* (Figs. 9.2, 9.3). This lizard is green in the dark-time of an LD 12:12 cycle. The rhythm persists in DD [1, 2, 3, 15, 16, 69] but is lost in LL. In the light (light-time of LD 12:12 or LL) the lizard can exhibit a variety of skin color patterns ranging from green to very dark brown depending upon the background.

Background adaptation and MSH   The background response is dependent upon the lateral eyes—blinding results in dark-colored fish, for example. Removing the pituitary gland (hypophysectomy) causes frogs or tadpoles to be pale (Fig. 9.4). Pieces of lizard skin exposed to a homogenized pituitary (e.g., from a rat) turn dark. The darkening factor appears to be the peptide hormone MSH (melanophore stimulating hormone). When the lateral eyes perceive a dark-colored

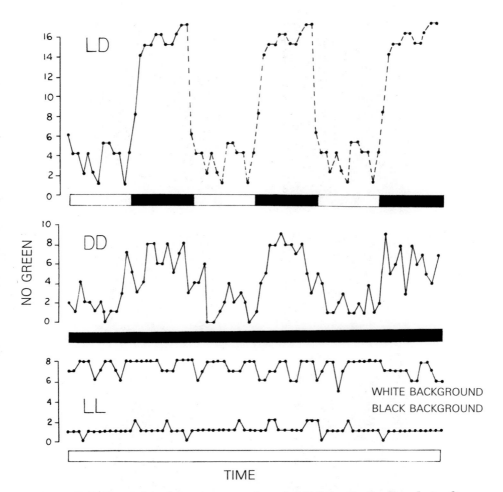

Figure 9.2 Skin color changes versus time and lighting in the lizard, *Anolis carolinensis*. In a light-dark cycle the lizards were green in the dark-time (the dashed line is duplicated data for comparison with DD and LL); the rhythm persisted in DD but was abolished by LL. In LL, the lizards' color was dependent upon background. Subcutaneous implantation of capsules (made of Silastic brand silicon) containing melatonin kept the lizards green [12]. Single serotonin injections turned the lizards brown. Melatonin is high at night in the pineal (but not the retina) of this species [87].

background, a neural signal is sent to the hypothalamus, which in turn signals the pituitary to release MSH. MSH travels to its target cells, chromatophores in the skin, via the bloodstream. Serotonin was suggested for the signal from the hypothalamus to the pituitary; injecting serotonin into *Anolis carolinesis* turns them dark [44, 84]. There is no evidence that melatonin and the pineal gland play a role in background adaptation.

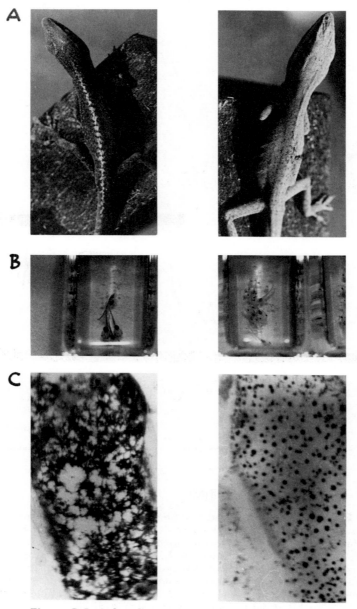

Figure 9.3 Color changes in *Anolis carolinensis* (A) and *Xenopus* tadpoles (B, C). The lizard (A) was dark brown (*left*) on a black background in the light but bright green in the dark-time or at any time when implanted with a melatonin capsule as here. *Xenopus* tadpoles exhibit skin with punctate melanophores in the dark-time (B and C). The production of punctate melanophores by melatonin was the basis for a bioassay [68]. The tadpoles kept in light on a dark background have dispersed pigment in their melanophores. (Photos courtesy of Binkley, Reilly, and White.)

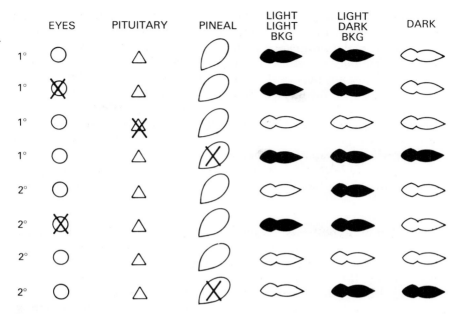

	EYES	PITUITARY	PINEAL	LIGHT LIGHT BKG	LIGHT DARK BKG	DARK
1°						
1°						
1°						
1°						
2°						
2°						
2°						
2°						

Figure 9.4 Diagrammatic representation of the probable effects of surgeries, lighting, and background on color change in lower vertebrates. There is a primary stage (1°) in which removing the pituitary abolishes darkening and removing the pineal abolishes blanching. There is a secondary stage (2°) in which removing the pituitary abolishes background adaptation and removing the pineal abolishes nighttime blanching. In this model the pineal ability to cause dark-time pallor precedes in development or evolution the ability to background-adapt which is mediated by the pituitary.

Dark-time pallor and melatonin   Blind, dark-colored fish (e.g., *Fundulus*) become pale (contracted or punctate melanophores) in the dark so the eyes are apparently not responsible for dark-time pallor. The pineal may be responsible.

Melatonin was named for the fact that it lightens melanophores of tadpoles [41, 42]. McCord and Allen [48] produced lightening in frogs and tadpoles by feeding them mammalian pineal glands. Investigators have observed that the blanching reaction is seen first in the pineal region of tadpoles [1, 2, 3]. The paling response to melatonin exhibited by tadpoles (*Xenopus laevus*, Fig 9.3 B, C *Rana pipiens*) has, in fact, been used for a melatonin bioassay [68]. Melatonin is produced in a lizard pineal (*Anolis carolinensis*) in the dark-time in a rhythmic fashion; the rhythm can be synchronized by light-dark or temperature cycles [87]. The lizards have a rhythm in color change (being green at night); melatonin implants keep the lizards green [12]. Lizard pineals are capable of self-sustained melatonin secretion rhythms in superfusion culture [50].

Studies in a lamprey (*Geotria*) support the idea that nocturnal melatonin production is responsible for nighttime paling: pineal implants or melatonin cause paling, and pinealectomy abolishes the daily color change rhythm. Dark-time color patterns result in pencilfish [69] and guppies [54] when melatonin is added to the water in which they swim. Kavaliers, Firth, and Ralph [36] concluded that the pineal controls the circadian color change rhythm in killifish.

However, light sensitivity and dark-time pallor are not completely abolished by pinealectomy (or by pinealectomy plus blinding) in some species, and some species do not blanch in response to melatonin. It is possible that the light sensitivity and paling response is not wholly pineal mediated; portions of the diencephalon or the skin itself may be involved.

Color change hypothesis A model similar to that suggested for the pineal role in circadian locomotor rhythms and in reproduction may explain dark-time pallor. The pineal gland produces melatonin at night under the direction of a biological clock (probably self-sustaining); light synchronizes the cycle (via extraretinal and/or pineal photoreceptors); melatonin in the blood causes nocturnal paling. Melatonin may affect chromatophores themselves; however, it is also possible that another target is the hypothalamus and/or pituitary; there may be a rhythm because more MSH is in the pituitary in the late light-time in nocturnal rats [55, 86]. Since the pineal uses serotonin as a substrate for melatonin production, it is possible that decreased serotonin availability (due to its conversion to melatonin) contributes to reduction of MSH.

9.2.2 Higher vertebrates

The possibility of color dependency on melatonin in higher vertebrates has been studied in animals that exhibit white winter pelage (Table 9.1). In one of these animals, the weasel, melatonin implants resulted in the prevention of the normal spring molt from winter white fur to brown fur [77]. Another experimental subject was the Djungarian hamster (*Phodopus*). When the hamsters were implanted with melatonin, the change from winter to summer fur was retarded; as might be expected, pinealectomy prevents the molt to white winter pelage [30]. Hair follicles from this species (LD 14:10, pigmented summer coat) were cultured with α-MSH, which stimulates melanogenesis (pigment formation). Melatonin and cGMP inhibited melanogenesis and blocked stimulation by cAMP and α-MSH [94].

9.3 Interactions with the Eyes

The role of the eye in pineal function is not limited to photoreception. In a number of species, the retina is capable of rhythmic melatonin

TABLE 9.1 Hair color change in weasels and hamsters

Species	Conditions	Hair Color
Weasel	Summer Melatonin in beeswax	White
	Summer Untreated, beeswax	Brown
	Winter Melatonin in beeswax	White
	Winter Untreated, beeswax	Brown
Djungarian hamster	LD 16:8	Brown
	LD 8:16	White
	LD 8:16 Pinealectomized	Brown

Sources: Based on data in Hoffman [30]; Reiter [70]; and Rust and Meyer [77].
Note: Changes are related to photo period in weasels and to pineal function in hamsters. These animals normally molt from brown summer pelage to white winter coats.

synthesis. Retinal melatonin may be an auxiliary source of circulating melatonin (making the retina a source of hormones) and/or retinal melatonin may play a role within the retina that is reminiscent of the changes caused by melatonin upon skin color. Retinal melatonin confounds studies of pineal function. When the interactions of the eyes and pineal were studied, the eyes were independent of each other and of the pineal [13, 14]. Retinal melatonin production is affected by environmental lighting and has circadian rhythms.

9.3.1 Retinal melatonin secretion

The retinas of some species are capable of substantive melatonin production. Melatonin rhythms are found in the retinas (including humans); N-acetyltransferase (NAT) rhythms are found in the retinas, and hydroxyindole-O-methyltransferase (HIOMT) activity is present [9, 13, 14, 26, 62, 95]. Eyecups of a frog, *Xenopus*, are capable of NAT cycles in vitro [7]. Melatonin is found in the outer nuclear layer with immunohistology (fish, tortoise, lizard, snake, rat, mouse, hamster) [92]. The amount of melatonin synthesis in the eye may be almost nil (as in rats, hamsters, sparrows, and lizards) or it may be comparable to that in the pineal (chickens and quail) [9, 75, 88, 95, 96].

Melatonin synthesized in the eye is found in the circulation. In the chick about 20% of dark-time circulating melatonin comes from the eyes; in the quail, about 50%. Ocular melatonin is regulated by light and dark in the same manner as pineal melatonin: it peaks in the dark-time; it entrains to LD cycles; there is a rapid plummet; and LL damps the cycle. The eyes respond to light and dark independently of each other and of the pineal gland.

Thus, at least in these species, the eye could be functioning as an endocrine gland. Yu, Pang, and Tang [97] proposed for rats that there is compensatory production of melatonin by the eyes of pinealectomized rats. Ocular melatonin production, especially if there is compensation in pinealectomized rats, could account for the failure of pinealectomy to produce results in many experiments. However, the pineal is the primary source of circulating dark-time melatonin. Presumably, if circulating melatonin has any functions, they are similar whether the origin is the eye or the pineal.

9.3.2 Intraocular melatonin

If the eyes make only a minor contribution to circulating melatonin, it seems possible that the role of intraocular melatonin production is in the eye itself. In view of the fact that the eye adapts for day and/or night vision, it is not surprising to find circadian rhythms in eye function. Furthermore, it is logical to suggest that melatonin rhythms may play a role in controlling the rhythms in ocular physiology. Because melatonin controls skin color in some animals, it seems reasonable to expect that melatonin may function in eyes to regulate pigment movement (e.g., within retinal melanocytes as it does in skin color). Four possible roles have been suggested for melatonin in the eyes: (1) disk shedding, (2) photoreceptor cell elongation, (3) pigment migration, and (4) ocular fluid regulation. In considering an intraocular role for melatonin, it is also possible that the role is indirect, involving production or removal of a metabolite (serotonin or N-acetylserotonin). Experimentally, rabbit retina sequestered serotonin but not melatonin [19].

Circadian rhythms have been observed in rod photoreceptor disk shedding [4, 5, 6, 7, 38, 39, 43, 85]. Peak shedding in rat and frog retina occurs just after lights-on. A persistent circadian cycle in phagosome (a structure indicative of shedding) counts was measured in *Xenopus* frog retina in vitro [22].

In *Midas cichlid*, a teleost fish, retinal cones elongate 69 μm in the dark and shorten in the light (Fig. 9.5) [43]. The rhythm of cone elongation persists in DD and it is damped in LL. Elongation can be elicited with dibutyryl cAMP [43].

Pigment migration may also occur in retinal melanin-containing cells of guinea pigs—the melanin aggregates in the dark and disperses in the light. Melatonin aggregates the pigment [58]. Melatonin also concentrated the retinal pigment of dark-adapted fish; serotonin dispersed the pigment in *Ciprinus carpio* [17].

Rat retinas degenerate under the influence of LL. Melatonin in-

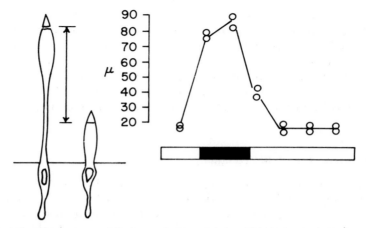

Figure 9.5 The cones of retinas of some fish exhibit a rhythm of elongation. The rhythm is shown on the right (data points for 2 fish); the change that was measured in microns is shown in the diagram at the left with the dark elongated cone represented at the far left. Dibutyryl cAMP elongated the cones but melatonin had no effect. (After Levinson and Burnside [43].)

creased the degeneration [40], but it did not damage the retina in the absence of high-intensity illumination.

9.4 Electrophysiology and the Pineal

Rhythms and effects of environmental light have been found in the electrophysiology of the pineal; melatonin and the pineal affect neurophysiology.

9.4.1 Rhythms

Rhythms are to be expected in pineal electrophysiology, especially in mammals, because of the sympathetic innervation and responses to norepinephrine. Semm and Vollrath [82] made extracellular recordings from guinea pig pineal glands in situ and found two populations of cells. The first population comprised cells that receive sympathetic input. They could be stimulated with electrical input from the optic chiasma, and they exhibited spontaneous alternating high and low activity that was abolished by sympathectomy. These cells responded to light and dark. The second population comprised constantly firing cells that receive a central input possibly from the limbic system via the habenular nuclei.

Semm further classified the first population of sympathetically innervated cells into two subcategories: (1) light-activated cells exhibited more spontaneous activity in the daytime and increased their firing rate in light; (2) darkness-activated cells were active at night. The rhythmicity observed in the spontaneous activity of the cells was also seen in their response to iontophoretically applied melatonin, norepinephrine, and thyroxine [75]. Semm noted that the dark-activated cells have properties that parallel those for pineal melatonin biosynthesis and NAT activity. The presence of rhythms in pinea-locytes has been found in rats, guinea pigs, and pigeons [76, 78, 80, 82].

9.4.2 Pineal responses to light

In Semm's studies of guinea pigs, there was a differential response of pineal cells to light and dark (Fig. 9.6). Darkness-activated cells decreased electrical activity in response to 1 minute of light at night but were not responsive in the subjective daytime. Light-activated cells responded to 10 minutes of dark in the daytime but did not respond in the subjective night. The guinea pig responses are presumably elicited by light acting on the eyes.

Measurements of electrical responses to light have also been made in isolated pineals. Intracellular recordings from lamprey pinea-locytes exhibited hyperpolarization in response to light [47]. The investigators considered the responses to sinusoidal modulated light stimuli similar to the photoreceptor response of the vertebrate lateral eye. In contrast, dissected pineal glands of quail and house sparrows

Figure 9.6 Three kinds of daily electrical patterns measured from guinea pig pineal glands have been observed. Cells were dark- or light-activated or did not respond to light. L/D = light-to-dark transition. (After data provided by Semm [79]).

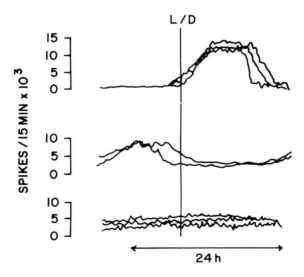

did not respond to light [66]. Frog (*Rana catesbeiana* and *Rana esculenta*) pineals responded to light when they were studied in anesthetized, blinded frogs [47, 49, 51, 52]. The scientists considered the response they measured (the early receptor potential) to be similar to retinal responses to light.

9.4.3 Pineal responses to magnetism

Semm exposed guinea pigs and homing pigeons to magnetic fields comparable to the strength of the earth's magnetic fields. The electrical activity of 21–30% of the pineal cells studied was altered by the fields [79, 81].

9.4.4 Brain responses to melatonin

Semm and Vollrath [82] applied melatonin to Purkinje cells in the brains of urethane-anesthetized homing pigeons and guinea pigs. Melatonin altered Purkinje cell activity but the responses were variable.

Melatonin (0.01–0.06 mg/g, intraperitoneal injection) induced a sleep state in 2- to 15-day old chicks that was characterized by EEG activity similar to slow wave sleep. The sedative and hypnotic effect began 1–2 minutes after the injection and lasted 30-60 minutes [29]. The results were supported by another study of 10- to 16-week-old chickens in which (melatonin produced high amplitude—low frequency EEGs characteristic of sleep. In addition, pinealectomy had the opposite effect to that of melatonin; pinealeactomy produced brain wave desynchronization [57]. Cats injected in the brain with melatonin or AVT exhibited sleep changes [47, 60]. Delta-sleep-inducing peptide attenuated the dark-time rise in rat pineal NAT [24].

9.4.5 Convulsions

Since 1938 there have been reports that pinealectomized animals may convulse following the operation [61]. Rats in particular convulse after pinealectomy when it is combined with parathyroidectomy. Nine of ten gerbils convulse after pinealectomy. The symptoms are wild running, clonus, tonus, and frequent death. Normal levels of serotonin, norepinephrine, and dopamine prevent seizures so the decrease in norepinephrine from 293 to 170 ng/g following pinealectomy may account for pinealectomy promotion of convulsions.

9.5 Thermoregulation

The pineal has been associated with thermoregulation, the control of body temperature [65, 67]. Here again, the possibilities of circadian

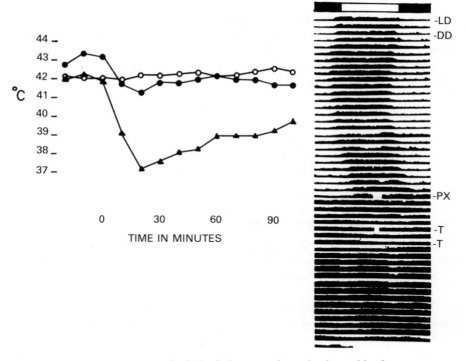

Figure 9.7 Pinealectomy abolished the circadian rhythm of body temperature in sparrows. Each line represents 24 hours of temperature recording; the lines are arranged vertically in chronological order. The sparrow was transferred from the LD 12:12 cycle shown in the bar over the record to constant dark (*DD*) and pinealectomized and returned to DD at *PX*. T = 2 days of technical problems. (From Binkley, Kluth, and Menaker [11] and Binkley [8].)

rhythms, environmental lighting control, and brain and endocrine interaction arise. An intriguing observation that could relate to pineal function in thermoregulation is the fact that species of lizards in which the parietal eye is absent tend to occur at low latitudes (warm equatorial regions). Parietal eyes are more common at higher latitudes where there are greater seasonal swings in photoperiod and temperature [64].

9.5.1 Core body temperature

Most species have daily temperature cycles either imposed by the environment (poikilothermy) or imposed from within (homeothermy). Pinealectomy abolished the 3°–4.5°C circadian rhythm of deep body temperature in house sparrows (Fig. 9.7) [11]. Melatonin injections 1.2–2.5 mg/bird) induced roosting and lowered body temperature 4.7°C in sparrows [8]. Pinealectomy did not abolish the rhythm in pigeons (possibly due to ocular melatonin synthesis), but it did raise

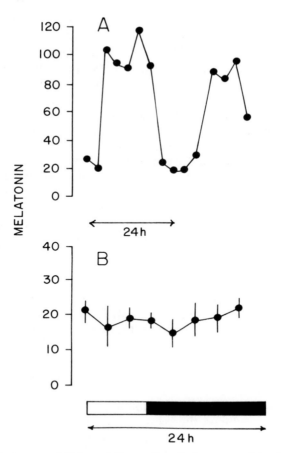

Figure 9.8 Marmots exhibit a daily cycle of plasma melatonin (A) that is abolished during hibernation (B). (After data of Florant et al. [23].)

the body temperature (hyperthermia) unless melatonin implants were present [31]. Pinealectomy raised the body temperatures of goldfish 2°–4°C [33, 36].

9.5.2 Hibernation

Melatonin was measured in hibernating marmots (Fig. 9.8), ground squirrels, and hamsters with the same result: the melatonin rhythm was lost in the presence of a light-dark cycle, apparently by diminution of the dark-time peak so that melatonin levels were not particularly high. Melatonin rose with arousal irrespective of whether the arousal occurred in the day or night [23, 83, 89, 90]. The melatonin results agree with pinealocyte size reduction noticed in pineals during hibernation [65].

Ralph [65] summarizes effects of pinealectomy on hibernation in ground squirrels: they range from no effect [27], to effects the first or second year after surgery. The timing, not the occurrence, of hibernation was affected; similarly, Zucker [98] found that the circannual body weight rhythm was 27 days shorter in the first year after pinealectomy and 58 days shorter the second year after surgery. But daily melatonin administration increased the duration and the incidence of hibernation [56]. Pinealectomy reduced and melatonin increased the incidence of torpor in mice [46]. Investigators have connected the photoperiodic regulation of thermogenic brown fat and nonshivering thermogenesis with the pineal gland [28, 65]. The possibility that the eyes may synthesize melatonin, and that there may be compensatory ocular melatonin synthesis in some species after pinealectomy, makes it difficult to rule out the possibility that melatonin is important to the physiology of hibernation.

9.5.3 Behavioral thermoregulation

The effects of pinealectomy on selection of preferred environmental temperature has been tested with fish [34–37] and lizards [65]. The preference for a lower daytime temperature exhibited by white suckers was eliminated by pinealectomy [37]. Shielding the pineal region from light resulted in more time spent in the warmer and/or more illuminated portions of the test apparatus [34]. Severing the parietal nerve caused collared lizards to select higher temperatures, but pinealectomy resulted in selection of lower temperatures [21]. Parietalectomy reduced the panting threshold in a species of lizard [20]; moreover, the daily cycle in the panting threshold (higher day threshold) was eliminated by parietalectomy, by eye shielding, and by melatonin or serotonin administration.

The region of the epithalamus of poikilotherms has a variable anatomy that may include structures in addition to the pineal (e.g., parietal eye, parietal organ, stirnorgan, frontal organ) collectively referred to as "the third eye" [18, 65]. Conjectures as to the functional significance of third eyes relate to: (1) thermoreception, (2) production of vitamin D, (3) inhibition of sexual activity, (4) radiation dosimetry, (5) navigation, (6) secretion, (7) photoreception, (8) pigment control, (9) light detection for the circadian clock, and (10) predator detection.

9.6 Behavior

Effects on behavior in addition to the control of locomotor rhythms has sometimes been noticed. For example, there are some subtle effects of pinealectomy on rat behavior [73, 74]. The quantity of locomotor behavior has been lowered with pineal extracts. Aggression (fighting duration and latency) was reduced by pinealectomy. In one study, but not others, pinealectomy reduced ethanol preference. Melatonin inhibited the phobic responses of rats to the introduction of saccharin in their drinking water. Isolation and stress may stimulate pineal function and/or size. It is possible that behavioral changes are secondary to pineal involvement in rat reproduction.

9.7 Hypertension

Pinealectomy produces hypertension (high blood pressure, 20 mm Hg or more); and pineal extracts are hypotensive. Melatonin prevented pinealectomy-induced hypertension. Spontaneously hypertensive rats had 1.5–2 times the pineal NAT of normal rats [32, 73, 74, 91].

9.8 Endocrine system

Many of the functions associated with the pineal—reproduction, circadian rhythms, color change, and thermoregulation—potentially involve the endocrine system. The endocrine system can be organized into a series of hierarchies of glands (Table 9.2). The hierarchies may be explained by the potential for sequential amplification: a small number of molecules from the hypothalamus release a large number of molecules from the pituitary. In the traditional endocrine hierarchies, the hypothalamus is subject to neural input from brain regions. Neurosecretory cells in the hypothalamus (first level) produce hormones (hypophysiotropins) that are small peptides. These hormones are released at the anterior hypothalamus via blood (hypophyseal portal veins) via axons of neurosecretory cells. The release or inhibition of release of the hormones synthesized in the anterior pituitary (second level) and intermediate lobe is brought about by the hypothalamic hormones. In turn, some of the pituitary hormones stimulate yet other endocrine glands (third level).

When the pineal (a fourth level) is found to act upon some aspect also known to involve one of the endocrine hierarchies, potential actions are myriad. The pineal could act (1) independently; (2) upon the brain; (3) upon the hypothalamic neurosecretory cells which make the releasing and inhibiting neurohormones; (4) upon the pituitary; (5) upon the thyroid, adrenal, or gonads; or (6) some combination of effects. Pineal hormone(s) routes to targets may include the cerebrospinal fluid (CSF) as well as the bloodstream. In the ensuing discussion, a general viewpoint supporting an endocrine-inhibiting role for the pineal related to rhythms and light is presented. Possible feedback on the pineal by hypothalamic hormones is also suggested.

TABLE 9.2 Hierarchies for hormone systems that have the hypothalamus and pituitary as common components

PINEAL

Brain

1. Growth hormone
Hypothalamus
    Growth hormone releasing hormone (GRF)
    Somatostatin
Anterior Pituitary
    Growth hormone (GH)

2. Prolactin
Hypothalamus
    Prolactin releasing hormone (PRH)
    Prolactin inhibiting hormone (PIH)
Anterior Pituitary
    Prolactin (PRL)

3. Adrenal
Hypothalamus
    Corticotrophin releasing hormone (CRF)
Anterior Pituitary
    Adrenocorticotrophic hormone (ACTH)
Adrenal
    Corticosteroids

4. Thyroid
Hypothalamus
    TSH stimulating hormone (TRH)
Anterior pituitary
    Thyroid stimulating hormone (TSH)
Thyroid gland
    Thyroxine (T_4)
    Triiodothyronine (T_3)

5. Gonad
Hypothalamus
    Gonadotrophin releasing hormone (GnRH, LRH)
Anterior pituitary
    Luteinizing hormone (LH)
    Follicle stimulating hormone (FSH)
Gonads
    Testosterone
    Estrogen

6. Intermedin
Hypothalamus
    MSH releasing factor (MRF)
    MSH inhibiting factor(s) (MIF)
Intermediate Pituitary
    Melanophore stimulating hormone (MSH)

(Continued)

TABLE 9.2 (Continued)

7. Neurohormone
Hypothalamus
   Vasopressin
   Oxytocin
Posterior pituitary
   Vasopressin
   Oxytocin

Note: Much of the endocrine system falls under a hierarchical organization in which the brain and other factors regulate the hypothalamus [25]. The hypothalamus in turn controls the pituitary. The pituitary has mastery of the adrenal, ovaries, testes, and thyroid. The hormones may feed back on various structures in the hierarchy above.

9.8.1 Pineal and growth hormone

The pineal influence on growth hormone is still in question [73]. Growth hormone is released at night in humans and during the day in rats. The growth hormone reduction that resulted from blinding was prevented by pinealectomy in one study, but pinealectomy reduced daytime growth hormone in another study. Somatostatin was detected in guinea pig and rat pineal. If there is a role for the pineal, it is probably inhibitory.

9.8.2 Pineal and prolactin

Pinealectomy and constant light increased prolactin in the pituitary and decreased plasma prolactin in rats [71, 74]. Blinding and constant dark lowered pituitary prolactin but the reduction was prevented by pinealectomy. Pinealectomy may prevent the morning rise in prolactin. Melatonin increased circulating prolactin, and AVT inhibited the increase in pituitary prolactin that follows pinealectomy in rats. Ewes have an annual prolactin cycle (peak in the summer) but the levels of prolactin remained high after pinealectomy.

9.8.3 Pineal and adrenal cortex

Pinealectomy has been associated with adrenal hypertrophy in mice and rats, implying adrenocortical inhibition by the pineal [74]. Blinding and constant dark or replacement of pineal substances (extracts, melatonin, AVT) decreased adrenal weight and/or compensatory adrenal hypertrophy in rats and mice.

Aldosterone is a mineralocorticoid of the adrenal cortex that functions in electrolyte balance. The pineal inhibits aldosterone secretion.

Corticosterone is a glucocorticoid of the adrenal cortex that functions in carbohydrate metabolism. Melatonin lowers plasma corticosterone and pinealectomy raises it. The role of the pineal in the adrenal may depend on sex and age.

Since glucorcorticoids are controlled by adrenocorticotrophic hormone (ACTH), the effect of pinealectomy is of interest. Pinealectomy only affected ACTH in male rats with sensory deprivation (blinding plus olfactory bulbectomy) where it increased ACTH. Some effects of melatonin on the adrenal may be direct because melatonin stimulated adrenal 5-α-reductase and inhibited 17- and 21-hydroxylases in vitro.

The adrenal gland has circadian rhythms (e.g., in steroid production). Attempts to prove the rhythms were under pineal control (with pinealectomy, melatonin, or N-acetylserotonin) produced mixed results. Generally, most of the work supports an adrenal inhibitory role for the pineal gland inhibition of steroid production.

9.8.4 Pineal and thyroid hormones

An inhibitory role seems likely for the pineal in thyroid physiology [74, 93]. The iodine-containing thyroid hormones—thyroxine (T_4) and triiodothyronine (T_3)—function in metabolism, and increased metabolic rate is associated with increases in thyroid hormones. Thyroid involvement in body temperature regulation could mean that the thyroid acts in mediating the pineal effects on thermoregulation. Pinealectomy increases the rate of T_4 secretion. Melatonin decreases the rate of T_4 secretion and depresses plasma T_4. Thyroid hypertrophy is a consequence of pinealectomy. Moreover, melatonin and the low molecular weight fraction of rat pineals increase thyroid stimulating hormone (TSH), so one action of the pineal may be on the pituitary.

Rhythms occur in plasma levels of TSH and thyroid hormones (light-time rat T_4 peaked at 80 ng/100 ml serum; dark-time nadir was 55 ng/100 ml serum). Constant dark raises radioactive iodine uptake by the thyroid in mice, increases thyroid cAMP in rats, and depresses pituitary and plasma TSH in hamsters; blinding lowers hamster plasma T_4 levels. Constant light depresses rat pituitary TSH, but raises plasma TSH, plasma protein-bound iodine, and T_4—effects similar to pinealectomy.

The thyroid may provide feedback that regulates the pineal. Thyrotropin releasing hormone (TRH) inhibits pineal cAMP accumulation that is stimulated by norepinephrine; thyroid hormones increased pineal melatonin in rats. TRH has been found in bovine, ovine, and porcine pineals.

9.8.5 Pineal and reproductive hormones

Pinealectomy abolishes the dark-induced regression of the gonads of some species. Melatonin inhibits the reproductive system. Because of this, interactions with the hormones of reproduction are expected and found. However, in understanding the interactions, many factors enter into consideration, including time of day, season of year, sex, stage of female cycle, and age.

The testes develop in short days if both LRH (luteinizing hormone releasing hormone which stimulates luteinizing hormone, LH, and follicle stimulating hormone, FSH) and PRL (prolactin which increases LH receptors in the gonads) are present. Reiter [71] has proposed that LH, FSH, and prolactin are all necessary to achieve fully functional gonads in hamsters. Gonadotrophin releasing activity was reduced in hamsters kept in short days. Pinealectomy reverses at least the FSH releasing activity. However, RIA measurements of LRH showed no change in hamsters kept in long versus short photoperiods.

Melatonin or pineal fragments implanted into the hypothalamus or injected into ventricles of the brain reduced pituitary and plasma LH and/or FSH but increased prolactin. Serum and pituitary LH, FSH, and prolactin drop in short days but are higher if the animals are pinealectomized (Fig. 9.9).

LRH has been found in bovine, sheep, and rat pineals. Reproductive steroids, LRH, LH, FSH, and prolactin affect pineal activity. Castration reduces pineal melatonin synthesis; administration of gonadotrophins increases pineal HIOMT [72].

9.8.6 Pineal and intermedin

In the regulation of color change, the pineal has traditionally been supposed as the source of a skin lightening agent (melatonin) which aggregates melanosomes in melanophores. The pituitary intermediate lobe was viewed as the source of MSH (intermedin), which darkened skin by dispersing melanosomes in melanophores [3].

MSH release has variously been viewed as under control of neurotransmitters (stimulation by serotonin or acetylcholine, inhibition by dopamine or norepinephrine). The possibility that melatonin causes paling via MSH inhibition was rejected because hypophysectomized tadpoles placed in water containing melatonin show aggregation of melanosomes even when MSH was in the water.

9.8.7 Pineal and oxytocin and vasopressin

Oxytocin and vasopressin are nonapeptides synthesized in the hypothalamus and released in the posterior pituitary. The hormones function in parturition and water balance. They are of interest in considering the pineal because their "ancestral" nonapeptide is AVT (arginine vasotocin), and this molecule has been reported in pineal glands and suggested as a possible pineal secretion (see Chapter 11). AVT prevented the increase in pituitary prolactin that normally follows pinealectomy.

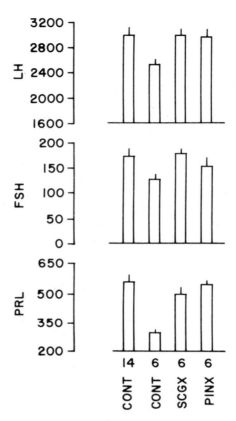

Figure 9.9 Hamster pituitary LH, FSH, and prolactin (PRL) content dropped in short days (LD 6:18) compared to long days (LD 14:10) in intact subjects (*Cont.*). The effect of short days was abolished by removal of the superior cervical ganglia (*SCGx*) or pinealectomy (*Pinx*). (After data of Reiter [71].)

9.8.8 Pineal and catecholamines

The hormones of the adrenal medulla are catecholamines (epinephrine and norepinephrine) whose release is associated with stress. Because NAT of some species is stimulated by adrenergic agents (isoproterenol, norepinephrine), it seemed likely that adrenal hormones would stimulate the pineal. NAT increases in rats stressed by swimming or immobilization [45, 59, 73].

The adrenal medulla has daily cycles in its physiology; for example, dopamine-β-hydroxylase increases sixfold within an hour after lights-off. The increase was prevented with constant light or pinealectomy [74]. Pinealectomy also changed the daily patterns that occur in vesicles of cells of the adrenal medulla.

Prostaglandins are found in the pineal gland and their release is augmented with norepinephrine [74].

9.8.9 Pineal and calcium-regulating hormones

Parathyroid glands secrete parathormone, which elevates blood calcium. Homeostasis of calcium is achieved with another hormone, calcitonin, from the thyroid, which lowers blood calcium.

In various investigations, pinealectomy has affected both parathyroid activity and the calcitonin-producing cells. The possibility was raised that the pineal gland has a calcium-lowering action but the opposite possibility was supported in other studies. Pinealectomy combined with parathyroidectomy resulted in convulsions in rats and gerbils but pinealectomy reduced convulsions in mice [74]. Such convulsions have been associated with altered levels of calcium in the blood.

9.8.10 Pineal and insulin

The pancreas is the source of insulin (which lowers blood sugar) and glucagon (which raises blood sugar). Blinding raises blood glucose and lowers insulin activity. Pinealectomy increased the insulin response to glucose in rats and lowered rat blood sugar. It also increased tyrosine uptake by the islets of Langerhans (insulin-producing cells).

Insulin secretion was decreased by melatonin. The effect was direct because it was obtained in vitro. Melatonin also inhibited insulin secretion in response to glucose. In monkeys, melatonin raised blood sugar. Pineal peptides reduced the enhanced glucose tolerance produced by pinealectomy. In sum, then, the pineal antagonizes the insulin function of the pancreas, possibly by direct action of pineal hormones on the pancreas [74].

Insulin is also of interest to pineal function. Various substances (including disulfides such as cystamine, and AVT) inhibit NAT in homogenates [10]. Insulin is the most potent such inhibitor [53].

9.9 Summary

In summarizing functions of the pineal, as stated in the introduction, general themes prevail. Environmental lighting affects (1) pineal and eye biochemistry and anatomy, (2) circadian rhythm, (3) reproduction, (4) color change, (5) brain neurophysiology, (6) thermoregulation, (7) behavior, and (8) the endocrine system. Circadian rhythms are involved in (1) pineal and eye biochemistry and anatomy, (2) measurement of photoperiod in reproduction, (3) color change, (4) locomotor behavior, and (5) the endocrine system. The relationships between the pineal and the neural and endocrine systems permits the pineal to have global effects.

REFERENCES

1. Bagnara, J. 1960. Pineal regulation of the body lightening reaction in amphibian larvae. *Science* 132:1481–1483.

2. Bagnara, J., and M. Hadley. 1970. Endocrinology of the amphibian pineal. *Amer. Zool.* 10:201–216.

3. ———. 1973. *Chromatophores and color change: The comparative physiology of animal pigmentation.* Englewoods Cliffs, N.J.: Prentice-Hall.

4. Basinger, S., R. Hoffman, and M. Matthes. 1976. Photoreceptor shedding is initiated by light in the frog retina. *Science* 194:1074–1076.

5. Besharse, J., and D. Dunis. 1983. Methoxyindoles and photoreceptor metabolism: Activation of rod shedding. *Science* 219:1341–1343.

6. Besharse, J., J. Hollyfield, and M. Rayborn. 1977. Turnover of rod photoreceptor outer segments II: Membrane addition and loss in relationship to light. *J. Cell Biol.* 75:507–527.

7. Besharse, J., and P. Iuvone. 1983. Circadian clock in *Xenopus* eye controlling retinal serotonin *N*-acetyltransferase. *Nature* 305:133–135.

8. Binkley, S. 1974. Pineal and melatonin: Circadian rhythms and body temperatures of sparrows. In *Chronobiology*, ed. L. Scheving, F. Halberg, and J. Pauly, pp. 582–585. Tokyo: Igaku Shoin.

9. Binkley, S., M. Hryshchyshyn, and K. Reilly. 1979. *N*-acetyltransferase activity responds to environmental lighting in the eye as well as in the pineal gland. *Nature* 281:479–481.

10. Binkley, S., D. Klein, and J. Weller. 1976. Pineal serotonin *N*-acetyltransferase activity: Protection of stimulated activity by acetyl-CoA and related compounds. *J. Neurochem.* 26:51–55.

11. Binkley, S., E. Kluth, and M. Menaker. 1971. Pineal function in sparrows: Circadian rhythms and body temperature. *Science* 174:311–314.

12. Binkley, S., K. Reilly, V. Hermida, and K. Mosher. 1987. Circadian rhythm of color change in *Anolis carolinensis*: Reconsideration of regulation, especially the role of melatonin in dark-time pallor. In *Pineal research reviews* V, ed. R. Reiter, pp. 133–151. New York: Alan R. Liss.

13. Binkley, S., K. Reilly, and T. Hernandez. 1980. *N*-acetyltransferase in the chick retina II: Interactions of the eyes and pineal gland in response to light. *J. Comp. Physiol.* 140:181–183.

14. Binkley, S., K. Reilly, and M. Hryshchyshyn. 1980. *N*-acetyltransferase in the chick retina I: Circadian rhythms controlled by environmental lighting are similar to those in the pineal gland. *J. Comp. Physiol.* 139:103–108.

15. Bogenshütz, H. 1964. Die beteiligung der epiphyse an der steuerung des tagesperiodischen farbwechsels bei amphibien. In *Deutschen gesellschaft für biophysik E.V. der Österreichischen gesellschaft für reine und angewandte biophysik un der schweizerischen gesellshaft für strahlenbiologie*, pp. 501–504.

16. ———. 1965. Investigations of the light-controlled color changes of tadpoles. *Z. Vergl. Physiol.* 50:598–614.

17. Chèze, G., and M. Ali. 1976. Rôle de l'épiphyse dans la migration du pigment épithélial retinien chez quelques Téléostéens. *Can. J. Zool.* 54:475–481.

18. Eakin, R. 1973. *The third eye.* Berkeley: Univ. of California Press.
19. Ehinger, B., and I. Floren. 1978. Quantitation of the uptake of indoleamines and dopamine in the rabbit retina. *Exp. Eye Res.* 26:1–11.
20. Firth, B., and H. Heatwole. 1976. Panting thresholds of lizards: The role of the pineal complex in panting responses in an Agamid, *Amphibolurus muricatus. Gen. Comp. Endocrinol.* 29:388–401.
21. Firth, B., C. Ralph, and T. Boardman. 1980. Independent effects of the pineal and a bacterial pyrogen in behavioral thermoregulation in lizards. *Nature* 285:399–400.
22. Flannery, J., and S. Fisher. 1984. Circadian disc shedding in *Xenopus* retina in vitro. *Invest. Ophthalmol. Vis. Sci.* 25:229–232.
23. Florant, G., M. Rivera, A. Lawrence, and L. Tamarkin. 1984. Plasma melatonin concentrations in hibernating marmots: Absence of a plasma melatonin rhythm. *Amer. J. Physiol.* 247:R1062–R1066.
24. Graf, M., A. Kastin, and G. Schoenenberger. 1985. Delta-sleep-inducing peptide and two of its analogs reduce nocturnal increase of N-acetyltransferase activity in rat pineal gland. *J. Neurochem.* 44:629–632.
25. Hadley, M. 1984. *Endocrinology.* Englewood Cliffs, N.J.: Prentice-Hall.
26. Hamm, H., and M. Menaker. 1980. Retinal rhythms in chicks: Circadian variation in melatonin and serotonin N-acetyltransferase. *Proc. Natl. Acad. Sci. USA* 77:4998–5002.
27. Harlow, H., J. Phillips, and C. Ralph. 1980. The effect of pinealectomy on hibernation in two species of seasonal hibernators, *Citellus lateralis* and *C. richardsonii. J. Exp. Zool.* 213:301–303.
28. Heldmaier, G., S. Steinlechner, J. Rafael, and P. Vsiansky. 1981. Photoperiodic control and effects of melatonin on nonshivering thermogenesis and brown adipose tissue. *Science* 212:917–919.
29. Hishikawa, Y., H. Cramer, and W. Kuhlo. 1969. Natural and melatonin-induced sleep in young chickens: A behavioral and electrographic study. *Exp. Brain Res.* 7:84–94.
30. Hoffman, K. 1981. Pineal involvement in the photoperiodic control of reproduction and other functions in the Djungarian hamster *Phodopus sungorus*. In *The pineal gland II: Reproductive effects*, ed. R. Reiter, pp. 83–102. Florida: CRC Press.
31. Hogben, L., and D. Slome. 1931. The pigmentary effector system VI: The dual character of endocrine coordination in amphibian color change. *London, Proc. Roy. Soc. B* 108:10–53.
32. Illnerová, H., and I. Albrecht. 1975. Isoproterenol induction of pineal serotonin N-acetyltransferase in normotensive and spontaneously hypertensive rats. *Experientia* 31:95–96.
33. John, T., S. Itoh, and J. George. 1978. On the role of the pineal in thermoregulation in the pigeon. *Hormone Res.* 9:41–56.
34. Kavaliers, M. 1982a. Effects of pineal shielding on the thermoregulatory behavior of the white sucker, *Catostomus commersoni. Physiol. Zool.* 55:155–161.
35. ———. 1982b. Pinealectomy modifies the thermoregulatory effects of bombesin in goldfish. *Neuropharmacology* 21:1169–1182.
36. Kavaliers, M., B. Firth, and C. Ralph. 1980. Pineal control of the circadin rhythm of color change in the killifish. *Can. J. Zool.* 58:456–460.

37. Kavaliers, M., and C. Ralph. 1980. Pineal involvement in the control of behavioral thermoregulation of the white sucker, *Catostomus commersoni. J. Exp. Zool.* 212:301–303.

38. Lavail, M. 1976. Rod outer segment disc shedding in the rat retina: Relationship to cyclic lighting. *Science* 194:1071–1074.

39. ———. 1980. Circadian nature of rod outer segment disc shedding in the rat. *Invest. Ophthalmol. Vis. Sci.* 19:407–420.

40. Leino, M. 1984. Effects of melatonin and 6-methoxy-tetrahydro-β-carboline in light induced retinal damage: A computerized morphometric method. *Life Sci.* 35:1997–2001.

41. Lerner, A., and J. Case. 1959. Pigment cell regulatory factors. *J. Invest. Derm.* 32:211–221.

42. Lerner, A., J. Case, and Y. Takahashi. 1958. Isolation of melatonin, the pineal gland factor that lightens melanocytes. *J. Amer. Chem. Soc.* 80:2587.

43. Levinson, G., and B. Burnside. 1981. Circadian rhythms in teleost retinomotor movements: A comparison of circadian rhythm and light condition on cone length. *Invest. Ophthal. Mol. Vis. Sci.* 20:294–303.

44. Levitin, H. 1980. Further evidence that serotonin may be a physiological melanocyte-stimulating hormone-releasing factor in the lizard *Anolis carolinensis. Gen. Comp. Endocrinol.* 40:8–14.

45. Lynch, H., M. Hsuan, and R. Wurtman. 1975. Sympathetic neural control of indoleamine metabolism in the rat pineal gland. *Adv. Exp. Med. Biol.* 54:93–114.

46. Lynch, R., K. Sullivan, and S. Gendler. 1980. Temperature regulation in the mouse, *Peromyscus leucopus*: Effects of various photoperiods, pinealectomy and melatonin administration. *Int. J. Biometeorol.* 24:49–55.

47. Marczynski, T., N. Yamaguchi, G. Ling, and L. Grodzinska. 1964. Sleep induced by the administration of melatonin to the hypothalamus in unrestrained cats. *Experientia* 20:435–437.

48. McCord, C., and F. Allen. 1917. Evidences associating pineal gland function with alterations in pigmentation. *J. Exp. Zool.* 23:207–224.

49. Meissl, H., and S. George. 1984. Electrophysiological studies on neuronal transmission in the frog's photosensory pineal organ. *Vision Res.* 24:1727–1734.

50. Menaker, M., and S. Wisner. 1983. Temperature-compensated circadian clock in the pineal of *Anolis. Proc. Nat. Acad. Sci. USA* 80:6119–6121.

51. Morita, Y., and E. Dodt. 1975. Early receptor potential from the pineal photoreceptor. *Pflugers Arch.* 354:273–280.

52. Morita, Y., K. Segi, M. Samejima, and T. Nakamura. 1984. Intracellular dynamic response characteristics of pineal photoreceptors. *Ophthalmic Res.* 16:119–122.

53. Namboodiri, M., J. Weller, and D. Klein. 1981. Pineal N-acetyltransferase is inactivated by disulfide-containing peptides: Insulin is the most potent. *Science* 213:571–573.

54. Nayuda, P. and C. Hunter. 1979. Cytological aspects and differential response to melatonin of melanophore-based color mutants in the guppy. *Copeia* 2:232–242.

55. O'Donohue, T., R. Miller, R. Pendleton, and D. Jacobowitz. 1980.

Demonstration of an endogenous circadian rhythm of α-melanocyte stimulating hormone in the rat pineal gland. *Brain Res.* 186:145–155.

56. Palmer, D., and M. Riedesel. 1976. Responses of whole-animal and isolated hearts of ground squirrels, *Citellus lateralis* to melatonin. *Comp. Biochem. Physiol.* 53C:69–72.

57. Pang, S., C. Ralph, and J. Petrozza. 1976. Effects of melatonin administration and pinealectomy on the electroencephalogram of the chicken brain. *Life Sci.* 18:961–966.

58. Pang, S., and D. Yew. 1979. Pigment aggregation by melatonin in the retinal pigment epithelium and choroid of guinea pigs, *Cavia procellus*. *Experientia* 35:231–232.

59. Parfitt, A., and D. Klein. 1976. Sympathetic nerve endings in the pineal gland protect against acute stress-induced increase in N-acetyltransferase activity. *Endocrinology* 99:840–851.

60. Pavel, S. 1979. Pineal vasotocin and sleep: Involvement of serotonin-containing neurons. *Brain Res. Bull.* 4:731–734.

61. Philo, R. 1982. Catecholamines and pinealectomy-induced convulsions in the gerbil (*Meriones unguiculatus*). In *The pineal and its hormones*. ed. R. Reiter, pp. 233–241. New York: Alan R. Liss.

62. Quay, W. 1965. Retinal and pineal hydroxyindole-O-methyltransferase activity in vertebrates. *Life Sci.* 4:983–991.

63. Rahn, H., and F. Rosendale. 1941. Diurnal rhythm of melanophore hormone secretions in *Anolis* pituitary. *Proc. Soc. Exp. Biol. Med.* 48:100–102.

64. Ralph, C. 1975. The pineal gland and geographical distribution of animals. *Int. J. Biometeorol.* 19:289–303.

65. ———. 1984. Pineal bodies and thermoregulation. In *The pineal gland*, ed. R. Reiter, pp. 193–218. New York: Raven Press.

66. Ralph, C., and D. Dawson. 1968. Failure of the pineal body of two species of birds to show electrical responses to illumination. *Experientia* 24:147–148.

67. Ralph, C., B. Firth, and J. Turner. 1979. The role of the pineal body in ectotherm thermoregulation. *Amer. Zool.* 19:273–293.

68. Ralph, C., and H. Lynch. 1970. A quantitative melatonin bioassay. *Gen. Comp. Endocrinol.* 15:334–338.

69. Reed, B. 1968. The control of circadian pigment changes in the pencil fish: A proposed role for melatonin. *Life Sci.* 7:961–973.

70. Reiter, R. 1972. The role of the pineal in reproduction. In *Excerpta medica monograph*, ed. H. Balin and S. Glasser, pp. 71–114. Amsterdam: Excerpta Medica.

71. ———. 1981. Reproductive effects of the pineal gland and pineal indoles in the Syrian hamster and the albino rat. In *The pineal gland II: Reproductive effects*, ed. R. Reiter, pp. 45–81. Boca Raton, Fla. CRC Press.

72. Reiter, R., B. Richardson, and T. King. 1983. The pineal gland and its indole products: Their importance in the control of reproduction in mammals. In *The pineal gland*, ed. R. Relkin, pp. 151–199. New York: Elsevier.

73. Relkin, R. 1976. The pineal, adrenals and hypertension. In *The pineal*, pp. 68–71. Montreal: Eden Press.

74. ———. 1983. Pineal-hormonal interactions. In *The Pineal Gland*, ed. R. Relkin, pp. 225–245. New York: Elsevier.

75. Reppert, S., and S. Sagar. 1983. Characterization of the day-night variation of retinal melatonin content in the chick. *Invest. Ophthalmol. Vis. Sci.* 24:294–300.

76. Reuss, S., and L. Vollrath. 1984. Electrophysiological properties of rat pinealocytes: Evidence for circadian and ultradian rhythms. *Exp. Brain Res.* 55:455–461.

77. Rust, C., and R. Meyer. 1969. Hair color, molt, and testis size in male short-tailed weasels treated with melatonin. *Science* 96:921–922.

78. Semm, P. 1982. Electrophysiology of the mammalian pineal gland: Evidence for rhythmical and non-rhythmical elements and for magnetic influence on electrical activity. In *Vertebrate circadian systems*, ed. J. Aschoff, S. Daan, and G. Groos, pp. 147–157. Berlin: Springer-Verlag.

79. ———. 1983. Neurobiological investigations on the magnetic sensitivity of the pineal gland in rodents and pigeons. *Comp. Biochem. Physiol.* 76A:683–689.

80. Semm, P., C. Demaine, and L. Vollrath. 1981. Electrical responses of pineal cells to melatonin and putative transmitters: Evidence for circadian changes in sensitivity. *Exp. Brain Res.* 43:361–370.

81. Semm, P., T. Schneider, and L. Vollrath, 1980. Effects of an Earth-strength magnetic field on electrical activity on pineal cells. *Nature* 288:607–608.

82. Semm, P., and L. Vollrath. 1984. Electrical responses of homing pigeon and guinea pig Purkinje cells to pineal indoleamines applied by microelectrophoresis. *J. Comp. Physiol.* 154:675–681.

83. Stanton, T., C. Craft, and R. Reiter. 1984. Decreases in pineal melatonin content during the hibernation bout in the golden-mantled ground squirrel, *Spermophilus lateralis*. *Life Sci.* 35:1461–1467.

84. Thornton, B. and I. Geschwind. 1975. Evidence that serotonin may be a melanocyte-stimulating hormone-releasing factor in the lizard, *Anolis carolinensis*. *Gen. Comp. Endocrinol.* 26:346–353.

85. Tierstein, P., A. Goldman, and P. O'Brien. 1980. Evidence for both local and central regulation of rat rod outer segment disc shedding. *Invest. Ophthalmol. Vis. Sci.* 19:1268–1273.

86. Tilders, F., and P. Smelik. 1975. A diurnal rhythm in melanocyte-stimulating hormone content of the rat pituitary gland and its independence from the pineal gland. *Neuroendocrinology* 17:296–308.

87. Underwood, H. 1985. Pineal melatonin rhythms in the lizard *Anolis carolinensis*: Effects of light and temperature cycles. *J. Comp. Physiol.* 157:57–65.

88. Underwood, H., S. Binkley, T. Siopes, and K. Mosher. 1984. Melatonin rhythms in the eyes, pineal bodies, and blood of Japanese quail. *Gen. Comp. Endocrinol.* 56:70–81.

89. Vaněček, J., L. Jansky, H. Illnerová, and K. Hoffman. 1984. Pineal melatonin in hibernating and aroused golden hamsters. *Comp. Biochem. Physiol.* 77A:759–762.

90. ———. 1985. Arrest of the circadian pacemaker driving the pineal

melatonin rhythm in hibernating golden hamsters. *Comp. Biochem. Physiol.* 80A:21–23.

91. Vaughan, G., R. Becker, J. Allen, and M. Vaughan. 1979. Elevated blood pressure after pinealectomy in the rat. *J. Endocrinol. Invest.* 2:281–284.

92. Vivien-Roels, B., P. Pévet, M. Dubois, J. Arendt, and G. Brown. 1981. Immunohistochemical evidence for the presence of melatonin in the pineal gland, the retina, and the Harderian gland. *Cell Tiss. Res.* 217:105–115.

93. Vriend, J. 1983. Pineal-thyroid interactions. In *Pineal research reviews I*, ed. R. Reiter, pp. 183–206. New York: Alan R. Liss.

94. Weatherhead, B., and A. Logan. 1981. Interaction of α-melanocyte-stimulating hormone, cyclic AMP and cyclic GMP in the control of melanogenesis in hair follicle melanocytes in vitro. *J. Endocrinol.* 90:89–96.

95. Weichmann, A., D. Bok, and J. Horwitz. 1985. Localization of HIOMT in the mammalian pineal gland and retina. *Invest. Ophthalmol. Vis. Sci.* 26:253–265.

96. White, B., K. Mosher, and S. Binkley. 1984. Daily profiles of N-acetyl-transferase measured at a single time in rat pineal glands, retinas, and Harderian glands. *J. Pineal Res.* 1:129–137.

97. Yu, H., S. Pang, and P. Tang. 1981. Increase in the level of retinal melatonin and persistence of its diurnal rhythm in rats afer pinealectomy. *J. Endocrinol.* 91:477–481.

98. Zucker, I. 1985. Pineal gland influences period of circannual rhythms of ground squirrels. *Amer. J. Physiol.* 249:R111–115.

10

Pineal Hormone Secretion and Action

"Administration of melatonin can prevent the diurnal rhythm of serotonin concentration characteristic of the pineal organ. Whether or not such a change is induced depends upon the point of the photoperiod when the hormone is injected. This observation indicates that the action of melatonin is affected by the photic environment of the recipient."

V. M. Fiske and L. Huppert [15]

"In vitro studies of the skin-lightening activity of melatonin and related indoleamines were conducted on the frog, *Rana pipiens*. . . . indoleamines found to possess skin-lightening activity were ranked in approximate order of potency relative to melatonin, the most potent of the compounds studied. . . . the intrinsic activity of indolic compounds on the melatonin receptor is determined primarily by the moiety substituted on the 5th carbon atom, whereas, the affinity for the receptor binding site is determined primarily by the moiety substituted on the 3rd carbon atom of the indole nucleus."

C. Heward and M. Hadley [23]

10.1 Introduction

Because pineal hormones appear to have endocrine roles, the classical endocrine approaches for determining secretion mechanisms, routes of transport, target organs, and mechanisms of action have been sought. In the classic view, an endocrine gland synthesizes one or more hormones, usually as a consequence of some form of signal. The hormone may be stored, in which case the chemical form of hormone storage, the location of storage, and the mechanisms for placing the hormone in storage and recovering it for secretion are subjects of interest. The classical hormone is secreted into the bloodstream where it may be transported in dissolved form or where it may form an association with a more or less specific carrier molecule. Cells that selectively take up the hormone from the blood are potential "targets" upon which the hormone may act; however, cells may take up the hormone in order to excrete the hormone or for as yet undiscovered reasons. Studies of the binding distribution of radiolabeled hormone are useful in surveying potential sites of hormone action. The fundamental chemical manner in which a hormone achieves its effects upon target cells is the "mechanism of action"; most hormones use one of two types of mechanisms of action: (1) the mechanism typified by steroid hormones in which the hormone penetrates the target cell and stimulates synthesis of proteins characteristic of the target cells' functions, and (2) the mechanism typified by amine and protein hormones in which the hormone binds to receptor sites on the cell membrane and initiates a cascade of reactions through a second messenger molecule, such as cyclic AMP.

10.2 Hormone Secretion

It should be remembered that melatonin may not be the only hormone of the pineal gland; however, most investigators of the subject of secretion have focussed on secretion of melatonin. The pineal appears to secrete melatonin into the blood soon upon production; that is, melatonin is not stored for a long time by the pineal. The half-life of melatonin in the blood is short (less than an hour). There is evidence that melatonin may be secreted in a pulsatile fashion [32].

The blood is not the only conceivable recipient of pineal melatonin. There is a considerable rhythm of melatonin in the cerebrospinal fluid (CSF); as was pointed out in Chapter 3, the pineal is anatomically close to the cerebral spaces, so that investigators must consider how melatonin reaches the CSF.

10.2.1 Melatonin transport

Melatonin is present in plasma, urine, and cerebrospinal fluid (CSF) and is elevated in the dark-time as in the pineal gland. The simple conclusion is that the pineal gland secretes melatonin. Lynch [26] enumerated three potential routes for melatonin secretion based on the anatomy of the pineal: (1) into the subarachnoid space surrounding the pineal, (2) into ventricular CSF, and (3) into the blood via the pineal vessels.

10.2.2 Secretion and cytology

The secretory mechanisms of pinealocytes has been examined cytologically [11]. There may be two secretory modes, one for proteins and another for indoleamines.

Dense core vesicles In the mechanism proposed by Collin and Oksche [11] for protein secretion, amino acids are taken up by pineal cells. Proteins are synthesized on ribosomes and sequestered in the cisternal spaces of the rough endoplasmic reticulum. The proteins are concentrated in the Golgi complex and are stored in dense core vesicles (DCV) which have "three components: (1) a more or less conspicuous dense core, (2) a clear halo surrounding the fine granular core, and (3) a limiting membrane." Collin and Oksche suggest that the DCV migrate so that they end up in the cell processes near the perivascular space (with the synaptic ribbons and synaptic vesicles). The investigators propose a diffusion mechanism for secretion of the contents of the vesicles (molecular dispersion) but do not exclude an exocytotic process.

Indoleamines Indoleamine synthesis and secretion, as expected, involves a different mechanism [11]: The pineal cells take up tryptophan from the blood, and mitochondrial enzymes convert the amino acid to 5-HT (serotonin). The serotonin produced could have several fates: (1) uptake by dense core vesicles, (2) storage in cytosol of pinealocytes, (3) metabolism to form melatonin, and/or (4) metabolism by MAO to produce 5-hydroxyindole acetic acid (5-HIAA).

Lamellae, vacuoles, and concretions A secretory role for the concentric lamellae (membrane-whorls) associated with pinealocytes has been considered [34]. One reason is that there is variability in the whorls that is apparently associated with physiological differences. For example, the concentric lamellae are abundant in nocturnal animals, infertile diabetic mutant mice, and blind hamsters. The structures are also in high numbers during the season of reproductive decline in hedgehogs and during reproductive quiescence in dormice, and in blind hamsters. A sequential transformation from (1) vacuoles containing flocculent material to (2) a reticular structure (membranous lamellae with many vacuoles and flocculent material) to

(3) a lamellar whorl is suggested to be correlated with pineal antigonadotrophic activity.

Vacuolated pinealocytes (the vacuoles seem to originate from granular endoplasmic reticulum cisterns) appear in some species. They increase with age and their formation is prevented by superior cervical ganglionectomy. Moreover, the appearance of vacuoles is accompanied by an increase in calcareous concretions. Thus the possibility that concretion formation reflects pineal secretory activity has been put forward [34, 54].

Lipid droplets Lipid droplet numbers change in pineal cells with light and reproductive status. The droplets increase after injection of gonadotrophins or after male castration and decrease after hypophysectomy. Since melatonin is lipid soluble, the possibility that lipid droplets are involved in the pineal secretory process has been raised [34].

10.2.3 Melatonin in blood

Circulating melatonin levels are subject to a number of possible influences that affect half-life of the indoleamine.

TABLE 10.1 Melatonin in blood (pg/ml serum or plasma)

Class	Species	Day	Night
Birds	Chick	50	200
	Quail	10	400
	Sparrow	94	840
	Pigeon	20	858
Mammals	Rhesus monkey	32	88
	Rat	6	75
	Calf	19	200
	Sheep	10	240
	Human	23	97
	Donkey	24	108
	Pig	22	76
	Camel	29	221
Reptiles	Sea turtle	60	143
	Tortoise	20	180
	Scincid lizard	35	240
Amphibians	Tiger salamander	174	249
Fish	Trout	264	596

Sources: References are listed in Binkley [3] with added data for pigeons from Voisin et al. [51]; quail, Underwood et al. [46]; *Anolis*, Underwood [45]; rhesus monkeys, Brainard, Asch, and Reiter [6]; sparrows, Klein, Binkley, and Mosher [unpublished]; and tortoises, Vivien-Roels and Arendt [50].

TABLE 10.2 Estimated half-life of melatonin in serum or plasma

Species	Melatonin half-life (minutes)
Human	50
Rhesus monkey	30
Sheep	30
Rat	17–20
Mouse	2–35
Hamster	10

Sources: Data from Waldhauser et al. [53]; Reppert et al. [39]; Kennaway and Seamark [24]; Gibbs and Vriend [18]; Kopin et al. [25]; and Rollag and Stetson [41].

Amount and transport Levels of blood melatonin have been measured in many species in relation to time of day (Table 10.1). The low solubility of melatonin has implications for its transport in blood; in order to permit blood to carry more melatonin than can be dissolved, melatonin may be bound to plasma albumin [8, 26].

As Vollrath [52] points out, the "alleged mophological correlates of the secretory products are predominantly located in club-shaped endings of pinealocyte processes often lying in the immediate vicinity of blood vessels." The high rate of blood flow through the pineal (less than the kidney, the same as the pituitary, and more than most endocrine glands) supports secretion of products into the circulation [20]. The times of melatonin appearance in the various fluid compartments (measuring endogenous or radiolabeled melatonin) support secretion into the blood as a primary route [26].

Half-life The half-life (Table 10.2) of melatonin in the circulation has been estimated by examining radiolabeled or unlabeled melatonin introduced orally or by injection [25]. For example, humans were given crystalline melatonin (80 mg in a gelatin capsule) 4 hours after lights-on [52]. Serum melatonin rose from less than 100 pg/ml to over 100,000 pg/ml with peak values 60–150 minutes after the dose was administered. The high levels can be interpreted to mean that the carrying capacity for melatonin in the circulation is not a limiting factor that determines blood melatonin under normal conditions. Urine melatonin likewise shot up from less than 10 ng/hr to 60,000 ng/hr in the 4 hours following the melatonin ingestion. The urine melatonin correlated with the blood melatonin (r = correlation coefficient = 0.94). Melatonin in humans, and in some other species, has a biphasic disappearance: there is an initial very short half-life (e.g., 2 minutes during the first 10 minutes) where melatonin disappears rapidly; this phase is followed by a phase where the half-life is longer (e.g., 35 minutes).

The finding that melatonin has a short half-life is supported by the close correlation of the amounts of circulating melatonin with the amounts of pineal melatonin and the activity of N-acetyltransferase (NAT). That is, when NAT drops (at the end of the subjective night or when the lights are turned on), so does pineal and blood melatonin. Similarly, when melatonin was infused rhythmically into rats, its appearance in the urine was coincident with the times it was infused [27].

How is melatonin removed from an organism? The answer appears to be that it is excreted and that it may first be converted to other forms. The mechanism that has been proposed bears similarities to that for elimination of steroid hormones. In mice, melatonin was metabolized [27], probably by liver and kidney, by 6-hydroxylation followed by conjugation (e.g., with sulfate). Melatonin hydroxylating activity was found in liver microsomes.

10.2.4 Melatonin in cerebrospinal fluid

Melatonin rhythms have been measured in the CSF of a number of species [22, 26, 31, 35, 40]. As expected, melatonin was usually higher in the night than the daytime (Fig. 10.1; Table 10.3). The presence of a melatonin rhythm in CSF is intriguing because of the possibility that the brain (hypothalamus) is a melatonin target and the CSF could provide a direct route for bathing neural structures in pineal secretions. The anatomical relationship of the pineal to the CSF varies from

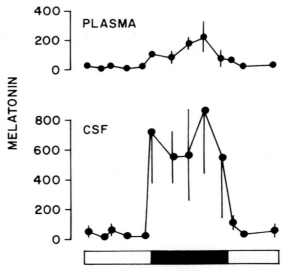

Figure 10.1 Melatonin profiles measured in blood (plasma) and cerebrospinal fluid (CSF) in 6- to 9-month-old Guernsey calves kept in LD 14:10. (After data in Hedlund et al. [22].)

TABLE 10.3 Melatonin in cerebrospinal fluid (pg/ml)

Species	Day	Night
Humans	29–118	—
Rhesus Monkey	2–10	9–50
Cat	5–15	50–80
Rat	14–20	33
Cattle	10–100	540–880
Sheep	10–100	10–300

Sources: Data from Reppert, Perlow, and Klein [38]; Reppert et al. [37]; and Withya-chumnarnkul and Knigge [55].

minimal contact in the area of the third ventricle between the habenular and posterior commissures to arrangements (such as in humans) where the pineal is "bathed in CSF" [52].

Transplanting the pineal to the anterior chamber of the eye did not change brain-serum melatonin ratios, which the investigators argue was evidence that melatonin was not secreted directly into the CSF from the pineal [31]. Moreover, in sheep, the rate of melatonin secretion into the circulation was 2–18 µg/min while the apparent rate of secretion into the CSF was less, 0.2–12 ng/min [40]. The estimated melatonin production was 1.5–5.0 mg/14-hr night (40–50 kg sheep) [40].

The possibility that the pineal is taking something out of (rather than secreting something into) the CSF deserves consideration. When substances (bromophenol blue; 3,6-diamino-acridinetrihydrochloride; fluorescein-labeled bovine serum proteins; radiolabeled phenylalanine) were injected into cerebral ventricles, they penetrated the pineal in as little as 1.5 minutes [52].

10.2.5 Melatonin in superfusion

Single pineals (from chicks, sparrows, starlings, and lizards) can be isolated in culture systems and continually supplied with fresh medium in a "flow-through" manner. Aliquots of the medium examined at successive time intervals exhibit circadian rhythms of melatonin (Fig. 10.2; Table 10.4). Thus, whatever the "secretion" process may be in pineals, it continues under in vitro conditions [2, 29, 42, 43, 44].

10.3 Target Tissues and Cells

In seeking targets for pineal hormones (mainly melatonin), five experimental directions have been pursued.

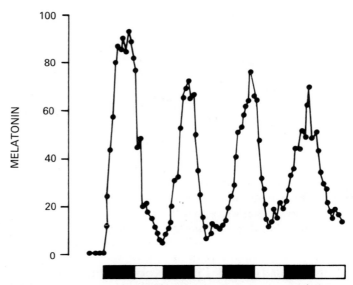

Figure 10.2 Melatonin measured from a single chick pineal gland in superfusion culture. The culture was in the LD 12:12 regimen illustrated by the bar below the record. (Unpublished data collected by Binkley, Muller, and Tamarkin replicating results obtained by Takahashi, Hamm, and Menaker [43].)

First, the binding of melatonin was studied by determining the distribution of radiolabeled melatonin in the body [56]. The pineal, eye, ovary, and sympathetic chain (in that order) accumulated the most 3H-melatonin when it was injected intravenously into cats and measured in tissues 1 hour later.

Second, if a function is affected by the pineal and/or melatonin, then some structure related to the carrying out of that function is a likely target; this is circumstantial evidence that a structure is a target of pineal hormones.

TABLE 10.4 Melatonin (ng/ml) in 60- or 90-minute samples of perfusate from single pineal glands

| Species | First cycle | | Second cycle | |
	Nadir	Peak	Nadir	Peak
Chicken	2	28	3	15
Chicken	10	170	20	200
Starling	2^{-3}	20^{-3}	2^{-3}	12^{-3}
Sparrow	0.5^{-3}	8^{-3}	5^{-3}	2.5^{-3}
Lizard	0.08^{-3}	1.5^{-3}	0.05^{-3}	0.7^{-3}

Sources: Data from Menaker and Wisner [29]; Takahashi [42]; and Binkley [2].

Third, several attempts have been made to locate melatonin "receptors" (molecules that bind melatonin specifically).

Fourth, in assuring that a potential target is not being affected indirectly, in vitro experiments that correlate with in vivo results provide direct evidence that a potential target responds to pineal extracts or hormones.

Fifth, responses to localized small melatonin implants have been used in seeking targets.

10.3.1 Pineal

The evidence for pineal effects on the pineal itself is indirect from in vivo studies. Pineal glands bind more 3H-melatonin than any other tissue; this could be evidence that the pineal can sequester melatonin. Moreover, administration of melatonin and pineal extracts affects pineal morphology. Variable effects or no effects at all have been reported for melatonin on parameters of melatonin biosynthesis—serotonin, NAT, or HIOMT [52]. Pavel [33] showed that melatonin raised cat CSF arginine vasotocin (AVT). When Fiske and Huppert [15] measured the effects of timed melatonin injections on pineal serotonin in rats, they found that melatonin injections at 8 hours of light reduced the light-dark serotonin by 43 ng/gland; melatonin injections after 14 hours of light did not reduce the light-dark serotonin difference).

10.3.2 Brain

The brain is the principal candidate for a target of the pineal because of the global nature of pineal or melatonin effects on behavior, circadian rhythms, sleep, convulsions, Purkinje cells, thermoregulation, and endocrine functions.

Evidence for the brain as a target is partially indirect from in vivo studies. The brain did not take up much tritiated melatonin; however, that does not preclude the possibility that small numbers of specialized cells in the brain are melatonin targets or the possibility that melatonin exerts action on brain cells without being sequestered by them. The hypothalamus is a prime candidate for a site of pineal hormone action because many of the potential endocrine targets are under hypothalamic control (pituitary, gonads, thyroid, adrenal, chromatophores). Melatonin can be found in the hypothalamus. Melatonin administration changed many hypothalamic parameters: it increased serotonin, increased GABA, decreased protein synthesis, decreased microtubule protein, increased or decreased δ-4-reductase activity, decreased MAO activity, increased number of LRH immunoreactive cells, increased cGMP, increased guanylate cyclase activity, and decreased cAMP [47, 49, 52]. Pinealectomy altered the hypothalamus:

it increased protein synthesis, increased MAO activity, decreased 5-HT uptake by synaptosomes, and altered nuclear diameters in supraoptic and paraventricular nuclei. If the hypothalamus is a target on which the pineal exerts its endocrine effects, the expectation would be for substantive changes in the time profiles of hypothalamic release and inhibiting hormones after pinealectomy or melatonin administration. A few investigators have looked at the hypothalamic hormones and found changes in LRH (luteinizing hormone releasing hormone), PIH (prolactin release inhibiting hormone), PRH (prolactin releasing hormone), and FSH-RH (follicle stimulating hormone releasing hormone) [52] after pineal related manipulations.

More direct evidence for target sites within the brain is from studies of mice. The brain loci of melatonin action were investigated in female white-footed mice [19] by implanting melatonin in various brain regions and measuring reproductive tract weight, vaginal perforation, and ovarian follicles after 7 weeks. Implants that released 45 ng/day caused gonad regression when they were placed in the medial preoptic and supra- and retrochiasmatic areas of the hypothalamus.

Direct evidence that melatonin can affect the hypothalamus comes from studies of rat hypothalamic tissue sections in vitro [57]. The sections were incubated in radiolabeled dopamine; electrical stimulation of the sections released 8–12% of the labeled dopamine; melatonin inhibited dopamine release (30%) from hypothalami obtained in the early light-time, but melatonin had minimal effect (1%) on hypothalami obtained at lights-out. The data constitute evidence that there is a daily cycle in hypothalamic sensitivity to melatonin which develops in the first week of life.

10.3.3 Pituitary

The pituitary was fourth on the list of tissues that acquire 3H-melatonin. The pituitary is a candidate for a pineal target because of pineal functions in the endocrine system, especially the regulation of the gonads and also the thyroid and adrenals. The neonatal rat pituitary responds to melatonin in vitro where melatonin inhibits LH release by LRH [28]. Incubation of pituitaries with pineal fragments or extracts blocks FSH release [52].

Pineal extracts or melatonin affect the pituitary: they increase the number of eosinophilic cells, increase thyrotroph (cells that produce TSH) activity, decrease protein synthesis, decrease MAO activity, increase leucine incorporation, increase thymidine incorporation, affect prolactin, affect LH, decrease MSH, and sometimes affect FSH. Melatonin increases serotonin levels in the pars intermedia. Pinealectomy may increase acidophils, decrease chromophobes, increase mitotic rate, increase MAO activity, increase estradiol uptake, increase MSH, and alter the appearance of gonadotropic cells.

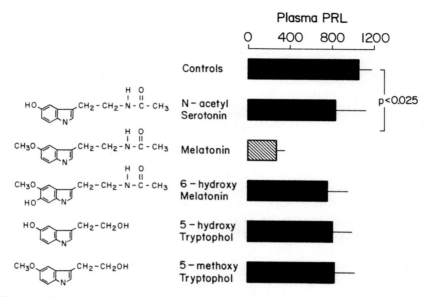

Figure 10.3 Melatonin was more effective than other indoles in suppressing plasma prolactin in adult male Syrian hamsters. (With permission from Vaughan et al. [48].)

Direct evidence that the pituitary is a pineal target is the finding that when rat hemipituitaries are incubated in vitro, prolactin release is elevated 285% when bovine pineal extract is present in the medium [4, 5]. When pituitaries are incubated in vitro with pineal fragments or extracts, FSH release is reduced [13, 30]. Effects on prolactin by melatonin in vitro is corroborated by in vivo findings: in the male hamster, melatonin injections (25 µg/day, 10 weeks, late afternoon) caused a decrease in pituitary and plasma prolactin (Fig. 10.3) as well as gonadal regression [48].

10.3.4 Gonads

When the striking melatonin uptake by ovaries is considered together with pineal function in reproduction, the gonads appear to be candidates for pineal targets. In one study of the effects of melatonin on rat ovarian granulosa cells in vitro, melatonin increased the levels of some estrogens by 40% [16]. Rat seminiferous tubules can be dissected from the testes and placed on a glass slide. Contractions of the tubule wall are measured by depression of the tubular diameter. When the rats were pretreated with daily 1 mg melatonin injections, the contractility of their seminiferous tubules was reduced—the diameter increased from 347 µm to 366 µm. Whether the effect by melatonin on the testes was direct or indirect has yet to be determined [14].

10.3.5 Endocrine glands

Evidence that other endocrine cells—those of the adrenal, thyroid, parathyroid, and islets of Langerhans—are pineal targets is indirect; but the possibility that they are pineal targets is supported by the fact that the pineal and/or its hormones has been linked to the functioning of these glands.

10.3.6 Retina

Evidence that melatonin produced in the retina has the retina as a target is as yet a matter of conjecture based on the finding of rhythmic retinal melatonin production via rhythmic NAT activity. The cat iris-choroid was second only to the pineal in 3H-melatonin uptake.

TABLE 10.5 Compounds that affected frog skin lightening in vitro ranked in order of potency (*top to bottom*)

Lightened

Melatonin
6-Hydroxymelatonin
6-Methoxyharmalan
5-Methoxytryptamine
5-Methoxyindole-3-acetic acid
5-Methoxy-D,L-tryptophan
N-Acetylserotonin
5-Methoxy-N,N-dimethyltryptamine
5-Methoxyindole

No Lightening

N-acetyltryptamine
Harmine
Tryptamine
5-Hydroxyindole-3-acetic acid
Indole-3-acetic acid
Serotonin
6-Methoxyindole

Melatonin Blockers

N-acetyltryptamine
N-acetylserotonin

Source: Heward and Hadley [23].

10.3.7 Chromatophores

The skins of some lower vertebrates (e.g., *Rana pipiens*) pale in color in response to melatonin. In the usual test, the skins are first darkened with α-MSH (which disperses melanosomes in dermal melanophores and aggregates reflecting crystals in iridophores to decrease reflectance) for 30 minutes followed by exposure by melatonin (which partially relightens the skin by aggregation of melanosomes in the melanophores). In one study [23], skin was exposed to a variety of melatonin-like compounds. As little as 5×10^{-11} M melatonin lightened the skin. Other compounds were ranked by potency or by whether they blocked the skin-lightening response (Table 10.5). Hypotheses about the nature of a possible binding site were made by examining the structures of the molecules (Fig. 10.4).

10.3.8 Toad bladder

Toad bladders can be isolated in vitro by attaching them as sacs to tubing, filling them with a Ringer's solution, and suspending them in water. When arginine vasopressin (antidiuretic hormone) is added to the bathing solution, the bladders lose water and weigh 33% less at the end of 60 minutes. When melatonin is also added to the bathing water (4.3×10^{-6} M), the weight loss is only 20% [21].

10.4 Mechanism of Action

As discussed in the introduction, most hormones produce their effects on cells via one of two mechanisms of action involving protein receptors located either in cell membranes or in the cytoplasm of target cells. There have been some attempts to find evidence for melatonin effects on potential targets by these mechanisms; there is also work on the possibility that nontraditional mechanisms of action are used by melatonin. The possibility of multiple mechanisms of action has not been excluded.

10.4.1 Protein receptors in the plasma membrane

The first type of mechanism of action is common for peptide or amine hormones. In this mechanism the hormone (the first messenger) interacts with a protein of the cell membrane of a target cell—the hormone does not penetrate the cell. In turn, the information from the receptor is transduced into activation of a membrane enzyme such as adenyl cyclase. The adenyl cyclase catalyzes the production of cAMP (cyclic adenylic acid, the second messenger) from ATP (adenosine triphosphate). The cAMP, in turn, releases the catalytic enzymic subunit; the active enzyme in turn activates yet another enzyme; and so on, until the final action of the particular cell containing the hormone receptor is accomplished (a cascade of reactions that "amplifies" the original hormone signal since increasing numbers of molecules result at each step). The cAMP is removed by breakdown to 5'-AMP by another enzyme, phosphodiesterase, which is inside the cell. In an alternate mechanism, cGMP acts as the second messenger and the enzyme is guanylate cyclase.

Membrane receptors for melatonin were sought in beef brain [9]. Using a rapid filtration technique, the investigators found melatonin binding to membranes of medial basal hypothalamus. Less binding was found in the occipital and cerebellar cortices (34–73% of that in hypothalamus). Binding was located in the 27,000-g pellet; binding site concentration was estimated at 8–14 fmol/mg protein.

For the second messenger mode of action, the hormone should alter cyclic nucleotides in the target. In 10 minutes, melatonin (10^{-8} M) increased cGMP (from 0.226 to 0.342 pmol/mg protein) and decreased cAMP (from 119 to 68 pmol/mg protein) in rat medial basal hypothalamus in vitro. Melatonin increased guanylate cyclase in homogenates of rat anterior pituitary, thyroid, testis, ovary, liver, and small intestine [49].

A model has been proposed for melatonin action on melanophores in pieces of frog skin whose melanophores were dispersed with MSH which involves melatonin [23]. The investigators studied a variety of analogs and came up with the proposition that the methoxy group of melatonin was required for melanosome aggregation and the N-acetyl group was required for binding of melatonin to the receptor. They defined a melatonin receptor pharmacologically by potency (melatonin > 5-methyoxytryptamine > 5-methoxyindole > serotonin) and by susceptibility to specific blockade by N-acetyltryptamine.

10.4.2 Protein receptors in the cytoplasm

The second mechanism is common for steroid hormones. In this mechanism, the hormone penetrates the cell and is recognized by interaction with a protein receptor that is in the cytoplasm. The interaction results in a change in molecular shape (a conformational change called transformation) and in movement of the molecule (translocation) to the nucleus. There the hormone receptor complex causes production of messenger RNA, which exits the nucleus and causes the cell to produce protein characteristic of the cell.

Evidence for a cytoplasmic receptor for melatonin was sought in ovaries of hamsters, rats, and humans [10]. Specific binding of 3H-melatonin (based on the difference in 3H-melatonin bound to protein of ovary homogenates in the presence and absence of excess melatonin) was found in a fraction of the supernatant (105,000–g). Binding was also noted in the testis, uterus, skin, and liver of rodents. The

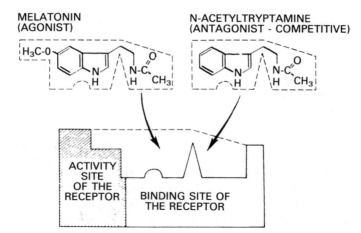

MELATONIN RECEPTOR

Figure 10.4 A diagrammatic conceptualization of the melatonin receptor in chromatophores. The diagram is based on binding studies with a series of analogs. (Redrawn from Heward and Hadley [23].)

authors estimated the number of binding sites in hamster ovaries (250–656 fmol/mg protein) and rat uteri (156–1004 fmol/mg protein). The results are evidence for direct action of melatonin on reproductive targets. There is also evidence that melatonin affects cytoplasmic estrogen receptors in immature hamster uterus in vitro [12]: melatonin increased the unoccupied estrogen receptor activity 83% (from 41.3 to 75.4 fmol/mg protein).

10.4.3 Other possibilities

It is also possible that melatonin acts by yet some other mechanism. For example, Cardinali [7] discusses a "microtubule hypothesis of melatonin action": melatonin "binds to the protein tubulin at the colchicine binding site and thereby prevents the assembly of the 6S tubulin dimer into microtubules." Tubulin is a protein subunit that polymerizes to form microtubules. Microtubules are organelles found in the cytoplasm which play roles in mitosis, cell motility, cell shape, and intracellular transport. Tubulin is ubiquitous in cells but is especially high in the brain where it is believed to be involved in neuroendocrine hormone secretion and axonal transport. Colchicine is one of many drugs that disrupt microtubules. There are a number of pineal- and/or melatonin-related effects that also involve microtubules.

First, melanosome movements are influenced by melatonin in the blanching response and are believed to involve microtubules and microfilaments. Second, retinas, depending on species, exhibit pigment migration and cell elongation which also involve microtubules and microfilaments. Third, mitosis is another process that involves microtubules and microfilaments. Melatonin caused mitotic arrest in onion root [1] and delayed oral band development in a ciliate, *Stentor*; neither effect was obtained with N-acetylserotonin (NAS) or 5-HT. Melatonin (10^{-4} M) reduced the mitotic index that was produced with colchicine in HeLa cells [17]. However, the in vitro assembly of brain microtubules, the inhibition of colchicine binding in purified tubulin, mitoses of Chinese hamster ovary cells, and neurite formation of neuroblastoma cells in culture were unaffected by melatonin [36]. Fourth, pinealectomy or ganglionectomy reduced hypothalamic tubulin in rats [7]. Injecting rats with melatonin (100 μg, two times a day, 10 days) reduced tubulin in the hypothalamus. Fifth, melatonin reduced axonal transport in rabbit optic tracts and nerves, rat sciatic nerves, and frog sciatic nerves [7]. Even if microtubules are affected by the pineal, the effects could be indirect.

REFERENCES

1. Banerjee, S., and L. Margulis. 1973. Mitotic arrest by melatonin. *Exp. Cell Res.* 78:314–318.

2. Binkley, S. 1980. Functions of the pineal gland. In *Avian endocrinology*, ed. A. Epple and M. Stetson, pp. 53–74. New York: Academic Press.

3. ———. 1981. Pineal biochemistry: Comparative aspects and circadian rhythms. In *The pineal gland I: Anatomy and biochemistry*, ed. R. Reiter, pp. 155–172. Boca Raton, Fl.: CRC Press.

4. Blask, D., and G. Vaughan. 1976. PRF and PIF activity in the bovine, rat and human pineal gland. *Anat. Rec.* 184:361.

5. Blask, D., M. Vaughan, R. Reiter, L. Johnson, and G. Vaughan. 1976. Prolactin-releasing and release-inhibiting factor activities in bovine, rat, and human pineal gland: In vitro and in vivo studies. *Endocrinology* 99:152–162.

6. Brainard, G., R. Asch, and R. Reiter. 1981. Circadian rhythms of serum melatonin and prolactin in the rhesus monkey. *Biomed. Res.* 3:291–297.

7. Cardinali, D. 1980. Molecular biology of melatonin: Assessment of the "microtubule hypothesis of melatonin action." In *Melatonin: Current status and perspectives*, ed. N. Birau and W. Schloot, pp. 247–256. Advances in the Biosciences 29. Oxford: Pergamon Press.

8. Cardinali, D., H. Lynch, and R. Wurtman. 1972. Binding of melatonin to human and rat plasma proteins. *Endocrinology* 91:1213–1218.

9. Cardinali, D., M. Vacas, and E. Boyer. 1979. Specific binding of melatonin in bovine brain. *Endocrinology* 105:437–441.

10. Cohen, M., D. Roselle, and B. Chabner. 1978. Evidence for a cytoplasmic melatonin receptor. *Nature* 247:894–895.

11. Collin, J., and A. Oksche. 1981. Structural and functional relationships in the nonmammalian pineal gland. In *The Pineal gland I: Anatomy and biochemistry*, ed. R. Reiter, pp. 27–67. Boca Raton, Fl.: CRC Press.

12. Danforth, D., L. Tamarkin, R. Do, and M. Lippman. 1983. Melatonin-induced increase in cytoplasmic estrogen receptor activity in hamster uteri. *Endocrinology* 113:81–85.

13. Ebels, L., A. Moszkowska, and A. Scemana. 1965. Étude in vitro des extraits épiphysaires fractionnés. Résultats préliminaires. *C.R. Acad. Sci.* (Paris) 260:5126–5129.

14. Ellis, L., and L. Buhrley. 1978. Inhibitory effects of melatonin, prostaglandin E_1, cyclic AMP, dibutyryl cyclic AMP and theophylline on rat seminiferous tubular contractility in vitro. *Biol. Reprod.* 19:217–222.

15. Fiske, V., and L. Huppert. 1968. Melatonin action on pineal varies with photoperiod. *Science* 162:279.

16. Fiske, V., K. Parker, R. Ulmer, C. Ow, and N. Aziz. 1984. Effect of melatonin alone or in combination with HCG or ovine LH on the in vitro secretion of estrogens or progesterone by granulosa cells of rats. *Endocrinology* 114:407–410.

17. Fitzgerald, T., and A. Veal. 1976. Melatonin antagonizes colchicine-induced mitotic arrest. *Experientia* 32:372–373.

18. Gibbs, F., and J. Vriend. 1981. The half-life of melatonin elimination from rat plasma. *Endocrinology* 109:1796–1798.

19. Glass, J., and G. Lynch. 1981. Melatonin: Identification of sites of antigonadal action in mouse brain. *Science* 214:821–823.

20. Goldman, H., and R. Wurtman. 1964. Flow of blood to the pineal body of the rat. *Nature* 203:87.

21. Haswell, M., W. Gern, and C. Ralph. 1980. Melatonin inhibition of vasopressin-stimulated water transport in the toad urinary bladder. *J. Exp. Zool.* 211:407–409.

22. Hedlund, L., M. Lischko, M. Rollag, and G. Niswender. 1977. Melatonin: Daily cycle in plasma and cerebrospinal fluid of calves. *Science* 195:686–688.

23. Heward, C., and M. Hadley. 1978. Structure-activity relationships of melatonin and related indoleamines. *Life. Sci.* 17:1167–1178.

24. Kennaway, D., and R. Seamark. 1980. Circulating levels of melatonin following its oral administration or subcutaneous injection in sheep and goats. *Aust. J. Biol. Sci.* 33:349–353.

25. Kopin, I., C. Pare, J. Axelrod, and H. Weissbach. 1961. The fate of melatonin in animals. *J. Biol. Chem.* 236:3072–3075.

26. Lynch, H. 1983. Assay methodology. In *The Pineal Gland*, ed. R. Relkin, pp. 129–150. New York: Elsevier.

27. Lynch, H., R. Rivest, and R. Wurtman. 1980. Artificial induction of melatonin rhythms by programmed microinfusion. *Neuroendocrinology* 31:106–111.

28. Martin, J., and D. Klein. 1976. Melatonin inhibition of the neonatal pituitary response to luteinizing hormone-releasing factor. *Science* 191:301–302.

29. Menaker, M., and S. Wisner. 1983. Temperature-compensated circadian clock in the pineal of *Anolis*. *Proc. Natl. Acad. Sci. USA* 80:6119–6121.

30. Moszkowska, A. 1967. Étude des extraits épiphysaires fractionnés. *Physiologie Biol. Med.* 56:403–412.

31. Pang, S., and C. Ralph. 1975. Mode of secretion of pineal melatonin in the chicken. *Gen. Comp. Endocrinol.* 27:125–128.

32. Pang, S. 1986. Personal communication.

33. Pavel, S. 1973. Arginine vasotocin release into cerebrospinal fluid of cats induced by melatonin. *Nature (New Biol.)* 246:183–184.

34. Pévet, P. 1981. Ultrastructure of the mammalian pinealocyte. In *The pineal gland I: Anatomy and biochemistry*, ed. R. Reiter, pp. 121–154. Boca Raton, Fl.: CRC Press.

35. Poffenbarger, M., and G. Fuller. 1976. Is melatonin a microtubule inhibitor? *Exp. Cell Res.* 103:135–141.

36. Ralph, C. 1976. Correlations of melatonin content in pineal gland, blood and brain of some birds and mammals. *Amer. Zool.* 16:35–43.

37. Reppert, S., R. Coleman, H. Heath, and H. Keutmann. 1982. Circadian properties of vasopressin and melatonin rhythms in cat cerebrospinal fluid. *Amer. J. Physiol.* 243:E489–E498.

38. Reppert, S., M. Perlow, and D. Klein. 1980. Cerebrospinal fluid melatonin. In *Neurobiology of cerebrospinal fluid*, ed. J. H. Wood, pp. 579–589. New York: Plenum.

39. Reppert, S., M. Perlow, L. Tamarkin, and D. Klein. 1979. A diurnal melatonin rhythm in primate cerebrospinal fluid. *Endocrinology* 104:295–301.

40. Rollag, M., R. Morgan, and G. Niswender. 1978. Route of melatonin secretion in sheep. *Endocrinology* 102:1–7.

41. Rollag, M., and M. Stetson. 1982. Melatonin injection into Syrian hamsters. *Prog. Clin. Biol. Res.* 92:143–152.

42. Takahashi, J. 1981. Neural and endocrine regulation of avian circadian systems. Ph.D. diss., Univ. of Oregon.

43. Takahashi, J., H. Hamm, and M. Menaker. 1980. Circadian rhythms of melatonin release from individual superfused chicken pineal glands in vitro. *Proc. Nat. Acad. Sci. USA* 77:2319–2322.

44. Takahashi, J., and M. Menaker. 1984. Multiple redundant circadian oscillators within the isolated avian pineal gland. *J. Comp. Physiol. A* 154:435–440.

45. Underwood, H. 1985. Pineal melatonin rhythms in the lizard *Anolis carolinensis*: Effects of light and temperature cycles. *J. Comp. Physiol.* 157:57–65.

46. Underwood, H., S. Binkley, T. Siopes, and K. Mosher. 1984. Melatonin rhythms in the eyes, pineal bodies, and blood of Japanese quail. *Gen. Comp. Endocrinol.* 56:70–81.

47. Vacas, M., M. Sarmiento, and D. Cardinali. 1981. Melatonin increases cGMP and decreases cAMP levels in rat medial basal hypothalamus in vitro. *Brain Res.* 225:207–211.

48. Vaughan, M., A. Holtorf, J. Little, T. Champney, and R. Reiter. 1985. A survey of pineal indoles and analogues which affect prolactin secretion in the adult male Syrian hamster. In *Prolactin: Basic and clinical correlates*, ed. R. MacLeod, M. Thorner, and V. Scapagnini, pp. 143–150. Fidia Research Series 1. Padova: Liviana Press.

49. Veseley, D. 1980. Melatonin enhances guanylate cyclase activity in a variety of tissues. *Mol. Cell. Biochem.* 35:55–58.

REFERENCES

50. Vivien-Roels, B., and J. Arendt. 1980. Relative roles of environmental factors, photoperiod and temperature in the control of serotonin and melatonin circadian variations in the pineal organ and plasma of the tortoise, *Testudo Hermanni Gmelin*. In *Melatonin: Current status and perspectives*, ed. N. Birau and W. Schloot, pp. 401–406. Advances in the Biosciences 29. Oxford: Pergamon Press.

51. Voisin, P., M. Geffard, M. Delaage, and J. Collin. 1982. Melatonine dans l'organe pineal, la rétine et le plasma. Étude immunologique chez le pigeon. *Reprod. Nutr. Develop.* 22:959–971.

52. Vollrath, L. 1984. *The pineal organ*. Berlin: Springer-Verlag.

53. Waldhauser, F., M. Waldhauser, H. Lieberman, M. Deng, H. Lynch, and R. Wurtman. 1984. Bioavailability of oral melatonin in humans. *Neuroendocrinology* 39:307–313.

54. Welsh, M., and R. Reiter. 1978. The pineal gland of the gerbil, *Meriones unguiculatus*, I: An ultrastructural study. *Cell. Tiss. Res.* 193:323–336.

55. Withyachumnarnkul, B., and K. Knigge. 1980. Melatonin concentrations in cerebrospinal fluid, peripheral plasma and plasma of the confluens sinuum of the rat. *Neuroendocrinology* 30:382–388.

56. Wurtman, J., J. Axelrod, and L. Potter. 1984. The uptake of ^{3}H-melatonin in endocrine and nervous tissues and the effects of constant light exposure. *J. Pharmacol. Exp. Ther.* 143:314–318.

57. Zisapel, N., Y. Egozi, and M. Laudon. 1985. Circadian variations in the inhibition by dopamine release from adult and newborn rat hypothalamus by melatonin. *Neuroendocrinology* 40:102–108.

11

Other Substances That May Be Important to the Pineal

"The pineal nonapeptide hormone arginine vasotocin (AVT) is synthesized by the ependymal cells of the pineal recess and subcommissural organ. . . . AVT is first released into the cerebrospinal fluid (CSF) and reaches the blood only secondarily after its absorption from CSF. It displays a diurnal rhythm in the pineal and CSF. . . . Melatonin represents its releasing hormone. . . . AVT activat(es) serotonin neurotransmission in the brain with resultant inhibition of release of hypothalamic . . . hormones and induction of sleep. . . . AVT is a CSF hormone whose . . . site of action is the brain itself."

S. Pavel [12]

"When we were going flat out in trying to isolate melatonin from pineal glands we were constantly aware of the possibility that the fractions we threw away might contain natural products that would be more useful in medical science than the agent that we wanted to purify. This possibility is a real one. . . .

At least three active peptides are present in the pineal. In addition to arginine vasotocin . . . and angiotensin I . . . there is a peptide . . . with melanotrophic and lipotrophic activities . . .

I have complete confidence in the view that new and interesting molecules of biologic value will be found in the pineal gland."

A. B. Lerner [11]

"It is manifestly evident after 2 decades of research that the nonapeptide AVT directly or indirectly affects the reproductive system of all classes of vertebrates. Although most investigators ostensibly agree that an antigonadotrophic peptide compound is found in the pineal of mammals, considerable controversy still resounds over whether it is AVT, AVP, oxytocin, E_5, and/or as yet another unidentified peptide."

M. K. Vaughan [23]

11.1 Introduction

Most pineal work has centered around the production of melatonin as a pineal hormone. Production of melatonin may not be the only function of the gland. There may be other pineal hormones, and there may be other substances in the pineal of particular importance but which are not themselves hormones. The purpose of this chapter is to mention some of these substances.

11.2 Arginine Vasotocin

Arginine vasotocin (AVT) is believed to be the primordial molecule for a family of nonapeptides (9 amino acids) synthesized in the hypothalamus and stored in the posterior pituitary gland. The basis for the belief that the molecule evolved early is its presence in vertebrates and the potential for its evolution to the other structurally related neurohypophyseal peptides (vasopressin, oxytocin, lysine vasotocin, etc.) by changes in amino acid sequence [7]. The substance has also been found in the pineal. Structurally related molecules (vasopressin, oxytocin, and lysine vasotocin) have also been studied and will be mentioned here with the consideration of AVT.

11.2.1 Presence of AVT in the pineal

AVT levels have been measured by bioassay and radioimmunoassay (RIA) techniques (Table 11.1). One bioassay uses the eel ventral aorta [27]. Contractions of isolated aorta are used to detect AVT. Other bioassays are the rat antidiuretic assay and the frog bladder hydroosmotic assay. Investigators have had mixed results in attempting to demonstrate AVT in the adult mammalian pineal gland but have found it in fetal pineals [3]. AVT has been claimed to be present in bovine, rat, human, and porcine pineals. In rats, 10–40 pg/gland was detected with bioassay; 200 pg/gland was detected with an RIA [12]. AVT and related peptides (arginine vasopressin and oxytocin) were measured in human pineal glands obtained at autopsy; AVT was

TABLE 11.1 Arginine vasotocin (AVT) in the pituitary and pineal of various species (ng/gland)

Species	Pituitary AVT			Pineal AVT		
	RIA1	**RIA2**	**Bioassay**	**RIA1**	**RIA2**	**Bioassay**
Lamprey	6	11	8	ND	24	11
Trout	1315	594	488	124	193	136
Frog	228	244	NM	324	556	492
Tortoise	1640	1148	1120	181	247	314
Lizard	171	188	165	210	416	383
Snake	713	680	613	245	353	328
Quail	12	17	16	44	94	119
Chicken	33	40	33	31	189	163

Sources: Data from Holder et al. [8] and Vivien-Roels et al. [26, 27].
Note: Bioassay = eel aorta bioassay; ND = nondetectable; NM = not measured.

detected in 70% of the glands (44 pg/gland) [6]. A difficulty in interpreting the work results from the fact that structurally related molecules are also detected in the assays.

According to Pavel [12], AVT is found throughout the adult pineal but is only synthesized in secretory ependymal cells located in the pineal recess. A nearby organ, the subcommissural organ (SCO) also contains AVT. The pineal receives peptidergic fibers with a hypothalamic origin and these fibers may be the source of the AVT and related peptides detected in pineals by immunocytochemistry [15].

11.2.2 AVT synthesis

De novo synthesis of AVT (or a related peptide) by pineals is claimed on the basis of in vitro studies. In one study, human fetal pineal cells were placed in culture; the hydroosmotic and antidiuretic activity were assayed in the culture medium. The investigators found 10 times the pineal activity in medium from 38 days' incubation suggesting that the active agent was synthesized and secreted by the cells [13]. The same group also found chromatographic evidence for vasotocin synthesis by rat pineal cells in culture [14].

11.2.3 AVT secretion

Because of the suspected location of the AVT-producing cells, Pavel [12] proposed that AVT is secreted into the CSF and reaches the blood only secondarily. Human CSF had a bioassay activity ratio (frog bladder activity/uterus activity = 275) similar to that for AVT (260) and very different from the ratios for oxytocin (1) and vasopressin (1.4).

Chemical stimuli that may affect AVT secretion include melatonin, adrenergic agents, cholinergic agents, and releasing hormones (LRH,

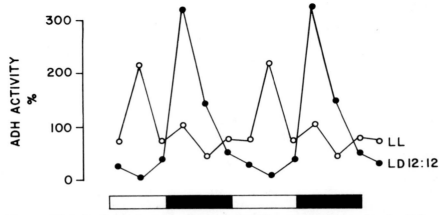

Figure 11.1 Daily cycle in antidiuretic (ADH) activity in rat pineals. (After data provided by König and Meyer [10].)

TRH, somatostatin, MIF). Melatonin is more effective in stimulating AVT (500 times) in the light-time than in the dark-time [3].

11.2.4 Daily and seasonal cycles

A daily cycle in rat pineal antidiuretic activity (bioassay water retention in male rats) has peak activity in the dark-time (3 hours after lights-out) [10] (Fig. 11.1). Four bioassays were used to measure antidiuretic and hydroosmotic activities of pineals from rats [5]. The midnight to noon estimates were 25:6 for rat antidiuresis and 430:996 for frog bladder. In this study, removing the pituitary abolished the antidiuretic cycle. A daily cycle with midnight nadir was reported for AVT [5]. The vasopressin daily cycle (peak in the light-time) was measured in cats [20, 21]; the possibility that vasopressin was directly secreted by the hypothalamic suprachiasmatic (SCN) region was suggested. Pavel has put forward an hypothesis of AVT secretion from the pineal into the CSF with brain targets because many of the studies in which AVT was effective involved intraventricular AVT injections. Presumably because of nighttime melatonin synthesis, Pavel expects human CSF AVT to be higher at night [12].

Laboratory rats (28–30 days old, 3–4 hours after lights-on of LD 16:8) exhibited a seasonal variation in AVT measured with an RIA (Fig. 11.2). AVT dropped to its nadir (2.15) in January but twice in August spiked to 1170–1720 pg/gland [16].

11.2.5 Functions of AVT

· In the model proposed by Pavel [12], AVT is a CSF hormone whose target is the brain.

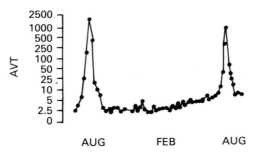

Figure 11.2 Annual cycle in arginine vasotocin (pg/gland) in rat pineals with August peaks. (After data provided by Prechel, Audhya, and Schlesinger [16].)

Direct evidence that the pituitary could be a target comes from studies where AVT stimulated luteinizing hormone (LH) and prolactin from anterior pituitary (rat, hamster) in vitro. This would make AVT a progonadotrophic hormone; however, antigonadotrophic properties have also been reported [3].

Antigonadotrophic activities for AVT include inhibition of gonadotrophin-stimulated reproductive organ growth and ovulation, lengthening of the estrous cycle, abortion, atrophy of mouse prostate and seminal vesicles, inhibition of compensatory ovarian hypertophy, and decrease in plasma LH [3]. Progonadotrophic activities for AVT have also been claimed, including augmentation of the preovulatory LH surge that occurs in immature rats with ovulation induced with pregnant mare's serum, and stimulation of LH and prolactin from rat and hamster anterior pituitaries in vitro [3, 25].

There may be some interaction between AVT and melatonin synthesis. First, an interaction of AVT with rat pineal N-acetyltransferase (NAT) was found in homogenates [2]. AVT contains the sequence (RHN-CH$_2$-CH$_2$-SR) necessary to protect dark-stimulated NAT. AVT that was reduced (disulfide bond opened with dithiothreitol) protected NAT and AVT itself was inhibitory. Second, when rat pineals were incubated with tryptophan and given norepinephrine (NE) to stimulate melatonin synthesis, AVT decreased melatonin synthesis [22]

Pavel [12] maintains that AVT has general effects of inhibition of the pituitary endocrine functions by affecting release and inhibiting hormones. AVT decreased plasma cortisol. Plasma prolactin normally increases 7 days after pinealectomy; AVT blocks the increase. AVT decreased pituitary stimulating hormone (MSH) and reversed the MSH increase that follows pinealectomy. A relationship of AVT and sleep has been proposed for cats [12]. AVT increases hypothalamic serotonin, induces slow wave sleep, and suppresses paradoxical sleep.

11.2.6 AVT targets

As mentioned, Pavel [12] has put forward an hypothesis of AVT secretion from the pineal into the CSF with brain targets. Many of the reported studies in which AVT was effective involved intraventricular AVT injections.

11.3 Hypophysiotropic Hormones

A group of hormones that are detectable in pineal glands includes the hypothalamic release and inhibiting hormones: LRH, TRH, somatostatin, PIF. These hormones are synthesized in the hypothalamus; they act on the pituitary gland to release or inhibit the release of hormones synthesized in the anterior pituitary. The possibilities for the origin of these molecules in the pineal are (1) intrapineal, by synthesis, and (2) extrapineal, by sequestering the molecules from CSF, neurons, or blood.

LRH is a hypothalamic decapeptide hormone that releases LH and FSH from pituitary glands. It has been detected in bovine, ovine, and porcine pineals [3] by immunological reactions and biological activity (ability of pineal extract to release FSH and LH from cultured pituitary cells). The amounts of LRH are estimated to be 185 ng/gland (pig) and 490 ng/gland (sheep). The molecule has not been detected in some pineals (mice). Seasonal variation was found in LRH of rat pineals (spring peak) and frogs. Pineal glands can take up LRH, so they may not synthesize it; the LRH is localized around blood vessels [1, 3, 12, 28].

TRH (thyroid stimulating hormone releasing hormone) is a tripeptide hormone of the hypothalamus. TRH was found in pineals of rats, cows, sheep and pigs [1, 3, 12, 28]. In some studies there was as much TRH in the pineal as in the hypothalamus. Rat pineal TRH was higher at noon than midnight [4].

Somatostatin (growth hormone inhibiting hormone) is a tridecapeptide hormone of the hypothalamus and pancreas. Somatostatin was found in pineals of guinea pigs and rats [3].

Prolactin release inhibiting hormone (PIF) and prolactin releasing hormone (PRF) activity were found in bovine, rat, and human pineal [3].

A putative MSH inhibiting hormone (MIF) is a hypothalamic tripeptide (pro-leu-gly-NH$_2$). When radiolabeled MIF was injected into rats it accumulated in the pineal and the pituitary [18].

11.4 Other Pineal Factors

There are a number of peptide and pineal fractions that have antireproductive activity. Moreover, some scientists feel that pineal melatonin production is insufficient to account for the pineal role in reproduction. The difficulty in the work with these fractions and peptides is that they are often available only in very small amounts. Several tests have commonly been employed to bioassay fractions of pineals. For example, injection of a gonadotropin (PMS or HCG) stimulates ovulation or ovarian hypertrophy in rats and mice. Inhibition of this response is a test for antigonadotropic activity in the presence of gonadotropin. Still other pineal-related molecules besides melatonin and peptides have been tested for possible mediation of pineal function, usually in reproduction. The efficacy of the indoles in blocking compensatory ovarian hypertrophy in mice revealed that other indoles besides melatonin were effective [25].

11.4.1 Pineal antigonadotropin

Pineal antigonadotropin (PAG) is a pineal fraction of an extract of sheep or cow pineals [1, 3]. The pineal fraction containing PAG does not have AVT or melatonin, but does have oxidized glutathione. The active molecule in PAG may be a peptide because it is inactivated with trypsin. The substance inhibits compensatory ovarian hypertrophy (COH) in mice (if one ovary is removed, the remaining ovary enlarges), and this response provides a bioassay for the putative peptide. PAG also lowers mouse ventral prostate weight, delays vaginal opening time in mice, reduces fertility in female mice, and inhibits ovulation in rats.

11.4.2 Threonylseryllysine

Threonylseryllysine (TSL) is a tripeptide with antigonadotropic activity isolated from one of three antigonadotropic fractions of bovine pineals. TSL inhibited COH, delayed the FSH surge in male rats treated with LRH, and lowered pituitary prolactin content in vitro [3].

11.4.3 E_5 peptide of Neascu

E_5 is a 14 amino acid peptide isolated from bovine pineals. E_5 depressed plasma LH and pituitary weight, lowered pituitary prolactin in normal and castrated male rats, and affected prolactin-secreting cells in vitro [3].

11.4.4 Serotonin

Serotonin (5-HT) is present in high concentrations in pineal gland. There are several potential explanations beyond the role that 5-HT has as a precursor of melatonin. Some effect on reproduction has been reported for 5-HT [19]. It lowered pituitary FSH when it was implanted in the hypothalamus, lowered male rat LH and FSH and increased prolactin when it was injected intraventricularly, and lowered LRH-induced LH release from incubated neonatal rat pituitaries.

11.4.5 *N*-acetylserotonin

N-acetylserotonin (NAS) inhibited COH but stimulated ova release in PMS-treated immature female rats. Intraventricular injection of NAS increased pituitary prolactin release [19].

11.4.6 5-Hydroxytryptophol (HTOH)

Injections of 5-hydroxytryptophol (HTOH) inhibited COH in mice, reduced PMS ovulation in immature rats, and lowered pituitary LH.

11.4.7 5-Methoxytryptophol

5-Methoxytryptophol (MTOH) is found in plasma (rat) and CSF (human) as well as in pineals (340 pg/gland, peak dark-time) [19]. Daily cycles in plasma MTOH have been observed in human and rat plasma (peak daytime, maximum detected 684 pg/ml).

11.4.8 5-Methoxytryptamine

5-Methoxytryptamine has been found in human and rat pineal glands and in human CSF [19]. Afternoon injections, like melatonin, regress the reproductive system of hamsters.

11.4.9 β-Carbolines

A group of molecules containing 6-methoxytetrahydroharman may be formed in the pineal by cyclodehydrogenation of 5-HT, 5-methoxytryptamine (5-MT), or melatonin [17]. The compound can raise brain 5-HT. There is a toxic syndrome characterized by excitation, tremors, and convulsions; 8 μmol/kg causes behavioral disturbances in rats. The molecule was detected in chicken pineal glands (8–43 nmol/g) with more in the glands at the time of lights-on than at the time of lights-off [9].

REFERENCES

1. Benson, B., and I. Ebels. 1978. Pineal peptides. *J. Neural Trans. Suppl.* 13:157–173.

2. Binkley, S., D. Klein, and J. Weller. 1976. Pineal serotonin N-acetyltransferase activity: Protection of stimulated activity by acetyl CoA and related compounds. *J. Neurochem.* 26:51–55.

3. Blask, D., M. Vaughan, and R. Reiter. 1983. Pineal peptides and reproduction. In *The pineal gland*, ed. R. Relkin, pp. 201–223. New York: Elsevier.

4. Brammer, G., J. Morley, E. Geller, A. Yuwiler, and J. Hershman. 1979. Hypothalamus-pituitary-thyroid axis interactions with pineal gland in the rat. *Amer. J. Physiol.* 236:E416–E420.

5. Calb, M., R. Goldstein, and S. Pavel. 1977. Diurnal rhythm of vasotocin in the pineal of the male rat. *Acta Endocrinol.* 84:523–526.

6. Geelen, G., A. Allevard-Burguburu, G. Gauquelin, Y. Xiao, J. Frutoso, C. Charib, B. Sempore, C. Meunier, and G. Augoyard. 1981. Radioimmunoassay of arginine vasopressin, oxytocin and arginine vasotocin-like material in the human pineal gland. *Peptides* 2:459–466.

7. Hadley, M. 1984. *Endocrinology*. Englewood Cliffs, N.J.: Prentice-Hall.

8. Holder, F., M. Schroeder, J. Guerne, and B. Vivien-Roels. 1979. A preliminary comparative immunohistochemical, radioimmunological, and biological study of arginine vasotocin (AVT) in the pineal gland and urophysis of some teleostei. *Gen. Comp. Endocrinol.* 37:15–25.

9. Kari, I. 1981. 6-Methoxy-1,2,3,4,-tetrahydro-β-carboline in pineal gland of chicken and cock. *FEBS Lett.* 127:277–280.

10. König, A., and A. Meyer. 1971. The effect of continuous illumination on the circadian rhythm of the antidiuretic activity of the rat pineal. *J. Interdiscipl. Cycle Res.* 2:255–262.

11. Lerner, A. 1978. Hormones in the pineal other than melatonin. *J. Neural Trans. Suppl.* 13:131–133.

12. Pavel, S. 1978. Arginine vasotocin as a pineal hormone *J. Neural Trans. Suppl.* 13:135–155.

13. Pavel, S., M. Dorcescu, R. Petrescu-Holban, and E. Ghinea. 1973. Biosynthesis of a vasotocin-like peptide in cell cultures from pineal glands of human fetuses. *Science* 181:1252–1253.

14. Pavel, S., R. Goldstein, E. Ghinea, M. Calb. 1978. Chromatographic evidence for vasotocin biosynthesis by cultured pineal ependymal cells from rat fetuses. *Endocrinology* 100:205–208.

15. Pévet, P. 1983. Anatomy of the pineal gland of mammals. In *The pineal gland*, ed. R. Relkin, pp. 1–75. New York: Elsevier.

16. Prechel, M., T. Audhya, and D. Schlesinger. 1983. A seasonal variation in arginine vasotocin immunoactivity in rat pineal glands. *Endocrinology* 112:1474–1478.

17. Quay, W. 1974. *Pineal chemistry*. Springfield, Ill.: Charles C Thomas.

18. Redding, T., A. Kastin, R. Nair, and A. Schally. 1973. Distribution, half-life, and excretion of [14]C- and 3H-labeled L-prolyl-L-leucyl-glycinamide in the rat. *Neuroendocrinology* 11:92–100.

19. Reiter, R., B. Richardson, and T. King. 1983. The pineal gland and its indole products: Their importance in the control of reproduction in mammals. In *The pineal gland*, ed. R. Relkin, pp. 151–199. New York: Elsevier.

20. Reppert, S., H. Artman, S. Swaminathan, and D. Fisher. 1981. Vasopres-

sin exhibits a rhythmic daily pattern in cerebrospinal fluid but not in blood. *Science* 213:1256–1257.

21. Reppert, S., R. Coleman, H. Heath, and H. Keutmann. 1982. Circadian properties of vasopressin and melatonin rhythms in cat cerebrospinal fluid. *Amer. J. Physiol.* 243:E489–E498.

22. Sartin, J., B. Bruot, and R. Orts. 1978. Interaction of arginine vasotocin and norepinephrine upon pineal indoleamine synthesis in vitro. *Mol. Cell. Endocrinol.* 11:7–18.

23. Vaughan, M. 1981. Arginine vasotocin and vertebrate reproduction. In *The pineal gland II: Reproductive effects.*, ed. R. Reiter, pp. 125–163. Boca Raton, Fla.: CRC Press.

24. Vaughan, M., D. Blask, G. Vaughan, and R. Reiter. 1975. Dose dependent prolactin releasing activity of arginine vasotocin in intact and pinealectomized estrogen-progesterone treated adult male rats. *Endocrinology* 99:1319–1322.

25. Vaughan, M., R. Reiter, G. Vaughan, L. Bigelow, and M. Altschule. 1972. Inhibition of compensatory ovarian hypertrophy in the mouse and vole: A comparison of Altschule's pineal extract, pineal indoles, vasopressin and oxytocin. *Gen. Comp. Endocrinol.* 18:372–377.

26. Vivien-Roels, B., J. Guerne, F. Holder, and M. Schroeder. 1979. Comparative immunohistochemical, radioimmunological and biological attempt to identify arginine-vasotocin (AVT) in the pineal gland of reptiles and fishes. In *The pineal gland of vertebrates including man*, ed. J. Kappers and P. Pévet, pp. 459–463. Progress in Brain Research 52. Amsterdam: Elsevier.

27. Vivien-Roels, B., P. Pévet, J. Guerne, F. Holder, A. Meiniel, J. Dogterom, and R. Buijs. 1981. On the presence of arginine vasotocin (AVT) in the pineal organ of non-mammalian vertebrates. In *Pineal function*, ed. C. Matthews and R. Seamark, pp. 185–197. Amsterdam: Elsevier/North-Holland.

28. Vollrath, L. 1981. *The pineal organ.* New York: Springer-Verlag.

12

Pineal Function in Humans

"In order to determine whether the human pattern of circulating melatonin resembles that previously described in lower animals, men 19–22 years old were exposed to a light-dark cycle with 14 hours of light per day (LD 14:10). . . . nocturnal (dark phase, sleeping) melatonin levels were almost always elevated to 0.05–0.1 ng/ml plasma compared with lower or undetectable levels during the day."

G. Vaughan et al. [48]

12.1 Introduction

In humans it has been possible to consider the pineal in relation to disease. For example, at the outset of the twentieth century, Heubner noted precocious sexual maturity in a young boy in whom a tumor had destroyed the pineal [60].

12.2 Anatomy

Human pineals, like those of some animals, exhibit calcification; the calcification is extensive enough to make the human pineal radiopaque. Therefore, the pineal is visible in procedures using X-rays—

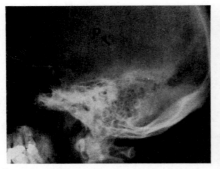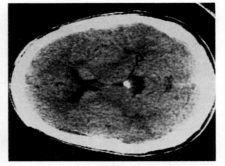

Figure 12.1 *A*, radiograph of the human head showing the pineal. *B*, scan of the human head obtained by computer-aided tomography (CAT) showing the transverse section containing the pineal gland. *(Photos courtesy of S. Binkley and H. R. Tatem)*

radiological studies and CAT scanning (computer-assisted tomography) (Fig. 12.1). It is not the only structure that can exhibit calcification; for example, the habenular commissure may also calcify [35].

12.2.1 Gross anatomy

The human pineal is usually located within 1–2 mm of the midline of the brain (Fig. 12.2). The normal central location has made the gland useful as a radiological marker of the midsagittal plane of the brain. Lesions that take space (tumors, hematomas, abscesses) displace the pineal from its normal position in a direction away from the mass; atrophy in a brain area displaces the pineal in the direction of the abnormality. The pineal lies at the posterior border of the third ventricle between the superior colliculi of the mesencephalon.

Vollrath [49] described a dual innervation of the human pineal. First, there is sympathetic innervation from the superior cervical ganglia (SCG) with the fibers forming the bilateral nervi conarii (0.1 mm thick with 150 fibers). When the nerve was followed from the posterior pole of the pineal, it coursed with the great vein of Galen. The nerve passed through a pia-arachnoid body (suprapineal body) to the dura mater of the tentorium cerebelli. In the pineal, the fibers terminate in the perivascular spaces accompanying the blood vessels. The fibers also terminate in the parenchyma (independent of blood vessels) in club-shaped boutons associated with pinealocyte cell membranes. Second, there are commissural fibers that reach the proximal pineal gland via the habenular and, to a lesser extent, the posterior commissures. These fibers may originate in the hypothalamus and may carry light information to the pineal.

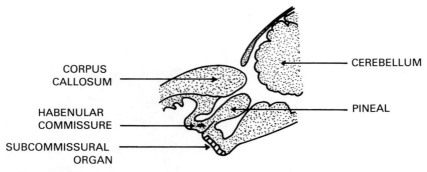

Figure 12.2 Diagram of the gross anatomy of the human pineal region in sagittal section.

12.2.2 Histology

The human pineal is composed of cords or lobules of cells that are set apart from each other by connective tissue septa that extend from the capsule. The cells observed are pinealocytes and neuroglia. The pinealocytes are "nerve-cell-like" with filament-containing cytoplasmic processes that terminate in, between, or near perivascular spaces, concretions, septa, pinealocytes, or the marginal glial plexus. Human pinealocytes are not usually considered to be "photoreceptor-like," but they are like the pinealocytes of animals in having organelles (elongated mitochondria, Golgi complex) concentrated in an "anuclear region . . . reminiscent of the inner segment of the photoreceptor" [49]. The neuroglia (astrocytes, interstitial cells) do not have an even distribution in the human pineal. They may surround pinealocytes in the human pineal and form glial patches in the periphery of the organ.

The fascinating sand-grain sized calcareous concretions (acervuli, corpora arenacea, brain sand) in the human pineal may be concentrated in the center of the gland [49]. The concretions have a curious mulberry shape (Fig. 12.3) and are composed of $Ca_3(PO_4)_2$, hydroxyapatite, and trace elements (magnesium, strontium). Some writers have compared the composition of the concretions to tooth enamel.

The degree of pineal calcification increases with age, leveling off at age 30. For example, in one study, the frequency of pineal calcification was 3% in the 1st year, 7.1% in the 10th year, and 33% in the 18th year [18]. However, when pineal serotonin, histamine, and enzymes were measured, no correlation was found between low values and calcification; thus calcification does not appear to be due to age deterioration. The incidence of calcification in Nigerian blacks was less than American blacks, which is half that in American whites [39, 44]. Because ganglionectomy reduced concretion formation in gerbils, the concretions could represent secretory activity in the pineal.

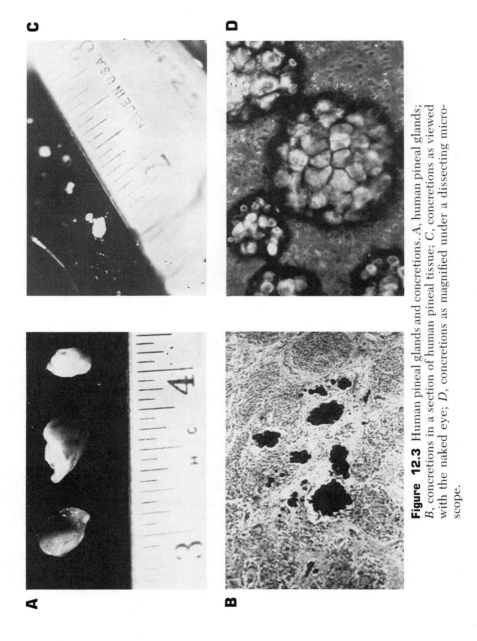

Figure 12.3 Human pineal glands and concretions. *A*, human pineal glands; *B*, concretions in a section of human pineal tissue; *C*, concretions as viewed with the naked eye; *D*, concretions as magnified under a dissecting microscope.

Lukaszyk and Reiter [26] hypothesize that pineal cells release a polypeptide that is a hormone-carrier protein complex. Calcium complexes with the carrier protein in exchange for hormone. The carrier-calcium complex is then the basis for concretion formation.

12.3 Biochemistry

In studying the biochemistry of the human pineal, there are some limitations. First, glands obtained at autopsy represent a range of time elapsed from time of death (e.g., 3–24 hours), which means that deterioration of enzyme activities may occur or there may be some continued metabolism or secretion beyond the moment of death. Some investigators have argued that indole amounts or enzymes are stable; however, postmortem losses could account for the fact that the evidence for human pineal nocturnal melatonin synthesis based on pineal measurements alone is weak. Second, pineals obtained at autopsy represent a variable population in terms of age, sex, racial background, cause of death, time of death, season of death, and so forth. These difficulties are not a problem in animal studies where the tissue can be obtained quickly and the characteristics of the population can be controlled.

12.3.1 Melatonin synthesis pathway

The pathway for melatonin biosynthesis in human pineals is likely to be the same as it is for other vertebrate species because of the presence of the necessary enzymes and substrates [40]. The data supporting a rhythm in a light-dark cycle are not wholly satisfying because the tissues were obtained at autopsy; thus, there could be problems with the measurements because the tissue was not equally fresh, lighting during the dying period is undefined, and disease/death may have introduced variation. Melatonin was detected in retinas of human donor eyes (347–1971 pg/g retina) [34].

Serotonin   Relatively large amounts of 5-HT (serotonin) were present in the human pineal (Fig. 12.4; 0.4–22.8 µg/g, exceeded only by the fur seal and swine pineals) [38]. Although serotonin is clearly present in the human pineal, caution must be observed in interpreting small, apparently significant differences which may be artifacts due to difficulties in controlling conditions (e.g., time from death to autopsy, environmental lighting conditions at time of death, etc.). Verification of the small apparent changes by replicate studies done by other investigators is needed.

Enzymes N-acetyltransferase (NAT) activity measured in one study (but not replicated in the data shown in Fig. 12.4) of postmortem

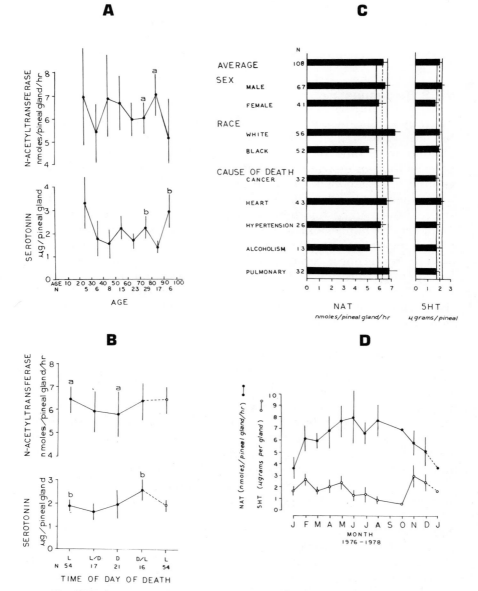

Figure 12.4 Amount of 5-HT and NAT measured in 108 human pineal glands obtained during autopsy and frozen (3–24 hours following the time of death). The data have been grouped according to (A) age, (B) time of day at death, (C) sex, race, and cause of death, and (D) month of year. There was considerable variation, probably due to the heterogeneity of the population, but most apparent differences among groups were statistically insignificant. (Unpublished data of Binkley, Reilly, Brammer, and Hoenig.)

human pineals was higher at night in pineals obtained at autopsy (1.6-fold, night 2200–0400, 1.1 nmol/hr/mg protein; 0.7 nmol/hr/mg protein [41, 42]). Hydroxyindole-O-methyltransferase (HIOMT) has been measured in human pineals [41, 42, 45, 59]. Highest HIOMT activity was found in January and July; lowest HIOMT activity was measured in March and October. Night HIOMT activity was 424-433 pmol/hr/mg protein; day HIOMT was 264-287 pmol/hr/mg protein. However, HIOMT is not limited to the pineal in humans; it has been found in red cells and the mucosa of inflamed appendices (presumably these were studied because of simple availability).

Melatonin   Melatonin (0.3 µg/g) was detected in human pinealoma [38] and in pineals (several studies, various methods with variable results: 45–613 pg/mg; 0.5–71 ng/pineal; 1–80 ng/pineal; 0.9–0.392 ng/pineal) [45]. The suggestion that human pineal melatonin increased at night and had a noon nadir has been made and challenged [17, 45]. Melatonin cycles with a dark-time peak have also been found in human fluids such as blood and saliva [30]. In humans, as other species, melatonin is believed to be metabolized by the liver; evidence for this is that oral doses of melatonin are eliminated more rapidly in normal subjects than in those whose livers are damaged with cirrhosis [22].

12.3.2 Other hormones

Hormones of the vasotocin family have been detected in human pineals with radioimmunoassay (RIA) [16]. Arginine vasopressin was detectable in 88% of the glands; the detectable amounts averaged 284 pg/pineal in women and 323 pg/pineal in men. Oxytocin was detected in 70% of the glands (4336 pg/pineal in women and 355 pg/pineal in men). Arginine vasotocin was found in 70% of the glands (42 pg/pineal in women and 46 pg/pineal in men). Histophysiological evidence for secretion of polypeptides was also found [26].

12.4 Physiology

Studies on the physiology of the human pineal involved measurement of blood and/or urine melatonin and melatonin administration (Fig. 12.5). Some studies supported roles for melatonin, some were equivocal, and some were negative. A more complete evaluation requires more attention paid to time of day and environmental illumination. Much of the work suggests directions that might be fruitful if more individual cases are studied. A study of human urinary melatonin led to the conclusion that human melatonin levels are inherited [56]. A study of melatonin in a population of 30 depressed individuals

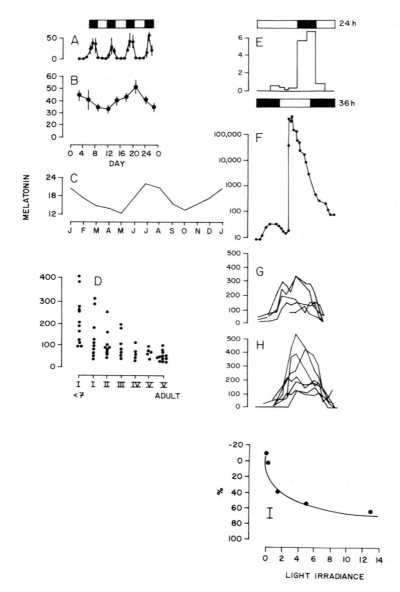

Figure 12.5 Human plasma and urine melatonin measured in various experiments. *A*, daily cycles of plasma melatonin (pg/ml, average for 5 men) [48]. *B*, plasma melatonin (pg/ml, average for 5 women, 9 A.M.) versus day of the menstrual cycle [3]; ovulation occurs about day 14. *C*, plasma melatonin (pg/ml, average for 6 men, 8 A.M.) versus month of the year [3]. *D*, dark-time melatonin (pg/ml; each point = one individual) versus stage of puberty [50]. *E*, daily cycle of urine melatonin (ng/4hr, 4 men) [27]; the bar over the graph is 24 hours long and shows where light and dark occurred. *F*, response of plasma melatonin (pg/ml) to an oral dose of 80 mg of melatonin [50]; the bar over the graph is 36 hours long and shows where light and dark occurred. *G*,

supported the conclusion that there was no difference in females versus males if body height was taken into account; melatonin correlated negatively with height [5].

12.4.1 Rhythms

Circadian rhythms in human pineal function and their regulation by environmental lighting have been studied for human melatonin. Taken together, the data for human blood (Fig. 12.5A) and urine melatonin (Fig. 12.5E) follow the pattern established for animals: synchronization by light-dark cycles, alteration of shape by photoperiod, possession of a refractory period, and suppression by light.

Daily cycle   The daily cycle in blood melatonin (Fig. 12.5A) has been well documented [36, 45, 48, 51]. The cycle was measured with bioassay in a light-dark cycle (LD 14:10); daytime melatonin was undetectable, nighttime melatonin was 40 pg/ml 5 hours after lights-out. The rhythm has also been measured with RIA with a typical noon level of 5–10 pg/ml and a typical midnight level of 90–115 pg/ml [3, 21, 27, 28, 50]. Occasional daytime maxima of 150 pg/ml and nighttime surges up to 500 pg/ml have been reported. Episodic release has been suggested [37, 51]. Melatonin daytime levels in human cerebrospinal fluid (CSF) range from undetectable up to 80 pg/ml [50]. Urinary melatonin levels in adult humans have been reported by bioassay (day 0–1.3 ng/4hr; night 0.55–7.75 ng/4hr) and with RIA (day 1.3–10.1 ng/4hr; night 4.3–38.2 ng/4hr) [27, 28].

Regulation by light and dark   Sleep/dark during the day did not increase melatonin in humans; this is consistent with the research in animals where it was found that stimulation of melatonin synthesis by dark was not possible in the early daytime (there is a refractory period) [45]. Awakening/light during the night did not produce the rapid plummet observed for melatonin in animals in the initial studies [45]. However, when the intensity of light was increased from 500 lux to 2500 lux, human plasma melatonin was suppressed (Fig. 12.5I) [24]. Phase shifting the light-dark cycle results in a gradual delay over 9–10 days of the melatonin peak to adjust to the new times of light and dark (resulting in high melatonin during some of the transient daytimes), so the melatonin rhythm can reset.

A study with constant light (LL) showed sleeping in the light did not lower plasma melatonin, but sleep deprivation and light obliter-

---

H, daily plasma melatonin (pmol/100 ml) profiles in individuals in summer (G) and winter (H) [19]. I, percent reduction in plasma melatonin in men 24–34 years old exposed to light of different intensities (brightest = 14) 3 hours after lights-out at 11 P.M. [10].

ated the plasma melatonin cycle in one man [52]. In another study, however, sleep deprivation did not abolish the urine melatonin cycle in 12 men sleep-deprived for 64 hours [52]. Studies of blind individuals (who sleep at night and may have high daytime melatonin) support the contention that melatonin and sleeping/waking are separable [41, 45, 53].

Shorter photoperiod (by addition of 4 hours of dark in the morning) shifted the melatonin peak so that its decline coincided with the new time of lights-on [53]. The data imply that human melatonin responds to photoperiod. Seasonal variation (Fig. 12.5G and H) has been reported with higher 8 A.M. plasma melatonin in winter-summer (22 pg/ml, July; 20 pg/ml, January) than in spring-fall (12 pg/ml, May; 14 pg/ml, October) [3, 4, 19, 45].

12.4.2 Surgical interventions and lesions

Tumor and surgical results have been evaluated in order to determine whether humans have a neural pathway for pineal regulation (e.g., as in rats).

Pineal tumors   Work with pineal tissue supports the presence of melatonin biosynthetic machinery in human pineal. Pineal tumor tissue has been found to have melatonin and HIOMT. Unusual serum melatonin values (e.g., high melatonin levels, elevated daytime melatonin, and early nocturnal rise in melatonin) have been found in patients with pineal tumors. Pinealocyte-like tumor cells produce melatonin in cultures [44, 45].

One to two percent of primary intracranial neoplasms are related to the pineal gland. Pineal tumors (pinealomas) may be of several types [9, 39]. Pineoblastomas (two-thirds of pineal parenchymal cell tumors) are malignant and are more undifferentiated tumors resembling medulloblastomas. This type of tumor was more common in young and in male individuals (average age 26). Pineocytomas have lobules like the pineal. The benign pineocytomas, found in older adults (one-third of pineal parenchymal cell tumors, average age 50) may contain cells in clusters or rosettes. The composition of the calcification found in pineal tumors was abnormal. The tumors are usually detected with radiographic techniques and may be accompanied by diabetes insipidus. The tumors are treated with surgery or radiotherapy.

Pineal ablation   Cases in which human pineal tissue has been damaged or removed support the idea that the pineal is the source of circulating melatonin in the human [45, 52]. Pineal tumors have been treated with combinations of radiation and surgery; pinealectomy and radiation abolished serum melatonin.

Superior cervical ganglia and hypothalamus Involvement of the SCG in regulation of human melatonin rhythms derives from two kinds of evidence [21, 45]. First, quadriplegics with cervical spinal cord transection had no blood melatonin rhythm. Second, victims of Shy-Drager syndrome have a preganglionic sympathetic lesion, low blood melatonin and no rhythm. Some patients with hypothalamic lesions had low melatonin and no melatonin rhythm. Vaughan et al. [48] offered the tentative conclusion that "melatonin secretion is controlled by a sympathetic pathway, the rhythm being reduced or eliminated by lesions of the pre- or postganglionic sympathetic nerves or their central origins and pathway (hypothalamus, brain stem, cervical cord)." Third, the daily cycle of melatonin was absent in some diabetics who had damaged autonomic systems (autonomic neuropathy) [33]. The principal evidence against the neural system of pineal control (as proposed for rats) is that adrenergic agonists have consistently failed to elevate human melatonin production, though adrenergic antagonists have reduced melatonin [46].

12.4.3 Pharmacology

Pineal pharmacology in humans has principally involved (1) attempts to establish a neurotransmitter control system for melatonin, and (2) determination of the effects of exogenous melatonin administration on various parameters in humans.

β-adrenergic stimulation and inhibition Adrenergic agonists that stimulate pineal NAT and melatonin in a few species (e.g. rats) have so far failed to stimulate human melatonin production [46]. Paradoxically, β-antagonists (e.g., atenolol, propranolol) block or reduce the nocturnal increase of melatonin in blood or urine in the human. For example, in one study, β-adrenoceptor blockers reduced midnight blood melatonin [12]. Human melatonin was unchanged by anticholinergics (e.g., scopolamine), dopamine agonists (bromocryptine, chloromethylergoline acetonitrile), and antidepressants that inhibit reuptake of norepinephrine (e.g., amitriptyline, maprotiline) [45, 50]. Human melatonin was increased by monoamine oxidase inhibiting compounds (also used as antidepressants) [31].

Melatonin Oral melatonin (80 mg) administration in the daytime dramatically increased blood melatonin from less than 100 pg/ml to over 100,000 pg/ml. Urine melatonin climbed from less than 10 ng/hr to more than 60,000 ng/hr [45, 50]. Modest amounts of oral melatonin (e.g., 2 mg) produced plasma melatonin in the day as high as or higher than night levels irrespective of the mode of administration (gelatine capsule, corn oil solution, slow-release pill); the melatonin increases lasted 3–4 hours and the half-life was estimated to be 0.54–0.67 hour [1].

Vaughan [45] discusses effects of melatonin administration on sedation, sleep, growth hormone, serotonin, pituitary function, epilepsy, depression, and cancer. Melatonin decreased alertness and increased sleepiness [25]. The inhibitory effect of melatonin on prolactin observed in animals has also been found in humans [30, 58]; when melatonin was injected intramuscularly into pubertal subjects in the afternoon, it decreased blood prolactin about 5 ng/ml [30]. In one study, daily melatonin (5 mg in gelatin lactose) reduced effects attributed to jet lag when traveling eight time zones [4].

12.4.4 Reproduction

The early historical association of precocious puberty and tumor destruction of the pineal and the involvement of the pineal in animal reproduction have focussed investigators' attention on the role of melatonin in human reproduction [45, 47].

Puberty There have been a number of attempts to confirm the hypothesis that melatonin from the pineal is antigonadal before puberty and that a melatonin decrease prompts or permits puberty to occur. Measurements of melatonin at various ages (Table 12.1) support a trend from higher values in youngsters to lower values in the aged [50, 60]. However, melatonin profiles measured at different stages of puberty and in precocious puberty were similar [12]. The suggestion has been made that the prepubertal lighter hair and skin color might be associated with melatonin [40]. Melatonin may act on reproduction by affecting prolactin; in that regard it may be important that morning melatonin infusions decreased prolactin in 2 of 9 prepubertal subjects and afternoon melatonin infusions in all 10 pubertal subjects [29].

Menstruation Several investigators have measured melatonin and excretion of its metabolite, 6-sulphatoxy melatonin, over the course of the menstrual cycle [3, 15, 54]. Only small changes in melatonin have been measured so far: morning melatonin was low (34 pg/ml) on the 12th (preovulatory nadir) and 25th day of the cycle and was high (45–52 pg/ml) on the 22nd (luteal phase rise) and 4th day of the cycle.

Pregnancy Melatonin cycles were compared in men and women and in pregnant women [20, 45]. Some higher melatonin values were found in women who were 33–39 weeks pregnant [20].

Light and human reproduction It has been tempting to seek human correlates of light regulation of reproduction [45]. There are so far

TABLE 12.1 Human melatonin (pg/ml) at successive ages

Tissue	Age	Time of measurement		
		Day	Unspecified	Night
Amniotic fluid	35–39 wk		102	
Amniotic fluid	Spontaneous term labor		262	
Plasma	Term cord	1.3		62
Plasma	1 yr	7		
Plasma	1–7 yr, precocious puberty	20		85
Plasma	9–13 yr, prepubertal	29		95
Plasma	13–15 yr	30		70
Plasma	Prepubertal			162
Plasma	Prepubertal			195
Plasma	Postpubertal			128
Plasma	Postpubertal			49
Plasma	25–34 yr			132
Plasma	21–37 yr	30		70
Plasma	26 yr	6		83
Plasma	40 yr	4		
Plasma	55–64 yr			30
Plasma	80 yr	3		
Plasma	85 yr	4		11

Sources: Data from Ehrenkranz et al. [14]; Vaughan [45]; and Waldhauser, Lynch, and Wurtman [50].
Note: The levels in the table are generally typical of the majority of studies; however there are miscellaneous reports of much higher melatonin values (e.g., 1508, 2300 pg/ml).

only sporadic reports here and there: (1) reduced reproduction in the blind, (2) cessation of menstruation in Eskimos in winter, (3) regularization of menstrual cycles with midcycle nocturnal illumination. If some of these effects are real actions of light on human reproduction, a pineal role would require further demonstration.

12.4.5 Sedation and sleep

Melatonin has been introduced by infusion, oral administration, and intranasal administration [37, 45]. Sedation, reduced sleep onset latency, increased rapid eye movement sleep, and increased sleep were reported in some of these studies.

12.4.6 Exercise

Plasma melatonin was measured in women exercising in a training program. During bouts of exercise, plasma melatonin increased (e.g., from 55 to 105 pg/ml in 60 minutes) [11]. In men 100-yard dashes did not change melatonin [45].

12.4.7 Pituitary function

Growth hormone (GH) has been found to have a daily cycle with peak levels during sleep. In some studies, the GH response to sleep was increased by melatonin and GH increases have been induced in awake individuals with melatonin [45]. Attempts to alter gonadotrophins (LH, FSH) or the response of gonadotrophins to LRH or testosterone levels with melatonin have been negative [45].

12.4.8 Mental health and behavior

Melatonin and pineal relationships to mental health (epilepsy, depression, schizophrenia, Parkinsonism, Huntington's chorea, headaches) have been studied [23, 45, 53].

Epilepsy   Some investigators have found a reduction in seizures with melatonin administration [45] which might agree with the work in gerbils (where pinealectomy produced seizures and melatonin attenuated them).

Depression   A type of seasonal depression syndrome (SAD, seasonal affective disorder) has been identified. Bright morning light (2500 lux or more) reduced winter depression in the individuals with this syndrome [24, 45, 57]. Other investigators have claimed alterations in the temporal organization of melatonin in individuals with mania and/or depression (e.g., higher plasma melatonin in manic patients). Melatonin administration to depressed patients exacerbated their illness [39]. However, when plasma melatonin daily profiles were measured in depressed patients, dark-time melatonin was reduced (e.g., from 78 pg/ml to 32 pg/ml [5, 13, 32, 55]. Melatonin measures may not be the only important factor; one investigator has suggested that the melatonin: cortisol ratio is important [55].

Schizophrenia   Melatonin and the pineal were evaluated for a possible role in schizophrenia [2, 7]. Melatonin values were low in some schizophrenic patients [45]. Alcohol abusers had low melatonin [52]. Melatonin reduced psychosis scores in some schizophrenic patients [39] but increased symptoms in some recovered schizophrenics. Administration of an extract of beef pineal ameliorated psychosis and the abnormalities in the carbohydrate metabolism of schizophrenic individuals [2]. Morning melatonin in human CSF was not different in normal versus schizophrenic individuals [6].

Headache   A patient with migraine had no melatonin cycle [52], but there are also reports of melatonin administration producing headaches [23].

12.4.9 Cancer

An oncostatic function of the pineal was proposed by Blask [8]. He notes that the evidence for an antimitotic action of melatonin is scant. Nevertheless, he cites studies in animals in which the pineal influenced cell growth and proposes that, in vivo, the gland may inhibit tumor growth and notes, in support of the idea, the rarity of pineal tumors. Enlarged pineal glands were found in breast and some other cancer patients; pineal HIOMT may be higher in cancer patients; cancer patients may have less pineal calcification [45].

Night urine melatonin may be less in breast cancer patients. When breast cancer patients were divided based on whether they had estrogen receptors in the tumor tissue, those with the receptors had a 29 percent reduction in peak melatonin [43, 45].

REFERENCES

1. Aldhous, M., C. Franey, J. Wright, and J. Arendt. 1985. Plasma concentrations of melatonin in man following oral absorption of different preparations. *Brit. J. Clin. Pharmacol.* 19:517–521.

2. Altschule, M. 1975. Effect of a pineal extract on carbohydrate metabolism in schizophrenic patients. In *Frontiers of pineal physiology*, ed. M. Altschule, pp. 197–203. Cambridge, Mass.: MIT Press.

3. Arendt, J. 1978. Melatonin assays in body fluids. *J. Neural Trans. Suppl.* 13:265–278.

4. Arendt, J., Aldhous, M., and V. Marks. 1986. Alleviation of jet lag by melatonin: Preliminary results of controlled double blind trial. *Brit. Med. J.* 292:1170.

5. Beck-Friis, J., D. von Rosen, B. Kjellman, J. Ljunggren, and L. Wetterberg. 1984. Melatonin in relation to body measures, sex, age, season and the use of drugs in patients with major affective disorders and healthy subjects. *Psychoneuroendocrinology* 9:271–277.

6. Beckman, H., L. Wetterberg, and W. Gattaz. 1984. Melatonin immunoreactivity in cerebrospinal fluid of schizophrenic patients and healthy controls. *Psychiat. Res.* 11:107–110.

7. Bigelow, L. 1975. Some effects of aqueous pineal extract administration on schizophrenia symptoms. In *Frontiers of pineal physiology*, ed. M. Altschule, pp. 225–263. Cambridge, Mass.: MIT Press.

8. Blask, D. 1984. The pineal: An oncostatic gland? In *The pineal gland*, ed. R. Reiter, pp. 253–284. New York: Raven Press.

9. Borit, A., and H. Schmidek. 1984. Pineal tumors and their treatment. In *The pineal gland*, ed. R. Reiter, pp. 323–343. New York: Raven Press.

10. Brainard, G., A. Lewy, M. Menaker, R. Fredrickson, S. Miller, R. Weleber, V. Cassone, and D. Hudson. 1985. Dose-response relationship between light irradiance and the suppression of plasma melatonin in human volunteers. *Ann. N.Y. Acad. Sci.* 453:376–378.

11. Carr, D., S. Reppert, B. Bullen, G. Skrinar, I. Beitins, M. Arnold, M.

Rosenblatt, J. Martin, and J. McArthur. 1981. Plasma melatonin increases during exercise in women. *J. Clin. Endocrinol.* 53:224–225.

12. Cowen, P., J. Bevan, B. Gosden, and S. Elliott. 1985. Treatment with β-adrenoceptor blockers reduces plasma melatonin concentration. *Brit. J. Clin. Pharmacol.* 19:258–260.

13. Claustrat, B., G. Chazot, J. Brun, D. Jordan, and G. Sassolas. 1984. A chronobiological study of melatonin and cortisol secretion in depressed subjects: Plasma melatonin, a biochemical marker in major depression. *Biol. Psychiat.* 19:1215–1228.

14. Ehrenkranz, J., L. Tamarkin, F. Comite, R. Johnsonbaugh, D. Bybee, D. Loriaux, and G. Cutler. 1982. Daily rhythm of plasma melatonin in normal and precocious puberty. *J. Clin. Endocrinol. Metab.* 55:307–310.

15. Fellenberg, A., G. Phillipou, and R. Seamark. 1982. Urinary 6-sulphatoxy melatonin excretion during the human menstrual cycle. *Clin. Endocrinol.* 17:71–75.

16. Geelen, G., A. Allevard-Burguburu, G. Gauquelin, Y. Xiao, J. Frutoso, C. Gharib, B. Sempore, C. Meunier, and G. Augoyard. 1981. Radioimmunoassay of arginine vasopressin, oxytocin and arginine vasotocin-like material in the human pineal gland. *Peptides* 2:459–466.

17. Greiner, A., and S. Chan. 1978. Melatonin content of the human pineal gland. *Science* 199:83–84.

18. Helmke, V. K., and P. Winkler. 1986. Die häufigkeit von pinealisverkalkungen in den ersten 18 lebensjahren. *Fortschr. Röntgenstr.* 144:221–226.

19. Illnerová, H., P. Zvolsky, and J. Vaněček. 1985. The circadian rhythm in plasma melatonin concentration of the urbanized man: The effect of summer and winter time. *Brain Res.* 328:186–189.

20. Kennaway, D., C. Matthews, R. Seamark. 1981. Pineal function in pregnancy: Studies in sheep and man. In *Pineal function*, ed. C. Matthews and R. Seamark, pp. 123–136. Amsterdam: Elsevier/North-Holland.

21. Kneisley, L., M. Moskowitz, and H. Lynch. 1978. Cervical spinal cord lesions disrupt the rhythm in human melatonin excretion. *J. Neural Trans. Suppl.* 13:311–323.

22. Lane, E., and H. Moss. 1985. Pharmokinetics of melatonin in man: First pass hepatic metabolism. *J. Clin. Endocrinol. Metab.* 61:1214–1216.

23. Lerner, A., and J. Nordlund. 1978. Melatonin: Clinical pharmacology. *J. Neural Trans. Suppl.* 13:339–347.

24. Lewy, A. 1983. Biochemistry and regulation of mammalian melatonin production. In *The pineal gland*, ed. R. Relkin, pp. 77–128. New York: Elsevier.

25. Lieberman, H., F. Waldhauser, G. Garfield, H. Lynch, and R. Wurtman. 1984. Effects of melatonin on human mood and performance. *Brain Res.* 323:201–207.

26. Lukaszyk, A., and R. Reiter. 1975. Histophysiological evidence for the secretion of polypeptides by the pineal gland. *Amer. J. Anat.* 143:451–464.

27. Lynch, H., D. Jimerson, Y. Ozaki, R. Post, W. Bunney, and R. Wurtman. 1978. Entrainment of rhythmic melatonin secretion in man to a 12-hour phase shift in the light/dark cycle. *Life Sci.* 23:1557–1564.

28. Lynch, H., Y. Ozaki, and R. Wurtman. 1978. The measurement of

melatonin in mammalian tissues and body fluids. *J. Neural Trans. Suppl.* 13:251–264.

29. Mauri, R., P. Lissoni, M. Resentini, C. De Medici, F. Morabito, S. Djemal, L. DiBella, and F. Fraschini. 1985. Effects of melatonin on PRL secretion during different photoperiods of the day in prepubertal and pubertal healthy subjects. *J. Endocrinol. Invest.* 8:337–341.

30. Miles, A., D. Philbrick, D. Shaw, S. Tidmarsh, and A. Pugh. 1985. Salivary melatonin estimation in clinical research. *Clin. Chem.* 31:2041–2042.

31. Murphy, D. 1985. Effects of antidepressants and other psychotropic drugs on melatonin release and pineal function. In *Melatonin in humans*, pp. 261–277. Cambridge, Mass.: Center for Brain Sciences and Metabolism Charitable Trust.

32. Nair, N., N. Hariharasubramanian, and C. Pilapil. 1984. Circadian rhythm of plasma melatonin in endogenous depression. *Prog. Neuro-Psychopharmacol. Biol. Psychiat.* 8:715–718.

33. O'Brien, I., I. Lewin, J. O'Hare, J. Arendt, and R. Corrall. 1986. Abnormal circadian rhythm of melatonin in diabetic autonomic neuropathy. *Clin. Endocrinol.* 24:359–364.

34. Osol, G., and B. Schwartz. 1984. Melatonin in the human retina. *Exp. Eye Res.* 38:213–215.

35. Paul, L., and J. Juhl. 1972. *The essentials of roentgen interpretation*, 3rd ed., pp. 340–341. Hagertown, Md.: Harper & Row.

36. Pelham, R., G. Vaughan, K. Sandock, and M. Vaughan. 1973. Twenty-four-hour cycle of a melatonin-like substance in the plasma of human males. *J. Clin. Endocrinol. Metab.* 37:341–344.

37. Penny, R. 1985. Episodic secretion of melatonin in pre- and postpubertal girls and boys. *J. Clin. Endocrinol. Metab.* 60:751–756.

38. Quay, W. 1974. *Pineal chemistry.* Springfield, Ill.: Charles C Thomas.

39. Relkin, R. 1983. The human pineal. In *The pineal gland*, ed. R. Relkin, pp. 273–311. New York: Elsevier.

40. Silman, R., R. Leone, R. Hooper, and M. Preece. 1979. Melatonin, the pineal gland and human puberty. *Nature* 282:301–303.

41. Smith, J., T. Mee, D. Padwick, and E. Spokes. 1981. Human post-mortem pineal enzyme activity. *Clin. Endocrinol.* 14:75–81.

42. Smith, J., J. O'Hara, and A. Schiff. 1981. Altered diurnal serum melatonin rhythm in blind men. *Lancet*, Oct. 24:933.

43. Tamarkin, L., D. Danforth, A. Lichter, E. DeMoss, M. Cohen, B. Chabner, and M. Lippman. 1982. Decreased nocturnal plasma melatonin peak in patients with estrogen receptor positive breast cancer. *Science* 216:1003–1005.

44. Tapp, E. 1982. The pineal gland in malignancy. In *The pineal gland III: Extra-reproductive effects*, ed. R. Reiter, pp. 171–188. Boca Raton, Fla.: CRC Press.

45. Vaughan, G. 1984. Melatonin in humans. In *Pineal research reviews II*, ed. R. Reiter, pp. 141–201. New York: Alan R. Liss.

46. ———. 1985. Human melatonin in physiologic and diseased states: Neural control of the rhythm. In *Melatonin in humans*, ed. R. Wurtman and F. Waldhauser, pp. 193–208. Cambridge, Mass.: Center for Brain Sciences and Metabolism Charitable Trust.

47. Vaughan, G., G. Meyer, and R. Reiter. 1978. Evidence for a pineal-gonad relationship in the human. *Prog. Reprod. Biol.* 4:191–223.

48. Vaughan, G., R. Pelham, S. Pang, L. Loughlin, K. Wilson, K. Sandock, M. Vaughan, S. Koslow, and R. Reiter. 1976. Nocturnal elevation of plasma melatonin and urinary 5-hydroxyindoleacetic acid in young men: Attempts at modification by brief changes in environmental lighting and sleep and by autonomic drugs *J. Clin. Endocrinol. Metab.* 42:752–764.

49. Vollrath, L. 1984. Functional anatomy of the human pineal gland. In *The pineal gland*, ed. R. Reiter, pp. 285–322. New York: Raven Press.

50. Waldhauser, F., H. Lynch, and R. Wurtman. 1984. Melatonin in human body fluids: Clinical significance. In *The pineal gland*, ed. R. Reiter, pp. 345–370. New York: Raven Press.

51. Weitzman, E., U. Weinberg, R. D'Eletto, H. Lynch, R. Wurtman, C. Czeisler, and S. Erlich. 1978. Studies of the 24 hour rhythm of melatonin in man. *J. Neural Trans. Suppl.* 13:325–337.

52. Wetterberg, L. 1978. Melatonin in humans: Physiological and clinical studies. *J. Neural Trans. Suppl.* 13:251–264.

53. ———. 1982. Psychiatric aspects of pineal function. In *The pineal gland III: Extra-reproductive effects*, ed. R. Reiter. pp. 219–227. Boca Raton, Fla.: CRC Press.

54. Wetterberg, L., J. Arendt, L. Paunier, P. Sizonenko, W. van Donelaar. 1976. Human serum melatonin changes during the menstrual cycle. *J. Clin. Endocrinol. Metab.* 42:185–188.

55. Wetterberg, L., J. Beck-Friis, B. Kjellman, and J. Ljunggren. 1984. Circadian rhythms in melatonin and cortisol secretion in depression. In *Frontiers of biochemical and pharmacological research in depression*, ed. E. Usdin, pp. 197–205. New York: Raven press.

56. Wetterberg, L., L. Iselius, and J. Lindsten. 1983. Genetic regulation of melatonin excretion in urine. *Clin. Genetics* 24:399–402.

57. Wirz-Justice, A., H. Fisch, and B. Woggon. 1986. How much light is antidepressant? *Psychiat. Res.* 17:75–77.

58. Wright, J., M. Aldhous, C. Franey, J. English, and J. Arendt. 1986. The effects of exogenous melatonin on endocrine function in man. *Clin. Endocrinol.* 24:375–382.

59. Young, I., R. Leone, P. Stovell, and R. Silman. 1985. Melatonin is metabolized to N-acetylserotonin and 6-hydroxymelatonin in man. *J. Clin. Endocrinol. Metab.* 60:114–119.

60. Young, I., and R. Silman. 1982. Pineal methoxyindoles in the human. In *The Pineal Gland III: Extra-reproductive effects*, ed. R. Reiter, pp. 189–218. Boca Raton, Fla.: CRC Press.

61. Zrenner, C. 1985. Theories of pineal function from classical antiquity to 1900: A history. In *Pineal Research Reviews III*, ed. R. Reiter, pp. 1–40. New York: Alan R. Liss.

13

Development and Aging

"The occurrence of pineal calcification in man is well known. . . . The incidence is negligible in the first decade of life; it approximates 25 percent in the second decade, and increases gradually from the third to eighth decades. No relation has ever been established between the occurrence of calcification and any functional status of the human pineal gland."

J. I. Kitay and M. D. Altschule [26]

"Changes in the pattern of melatonin production around puberty have long been sought to prove Marburg's hypothesis that the pineal regulates the onset of that event. Data on melatonin levels during development in animals have failed to show a consistent correlation between the ontogeny of the daily melatonin rhythm and the onset of sexual development. Although many investigations of the relation between melatonin secretion and puberty have been conducted in humans, the data are still equivocal."

L. Tamarkin [54]

13.1 Introduction

The data for the life cycle of the pineal gland comes mainly from three species: hamsters, rats, and chickens. Hamsters have been used because of the pineal role in reproduction; rats, because of the accessibility of fetal and neonatal rat pups; and chickens, because of the accessibility of the embryos in eggs.

The anatomy of the pineal at different ages has been examined. A useful feature of the developmental anatomy is the fact that the organization of the cells may be more readily seen in the developing glands. In examining the development, parallels between ontogeny (development) and phylogeny (evolution) have been sought because of the idea that ontogeny sometimes recapitulates phylogeny.

A problem of interest is the source of melatonin at various ages and pineal melatonin biosynthetic capabilities. For mammals, Reppert [46] has proposed a sequence for the origin of circulating melatonin in rats: prenatal melatonin comes from the mother by placental transport; in the first week of life, melatonin is acquired by pups through suckling the mother's milk; in the second and third weeks, by a combination of suckling and the pup's own pineal secretions; and postweaning, from the individuals' pineals. In old animals, melatonin synthesis is reduced [39, 41, 42].

The possibility that the pineal may function differently at different ages has been considered. The principal hypothesis has been that the pineal, especially in nonseasonal breeders and humans, might function in an antigonadal capacity prior to the onset of reproductive maturity, that is, in the embryo or young [54]. Pineal function in adults have been discussed in other chapters.

13.2 Embryonic Development

In embryos, the anatomy of the pineal and the ontogeny of melatonin synthesis in the pineal have been studied. In mammals, the relationship of the fetal pineal and the mother is a subject of interest as well as the mother-fetal interaction in synchronization of circadian rhythmicity.

13.2.1 Anatomy

The pineal develops from the diencephalon. The area of pineal origination is an ependymal area between the posterior and habenular commissures. The developmental patterns vary to some extent dependent upon the comparative anatomy of the species (Fig. 13.1).

The human pineal has been identified in the second month of gestation (6- to 8-mm embryos). Commissural fibers reach the pineal by day 60; sympathetic innervation reaches the pineal between 60 and 82 days; and there may be innervation connecting the pineal and the subcommissural organ (homologous to the pineal nerve of anurans, which passes the pineal on its way from the frontal organ to the

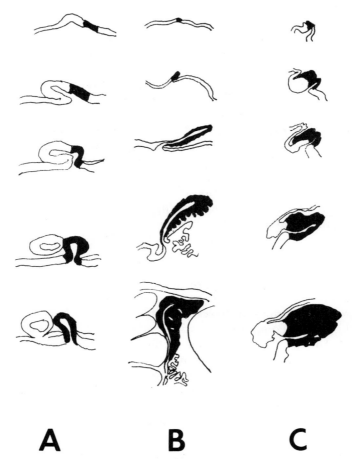

Figure 13.1 Sample developmental sequences (*top to bottom*) for pineal regions (black) of (*A*) lizards, (*B*) birds and (*C*) humans. (Redrawn from information provided by Calvo and Boya [11] and [60].)

subcommissural organ) [60]. The perivascular spaces are initially large and reduced in size. Human fetal pinealocytes are similar to adult mammal pinealocytes except that the fetal cells lack synaptic ribbons.

Rat pineal development has been described to have several phases, two of which are embryonic [60]. The first, the *morphogenetic phase* (when the cells form) begins day 12 of gestation, which coincides with the time that the evagination of the diencephalon between the commissures can be noticed. The second, beginning day 16 and ending a few days after birth, is the *cell proliferation phase*. There is an initial follicular organization that is lost by day 19. Commissural fibers appear at 18 days of gestation. Hamster pineal development begins at 12 days in a manner similar to that in rats.

Pineal development in birds may begin at 3 days of incubation [11, 12, 60]. The primary evagination elongates and has been called the *primary follicle*. Further follicular structures (*secondary follicles*) appear to bud off or are formed within the wall of the primary follicle. A connective tissue capsule was identified at 7 days of incubation; connective tissue proceeded to surround the follicles. Sympathetic nerves reach the pineal just before hatching. The occurrence of lymphocytes and vascularization was seen at 4 days.

In reptiles, controversy has surrounded the question of whether the parietal eye develops separately as a diencephalic evagination or together with the pineal. There may be species differences [60]. In amphibians such as *Xenopus*, the pineal was first seen in 2.4-mm embryos. At 10 mm, a separation of the frontal organ from the pineal was observed. New cells arise from the diencephalic area adjacent to where the pineal attaches (the orifice).

13.2.2 Maternal-fetal transport of melatonin

Maternal-fetal transport of melatonin was demonstrated by showing that fetal rats and primates (rhesus monkeys and baboons, 150 days gestation, near term) acquired 3H-acetyl-melatonin following injection of the tagged compound into the mother [27, 47]. In the primates, the labeled melatonin was found in the plasma 3 minutes after the injection; in amniotic fluid, 3–8 minutes after the injection; and the label was detected in the fetal cerebrospinal fluid (CSF). Moreover, melatonin infusion raised the primate fetal blood melatonin levels 12- to 21-fold. It is thus possible that periodic maternal melatonin signals could be used to synchronize rhythms of embryos.

13.2.3 Embryonic melatonin synthesis

Primate pineals (150 days gestation, near term) had N-acetyltransferase (NAT; 99–150 pmol/min/mg protein) and hydroxyindole-O-methyltransferase (HIOMT; 26–67 pmol/min/mg protein) [47]. NAT was detected in chick embryo pineals at 16–19 days of incubation (507–1158 pmol/pineal/hr); dark-time NAT was twice that in light-time in the embryos at 17 and 19 (but not at 16) days of incubation in LD 12:12 [3].

13.2.4 Suprachiasmatic nuclei

Because of the relationship of the pineal to the hypothalamus, development of rhythms in the hypothalamus is of interest. A daily cycle of metabolism in the suprachiasmatic nuclei (SCN) was measured in fetal rats using ^{14}C-deoxyglucose [49, 50]. Exposing pregnant rats to a 4-hour light extension increased the metabolism of the dam's SCN, but fetal SCN metabolism did not increase. Shifting the mother rat's light cycle during pregnancy shifted the embryonic SCN rhythm.

13.3 Neonatal, Preweaning, and Posthatch Development

Probably most of the work on the development of the pineal and its function has focussed on the first few weeks of life: birth to weaning (21 days) in the rat, and the first 3 weeks of life in chickens. In mammals, the interactions between dam and offspring have been accessible to study. In birds, the development of the pineal system is open to study in absence of maternal influence.

13.3.1 Anatomy

In most species studied, development of the pineal was not complete at birth or hatching but continued through the early weeks after birth or hatching.

Human pineals undergo histological changes following birth [60]. A change from homogeneous appearance of the cells to a mosaic pattern occurs 2–3 weeks after birth and persists to 6–9 months of age. The mosaic pattern is characterized by clumps of pineal parenchymal cells containing large, pale nuclei. The clumps are set apart by cells resembling lymphocytes.

Postnatal pineal development in the rat is characterized by the appearance of innervation beginning 1–2 days after birth and completed 10–21 days after birth [13, 60]. The size of the gland increases by mitosis for the first two weeks; the stalk forms. After the second week, pineal size increases are a consequence of hypertrophy of the cells rather than of continued mitosis. In rats, pineal size increases 3.5 times in the first 25–30 days and continues to grow for 8–12 weeks. Some investigators noted structures (apical knobs, cilia-bearing bulges) reminiscent of photoreceptor cell outer segments during 4–18 days of age. "Pseudo-rosettes" and "cords" of pinealocytes were noticed beginning at days 15–20 [13]. From days 0–10, ribosomes and endoplasmic reticulum increase; mitochondria increase up to 28 days. Two kinds of pinealocytes were observed by day 10 [13]. The pineal does not develop just by growth, but also by cell death (with resorption and phagocytosis) from days 3–21. In hamsters, the pineal gland receives innervation from the nervi conarii over days 1–5 and the adult state is reached by 15 days.

Bird pineals are subclassified into two structural patterns: (1) solid lobular (chickens), and (2) tubulofollicular (pigeons, ducks) [34]. Three kinds of cells are reported: pinealocytes, glia-like cells, and neuron-like cells. In chickens, the innervation that began in the egg on day 17 continued and became adult-like by day 10 after hatching

[11, 12, 60]. The whorl-like structures were attached to bulbous outer segments by 15 days, the adult pattern [33]. One investigator reported morphological changes in pineals of 1- and 2-month-old chicks kept in light-dark cycles. Ralph and Lane [36] describe anatomical progression of the pineal of the sparrow during the first 90 days of life from a "loose, highly folliculated" to a "compact, more solid-appearing" structure.

13.3.2 Melatonin synthesis

Early melatonin synthesis has been studied in pineals and deep pineals of young fowl, rats, and hamsters [3, 51, 55]. The onset of timing of pineal events has been determined (Fig. 13.2 maps these events). Generally, the day-night difference develops early and is present 1–15 days posthatch or birth. Adult levels are achieved rapidly in some species (in 3 weeks in rats and chicks). The melatonin and NAT rhythms develop from initial low values by increasing the dark-time levels (Fig. 13.3).

There was a rhythm in rat pineal serotonin in light-dark cycles as early as 1–2 days [21, 22, 23, 58, 70, 71] that was suppressed by light. Persistence of the rhythm in constant dark was observed at 30 days of age (the earliest age tested). A bimodal rhythm in chick pineal serotonin measured in 22- to 24-day-old chicks (the only age tested) [7].

The rhythm in NAT was measured in light-dark cycles in young rats as early as 4 days of age; the enzyme was present but not detectably rhythmic from 4 days before birth [18]. The NAT rhythm developed by increases in dark-time NAT and achieved adult daily excursions by 3 weeks of age (weaning age).

The rhythm in NAT was measured in light-dark cycles in young chicks on the first day after hatching, and as mentioned, for several days before hatching [3]. In chicks, as in rats, the rhythm developed by increases in dark-time NAT and achieved adult daily excursions by 18 days of age.

The development of HIOMT activity was studied in rat pineals [21, 70]. HIOMT was found as early as 3 days of age and rose to adult levels by 34 days. The development of HIOMT activity was studied in chick pineals [3]. HIOMT was found as early as 2 days of age (the earliest age tested). HIOMT climbed linearly and was still increasing at 56 days of age (the last age tested).

The development of melatonin in rats [53] follows a pattern similar to NAT in that a rhythm develops as a nocturnal increase. Melatonin was detectable in the first week but the day-night difference first appeared at 8 days. By 20 days, the daily excursion of melatonin was 80 percent of that of the adult. Developmental patterns of melatonin synthesis in hamsters were similar to those in rats except that

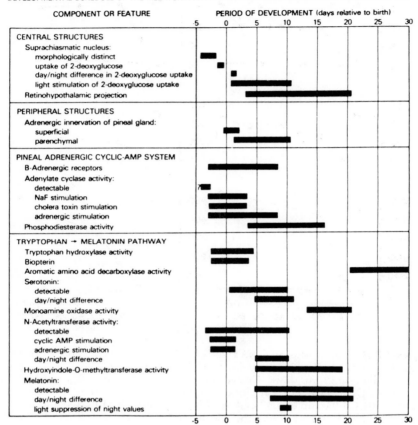

Figure 13.2 A map of the sequence of development of the melatonin system in the pineal of the laboratory rat. (Klein, Namboodiri, and Auerback [29] with permission.)

detectable day-night differences were not obtained until 12–15 days of age and at 20 days the amplitude of the daily cycle was only 50–60 percent of that of the adult [53].

13.3.3 Photoreception

Because of the presence of photoreceptor-like structures in pineals of neonatal rats, chicks, and other species, functional evidence for pineal light perception has been sought [4].

Evidence of extraretinal light perception per se was noticed in rat pups that were blind during the time at which photoreceptor-like structures are present in their pineals. In seeking the rat extraretinal light receptor, some investigators also turned to the Harderian glands

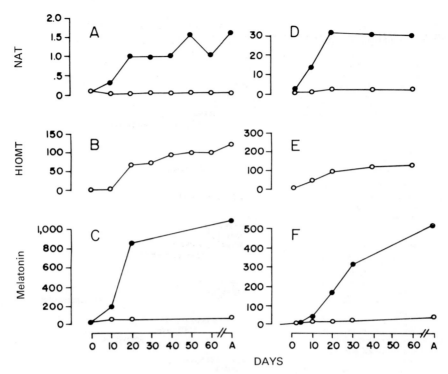

Figure 13.3 Graphs of pineal NAT activity, HIOMT activity, and melatonin content for rats (*A, B, C*) and chicks (*D, E, F*) versus age of the animals (from birth or hatching) in days. *Closed circles* = dark-time; *open circles* = light-time. Data have been replotted by taking numbers from the original graphs with a Bioquant image analysis system (Data from Binkley and Geller [3]; Ellison, Weller, and Klein [18]; Klein and Lines [28]; and Tamarkin et al. [55].)

[64, 65]. The Harderian glands are lacrimal glands located behind the eye; they are noted for their high porphyrin content, which results in red fluorescence when the glands are examined under uv light. Harderian gland removal from blinded 12-day-old rats abolished the light-stimulated increase in serotonin (5-HT) and abolished light inhibition of HIOMT; but constant light abolished the daily change in pineal 5-HT in 12-day-old rats from which the eyes and Harderian were removed [57, 71].

Pineal NAT of blind chicks exhibits dramatic responses to light and dark in vivo, and their pineal glands respond to light and dark in vitro [3, 5, 16, 53, 61].

13.3.4 Sympathetic regulation

The ontogeny of sympathetic regulation of the pineal has been sought in rats with a variety of techniques that denervate the pineal by interfering with the superior cervical ganglia: bilateral ganglionect-omy, immunosympathectomy, and injection of 6-OH dopamine [10, 17, 23, 30, 31]. These procedures abolished the serotonin rhythm (8- and 20-day-old rats) and abolished the NAT cycle (12- and 19- to 20-day-old rats) when they were done several days or more in advance of the chemical measurements.

The sympathetic regulation of the developing rat pineal has also been studied in 12- to 14-day-old rat pups with pharmacological agents [10, 17, 23]. Reserpine, propranolol, trimepranol, and cyclo-heximide blocked the dark-time rise in NAT when they were injected in vivo; the α-blocker phentolamine had no effect. Isoproterenol and epinephrine stimulated NAT in vitro and propranolol blocked in vitro stimulation. Rat pups were more sensitive to in vivo injection of isoproterenol than adults; rat pup pineals were not more sensitive to isoproterenol in vitro. The pineal glands of 2-day-old rats were stimulated by isoproterenol and desmethylimipramine and were in-hibited by propranolol and α-methyl-p-tyrosine [69]. Steroid and thyroxine treatments may alter the rate of development of the NAT responses to adrenergic agents [67, 68].

13.3.5 Biological clock

The presence of rhythm and/or timekeeping abilities within pineal glands has been demonstrated in adult lizards, adult birds, and 3-week-old chicks. Pineals from chicks as young as 9 days old [16] exhibit the clock properties. Pineal glands of 4- to 20-day-old rats are capable of generating a single cycle of NAT in vitro during the first 24 hours of culture [7, 8, 9, 10, 17]. The presence of the cycle is under sympathetic control: it does not occur in pineals from rat pups that were ganglionectomized, and it is blocked by propranolol. Similarly, in vivo, in rat pups whose pineal NAT was measured in the 24 hours immediately following ganglionectomy, NAT increased. In the pups, the ganglia are not required for the first cycle in vivo or in vitro, but are necessary for generation of subsequent cycles. Adult rat pineals did not have the capability for generation of even one cycle in vitro.

13.3.6 Maternal regulation

In rats, it has been possible to examine the interaction of dams and pups with regard to pineal responses to light and dark.

Melatonin is transferred in milk from mother rats to pups [48]. Labeled melatonin injected into the dams was recovered from the milk and from the pups (stomach contents). Neonatal rats given labeled melatonin by stomach tube had labeled melatonin in the plasma, intestine, liver, brain, viscera, and kidney in 15 minutes. Thus the dams could provide melatonin to their pups during the early days after birth when the melatonin rhythm has not fully developed. However, suckling in rats occurs primarily in the daytime. This behavior is probably imposed by the dams since the pups' feeding preference (judged by nipple attachment latency) is nocturnal [20].

The interaction of dams and pups was studied by measuring pineal NAT when the pups were 3 weeks old [15, 52]. When the pups were kept with their mothers, NAT in the mothers and pups peaked at the same time; when the pups were separated from their mothers, NAT peaked in the dark. Blinded pups were synchronized by their mothers but free-ran in the absence of maternal time cues.

Temperature may be a factor in regulation of pineal NAT in developing animals. Dark-time NAT was higher (484 pmol product/pineal/hr) in cool rat pups (b.t. = 27° C) than when they were very cold (b.t. = 7° C, 106 pmol product/pineal/hr) or at normal temperatures (b.t. = 33° C, 97–161 pmol product/pineal/hr) [57].

13.3.7 Reproduction and function

Antigonadal function of the pineal can be obtained in young animals. Rats blinded or injected with testosterone when 3 days old have testes at 72 days old that weigh 2508–2589 mg compared to 3110 mg in normal controls. Testicular inhibition due to blinding but not that caused by testosterone can be reversed by pinealectomy [40]. Testosterone treatment did not prevent an NAT cycle in rats [59]. Hamsters that were blinded delayed testis growth until they were 36 weeks old when growth occurred spontaneously, compared with early growth in controls and pinealectomized hamsters.

Rats (6 hours to 14 days old) were treated with white fluorescent light which reduced serum calcium 0.7–0.9 mg/dl. The effect was prevented by melatonin [19].

Tissue ability to retain melatonin is low in adult rats: the brain retains 61% and the liver retains 11% of labeled melatonin 30 minutes after injection. Five-day-old rats had longer tissue retention of melatonin, with 90% retained in brain and 73% retained in liver after 90 minutes [63]. Data such as these can be used to support the possibility that the pineal could exert differential effects on development by changes in the targets' responses to melatonin rather than by melatonin levels.

13.4 Puberty

There are two approaches that appear in the literature for investigating the possible relationships between the pineal and puberty (sexual maturation). The first approach has been to examine aspects of the pineal itself (e.g., anatomy, biosynthetic activity). The second has been to seek effects related to the pineal (e.g., via pinealectomy or melatonin administration) upon the occurrence or timing of sexual maturation. Both of these directions have been pursued under the hypothesis that the pineal provides a "brake" on sexual maturation, possibly by melatonin secretion. Many of the studies need to be redone or reconsidered in view of more current knowledge of circadian rhythms in pineal function and the possibility of rhythmic ocular formation of melatonin.

13.4.1 Pineal at sexual maturation

Human nocturnal melatonin has been reported to drop 75% by the end of puberty compared to levels in children 1–5 years old [62]. This kind of correlation and the association of pineal tumors with precocious puberty support a pineal role in the puberal process. Poth, Tetsuo, and Markey [35] looked at 6-hydroxymelatonin excretion in humans aged 3–16 years and found only an increase in nighttime melatonin at Tanner stage II of puberty in girls. The day-night increment in melatonin was compared in serum of subjects with early and late puberty and found to be lower (median 70 pg/ml) in the early puberty group and higher (median 115 pg/ml) in the delayed puberty group [2]. However, as discussed by Tamarkin [54], other investigators have failed to find differences between the 24-hour melatonin profiles of prepubertal, pubertal, and adult subjects.

13.4.2 Photoperiod, pinealectomy, and melatonin

The timing of sexual maturation is influenced by photoperiod in some species (e.g., in Djungarian hamsters, cotton rats, and field voles). For example, hamsters (*Phodopus*) raised in short days (LD 10:14) have a slowed rate of body growth, testis growth, less FSH, less LH, and less prolactin than in those raised in long days [66]. However, in other species (golden hamster, collared lemming), puberty is not dependent upon photoperiod [43]. The failure of short photoperiod to forestall sexual maturation in some species has been likened to the spontaneous reproductive recrudescence that occurs when they are maintained in short photoperiods which initially regress the testes.

Pinealectomy removes delaying effects of procedures, such as blinding, on the development of the reproductive system. For example, when female hamsters were blinded before puberty (25 days old) their uteri were atrophic and about one-fourth the normal weight; this inhibition was reversed by pinealectomy [37]. When female rats were blinded and made anosmic, the combined operations delayed reproduction in that their uterine weights were about one-third of the normal weight at 68–70 days of age; pinealectomy reversed the effect [39].

Melatonin administration to developing ewes kept in constant light delayed their normal puberty onset 21 weeks [24]. Melatonin inhibits the ability of rat pituitary cells (from 15-day-old rats) to respond (by releasing LH) to LRH in culture [32]. The investigators suggested that the neonatal pituitary is a target of melatonin.

13.5 Aging

Studies of pineal function in aging have mainly involved the formation of concretions (humans, gerbils), measurement of biosynthetic capabilities (hamsters, gerbils), and effects of pinealectomy and melatonin levels (hamsters).

13.5.1 Anatomy

Researchers who used several different techniques produced results that were quantitatively diverse, but the general trend was the same: pineal calcification increases with age in humans (Fig. 13.4) [26]. Ganglionectomized gerbils had fewer calcium concretions, which may mean that the calcification is a conseqence of secretory activity.

Anatomical changes besides those involving concretions have been described and attributed to age. For example, the area measurements of sparrow pineals decreased from 30 to 180 days of age [36]. Pineals of old (24–30 months) rats were compared to those of young (1-month-old) rats using transmission and scanning electron microscopy [1, 6]. Changes were noted in the glands from the aged rats:

1. An increase in overall thickness of the connective tissue
2. An increase in the number of connective tissue cells and fibers
3. An increase in the number of striated muscle fibers in the connective tissue capsule and parenchyma
4. Increased numbers of vacuoles, dense vesicles, and dense bodies in pinealocytes
5. Mitochondria with dense cores and longitudinally arranged cristae
6. Increase in size of cytoplasmic lipid droplets
7. Presence of myelin-like figures in the stalk
8. Increase in number and size of concretions
9. Nuclear infoldings and cytoplasmic lipofuscin deposits
10. Increase connective tissue fibers and remains of basement membranes in stroma

13.5.2 Melatonin synthesis reduction

Melatonin synthesis has been examined in old animals of several species (rats, gerbils, hamsters). Generally, old animals had reduced

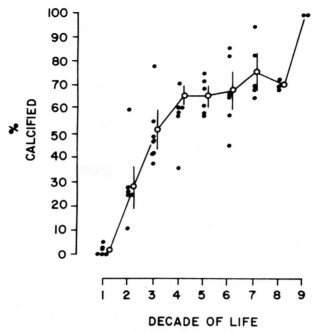

Figure 13.4 Human pineal calcification increases with age. Each closed circle represents the mean for a decade of life from a study by one investigator (70–2724 cases per study); the open circles with standard errors represent the means of the means of the different studies. (From data presented in Kitay and Altschule [26].)

dark-time peaks of pineal and serum melatonin and NAT [25, 42, 43, 56] and a reduction in serotonin. For example, in the golden hamster (with a life span of roughly 2 years) 18-month-old animals had low peak dark-time melatonin (200–300 pg/pineal) compared to pineal melatonin in 2-month-old animals (800–900 pg/pineal) (Fig. 13.5) [39, 42].

13.5.3 Pinealectomy and melatonin

Testes regression in response to natural short photoperiods was greater in young (3 months) than old (20 months) hamsters [44, 45] in one study. However, old (22–26 months) hamsters exhibited a larger testis inhibition response to melatonin injections, but the old hamsters had less weighty testes to begin with [14]. Retinal melatonin was also reduced in old hamsters [38].

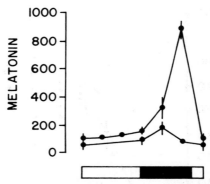

Figure 13.5 Melatonin in 18-month-old golden hamsters (*lower curve*) was reduced compared to that for 2-month-old hamsters. (After Reiter et al. [42].)

REFERENCES

1. Allen, D., L. DiDio, and E. Gentry. 1981. The aged rat pineal gland as revealed in SEM and TEM. *Age* 5:119–126.
2. Attanasio, A., P. Borrelli, R. Marini, P. Cambiaso, M. Cappa, and D. Gupta. 1983. Serum melatonin in children with early and delayed puberty. *Neuroendocrinol. Lett.* 5:387–392.
3. Binkley, S., and E. Geller. 1975. Pineal enzymes in chickens: Development of daily rhythmicity. *Gen. Comp. Endocrinol.* 27:424–429.
4. Binkley, S., S. MacBride, D. Klein, and C. Ralph. 1975. Regulation of pineal rhythms in chickens: Refractory period and nonvisual light perception. *Endocrinology* 96:848–853.
5. Binkley, S., J. Riebman, and K. Reilly. 1978. The pineal gland: A biological clock in vitro. *Science* 202:1198–1201.
6. Boya, J., and J. Calvo. 1984. Structure and ultrastructure of the aging rat pineal gland. *J. Pineal Res.* 1:83–89.
7. Brammer, M., and S. Binkley. 1979. Daily rhythms of serotonin and N-acetyltransferase in chicks. *Comp. Biochem. Physiol.* 63C:305–307.
8. ———. 1981. Pineal glands of immature rats: Rise and fall in N-actyltransferase activity in vitro. *J. Neurobiol.* 12:167–173.
9. Brammer, M., S. Binkley, J. Enrico, and M. Duffy. 1981. The rise and fall of pineal N-acetyltransferase in vitro: The influence of age. *Dev. Biol.* 86:256–258.
10. Brammer, M., S. Binkley, and K. Mosher. 1982. The rise and fall of pineal N-acetyltransferase in vitro: Neural regulation in the developing rat. *J. Neurobiol.* 13:487–494.
11. Calvo, J., and J. Boya. 1978. Embryonic development of the pineal gland of the chicken (*Gallus gallus*). *Acta Anat.* 101:289–303.
12. ———. 1979. Ultrastructural study of the embryonic development of the pineal gland of the chicken (*Gallus gallus*). *Acta Anat.* 103:39–73.
13. ———. 1983. Postnatal development of cell types in the rat pineal gland. *J. Anat.* 137:185–195.

14. Chen, H. 1981. Spontaneous and melatonin-induced testicular regression in male golden hamsters: Augmented sensitivity of the old male to melatonin inhibition. *Neuroendocrinology* 33:43–46.

15. Deguchi, T. 1977. Circadian rhythms of enzyme and running activity under ultradian lighting schedule. *Amer. J. Physiol.* 232:E375–E381.

16. ———. 1979. Circadian rhythm of serotonin N-acetyltransferase activity in organ culture of chicken pineal gland. *Science* 203:1245–1247.

17. ———. 1982. Sympathetic regulation of circadian rhythm of serotonin N-acetyltransferase activity in pineal gland of infant rat. *J. Neurochem.* 38:797–802.

18. Ellison, N., J. Weller, and D. Klein. 1972. Development of a circadian rhythm in the activity of pineal serotonin N-acetyltransferase. *J. Neurochem.* 19:1335–1341.

19. Håkanson, D., and W. Bergstrom. 1981. Phototherapy-induced hypocalcemia in newborn rats: Prevention by melatonin. *Science* 214:807–809.

20. Henning, S. 1980. Nocturnal feeding behavior in the neonatal rat. *Physiol. Behav.* 25:603–605.

21. Illnerová, H. 1972. The effect of light on the development of a diurnal rhythm in serotonin content and on the development of hydroxyindole-O-methyltransferase activity in the rat pineal gland. *Activ. Nerv. Sup.* (Praha) 14:130–131.

22. ———. 1975. The effect of constant light from birth on the appearance of diurnal rhythm in serotonin content in the rat epiphysis. *Devel. Biol.* 46:418–421.

23. Illnerová, H., and J. Škopková. 1976. Regulation of the diurnal rhythm in rat pineal serotonin N-acetyltransferase activity and serotonin content during ontogenesis. *J. Neurochem.* 26:1051–1052.

24. Kennaway, D. 1984. Pineal function in ungulates. In *Pineal research reviews II*, ed. R. Reiter, pp. 113–140. New York: Alan R. Liss.

25. King, T., B. Richardson, and R. Reiter. 1981. Age associated changes in pineal serotonin N-acetyltransferase activity and melatonin content in the male gerbil. *Endocrine Res. Comm.* 8:253–262.

26. Kitay, J., and M. Altschule. 1954. *The pineal gland.* Cambridge, Mass.: Harvard Univ. Press.

27. Klein, D. 1972. Evidence for the placental transfer of 3H-acetyl-melatonin. *Nature (New Biol.)* 237:117.

28. Klein, D., and S. Lines. 1969. Pineal hydroxyindole-O-methyltransferase activity in the growing rat. *Endocrinology* 84:1523–1525.

29. Klein, D., M. Namboodiri, and D. Auerbach. 1981. The melatonin rhythm generating system: Developmental aspects. *Life Sci.* 28:1975–1986.

30. Machado, C., A. Machado, and L. Wragg. 1969. Circadian serotonin rhythm control: Sympathetic and nonsympathetic pathways in rat pineals of different ages. *Endocrinology* 85:846–848.

31. Machado, C., L. Wragg, and A. Machado. 1969. Circadian rhythm of serotonin in the pineal body of immunosympathectomized immature rats. *Science* 164:442–443.

32. Martin, J. 1982. Melatonin effects on pituitary function during development. In *Melatonin rhythm generating system*, ed. D. Klein, pp. 232–249. Basel, Switzerland: Karger.

33. Omura, Y. 1977. Ultrastructural study of embryonic and post-hatching development in the pineal organ of the chick (Brown Leghorn, *Gallus domesticus*). *Cell Tiss. Res.* 183:255–271.

34. Oshima, K., and S. Matsuo. 1984. Functional morphology of the pineal gland in young chickens. *Anat. Anz. Jena* 156:407–418.

35. Poth, M., M. Tetsuo, and S. Markey. 1982. 6-Hydroxymelatonin excretion during childhood and puberty. In *Melatonin rhythm generating system*, ed. D. Klein, pp. 204–209. New York: Karger.

36. Ralph, C., and K. B. Lane. 1969. Morphology of the pineal body of wild house sparrows (*Passer domesticus*) in relation to reproduction and age. *Can. J. Zool.* 47:1205–1208.

37. Reiter, R. 1969. Growth of the endocrine organs of female hamsters blinded at 25 days of age. *Experientia* 25:751–752.

38. Reiter, R., C. Craft, J. Johnson, T. King, B. Richardson, G. Vaughan, and M. Vaughan. 1981. Age-associated reduction in nocturnal pineal melatonin levels in female rats. *Endocrinology* 109:1295–1297.

39. Reiter, R., and N. Ellison. 1970. Delayed puberty in blinded and anosmic female rats: Role of the pineal gland. *Biol. Reprod.* 2:216–222.

40. Reiter, R., J. Hoffman, and P. Rubin. 1968. Pineal gland: Influence on gonads of male rats treated with androgen three days after birth. *Science* 160:420–421.

41. Reiter, R., L. Johnson, R. Steger, B. Richardson, and L. Petterborg. 1980. Pineal biosynthetic activity and neuroendocrine physiology in the aging hamster and gerbil. *Peptides* 1:69–77.

42. Reiter, R., B. Richardson, L. Johnson, B. Ferguson, and D. Dinh. 1980. Pineal melatonin rhythm: Reduction in aging Syrian hamsters. *Science* 210:1372–1374.

43. Reiter, R., S. Sorrentino, and R. Hoffman. 1970. Early photoperiodic conditions and pineal antigonadal function in male hamsters. *Int. J. Fertility* 15:163–170.

44. Reiter, R., W. Trakulrungsi, C. Trakulrungsi, J. Vriend, W. Morgan, M. Vaughan, L. Johnson, B. Richardson. 1982. Pineal melatonin production: Endocrine and age effects. In *Melatonin rhythm generating system*, ed. D. Klein, pp. 143–154. Basel, Switzerland: Karger.

45. Reiter, R., J. Vriend, G. Brainard, S. Matthews, and C. Craft. 1982. Reduced pineal and plasma melatonin levels and gonadal atrophy in old hamsters kept under winter photoperiods. *Exp. Aging Res.* 8:27–30.

46. Reppert, S. 1982. Maternal melatonin: A source of melatonin for the immature animal. In *Melatonin rhythm generating system*, ed. D. Klein, pp. 182–192. Basel, Switzerland: Karger.

47. Reppert, S., R. Chez, A. Anderson, and D. Klein. 1979. Maternal-fetal transfer of melatonin in the non-human primate. International Pediatric Research Foundation, Inc. pp. 788–791.

48. Reppert, S., and D. Klein. 1978. Transport of maternal 3H-melatonin to suckling rats and the fate of 3H-melatonin in the neonatal rat. *Endocrinology* 102:582–588.

49. Reppert, S., and W. Schwartz. 1983. Maternal coordination of the fetal biological clock in utero. *Science* 220:969–971.

50. ———. 1984. The suprachiasmatic nuclei of the fetal rat: Characterization

of a functional circadian clock using ^{14}C-labeled deoxyglucose. *J. Neurosci.* 4:1677–1682.

51. Sheridan, M., and M. Rollag. 1983. Development and melatonin content of the deep pineal gland in the Syrian hamster. *Amer. J. Anat.* 168:145–156.

52. Takahashi, K., and T. Deguchi. 1983. Entrainment of the circadian rhythms of blinded infant rats by nursing mothers. *Physiol. Behavior* 31:373–378.

53. Takahashi, J., H. Hamm, and M. Menaker. 1980. Circadian rhythms of melatonin release from individual superfused chicken pineal glands in vitro. *Proc. Natl. Acad. Sci. USA* 77:2319–2322.

54. Tamarkin, L. 1984. Melatonin: A coordinating signal for mammalian reproduction. *Science* 227:714–720.

55. Tamarkin, L., S. Reppert, D. Orloff, D. Klein, S. Yellon, and B. Goldman. 1980. Ontogeny of the pineal melatonin rhythm in the Syrian (*Mesocricetus auratus*) and Siberian (*Phodopus sungorus*) hamsters and in the rat. *Endocrinology* 107:1061–1064.

56. Tang, F., M. Hadjiconstantinou, and S. Pang. 1985. Aging and diurnal rhythms of pineal serotonin, 5-hydroxyindoleacetic acid, norepinephrine, dopamine and serum melatonin in the male rat. *Neuroendocrinology* 40:160–164.

57. Ulrich, R., A. Yuwiler, L. Wetterberg, and D. Klein. 1973/74. Effects of light and temperature on the pineal gland in suckling rats. *Neuroendocrinology* 13:255–263.

58. Vaněcěk, J., and H. Illnerová. 1979. The regulation of pineal serotonin N-acetyltransferase activity in newborn rats. *Dev. Biol.* 68:287–291.

59. ———. 1982. Effect of photoperiod on the growth of reproductive organs and on pineal N-acetyltransferase rhythm in male rats treated neonatally with testosterone propionate. *Biol. Reprod.* 27:517–522.

60. Vollrath, L. 1981. *The pineal organ.* Berlin: Springer-Verlag.

61. Wainwright, S., and L. Wainwright. 1980. Regulation of the cycle in chick pineal serotonin-N-acetyltransferase activity in vitro by light. *J. Neurochem.* 35:451–457.

62. Waldhauser, F., H. Lynch, and R. Wurtman. 1984. Melatonin in human body fluids: Clinical significance. In *The pineal gland,* ed. R. Reiter, pp. 345–370. New York: Raven Press.

63. Weinberg, U. 1981. Evidence that melatonin retention by the neonatal rat is greatly increased as compared to the adult. A novel biochemical mechanism. *Brain Res.* 217:221–224.

64. Wetterberg, L., E. Geller, and A. Yuwiler. 1970. Harderian gland: An extraretinal photoreceptor influencing the pineal gland in neonatal rats? *Science* 167:884–885.

65. Wetterberg, L., A. Yuwiler, R. Ulrich, E. Geller, and R. Wallace. 1970. Harderian gland: Influence on pineal HIOMT in neonatal rats. *Science* 170:194–196.

66. Yellon, S., and B. Goldman. 1984. Photoperiod control of reproductive development in the male Djungarian hamster (*Phodopus sungorus*). *Endocrinology* 114:664–670.

67. Yuwiler, A. 1982. Sympathetic innervation of the pineal gland: Effect of

thyroxine and cortisol. In *Melatonin rhythm generating system*, ed. D. Klein, pp. 42–61. Basel, Switzerland: Karger.

68. Yuwiler, A., and G. Brammer. 1981. Neonatal hormone treatment and maturation of the pineal noradrenergic system: Hydrocortisone and thyroxine. *J. Neurochem.* 37:985–992.

69. Yuwiler, A., D. Klein, M. Buda, and J. Weller. 1977. Adrenergic control of pineal *N*-acetyltransferase activity: Developmental aspects. *Amer. J. Physiol.* 2:E141–E146.

70. Zweig, M. 1968. The development of serotonin and serotinin-related enzymes in the pineal gland of the rat. *Comm. Behav. Biol.* A1:103–108.

71. Zweig, M., S. Snyder, and J. Axelrod. 1966. Evidence for a nonretinal pathway of light to the pineal gland of newborn rats. *Proc. Nat. Acad. Sci. USA* 56:515–520.

14

Comparative Pineal Endocrinology: Mammals

"Long-term implants releasing a small quantity of melatonin (45 nanograms per day) were used to determine the brain sites of the hormone's antigonadal action in a photoperiodic species, the white-footed mouse (*Peromyscus leucopus*). Implants in the medial preoptic and supra- and retrochiasmatic areas elicited complete gonadal regression after 7 weeks. Implants in other brain regions had little effect on the animals' reproductive state."

J. Glass and G. Lynch [12]

"To determine which parameter of the day/night pattern of pineal melatonin secretion is the critical component signaling daylength information in the Djungarian hamster, we have developed a method for giving timed sc [subcutaneous] melatonin infusions in pinealectomized juvenile males. When given for 12 h daily as little as 10 ng melatonin (14 pg/min) consistently induced testicular regression within 12 days. However, 10 ng melatonin infused for 4 or 6 h daily did not inhibit gonadal development."

D. Carter and B. Goldman [9]

14.1 Vertebrates in General

14.1.1 Introduction

The pineal is an example of an endocrine system where the comparative anatomy and physiology have been particularly important to the discovery and understanding of its function [3, 4, 71]. This chapter and the one that follows contain summaries for selected species representing all the classes of vertebrates. Species were chosen for one or more of the following reasons: (1) they were useful in developing key information for pineal function; (2) they were representatives of a vertebrate class; and (3) they were extensively studied.

There are several reasons to consider the mammals separately from the birds and lower vertebrates. First, more species of mammals have been studied in detail so that there is a division by amount of information available for examination. Second, mammals generally lack pineal light sensitivity and their pineal circadian clock is driven by outside signals. In contrast, pineal light perception and circadian rhythm generation have been established for a number of birds and lower vertebrates.

For each of the species, a number of parameters may be considered: anatomy, chemistry, photoreception, neural regulation, biological clock, reproduction, and color. While there are only a few totally applicable generalizations, there are many features of anatomy, biochemistry, and function that are present in several species.

14.1.2 Some generalizations and observations

It may be helpful to point out a potpourri of generalizations and observations that have been made about the pineal gland, and, for some of these, to outline the exceptions to them. This exercise is more than academic since those attributes present in most pineal glands must be fundamental to its function. Moreover, the exceptions, like variations on a theme, must derive from the basic abilities of the gland.

One interesting comparative observation was made by Quay [45, 46] in a study of 28 species of rodents. There was a 90-fold difference between the highest and lowest pineal volumes and there was a correlation between pineal volume and latitude: more northerly species had greater pineal volumes (the volumes were adjusted for body weight).

A second idea is widely held, that the pineal has evolved from a more photoreceptor-like to a more endocrine-like gland. The generalization that a developmental sequence reflects evolutionary trends is encapsulated in the phrase "ontogeny recapitulates phylogeny." There are at least three instances where this generalization can be applied to the pineal. (1) Ontogeny appears to recapitulate phylogeny in the presence or absence of photoreceptor-like cells. In terms of evolution, there is evidence of more highly developed photoreceptor-like cells in the lower vertebrates but less evidence for photoreceptor-like structures (outer segments) in higher vertebrates. In terms of development, photoreceptor-like pinealocytes are seen in neonatal rats but not in adults. (2) Recapitulation of the phylogeny has been suggested by investigators attempting to demonstrate extraretinal light reception (found in birds and the lower vertebrates) in developing rats. (3) Pineals of birds and lizards are capable of generating N-acetyltransferase (NAT) and melatonin cycles in vitro. Adult rat pineals do not have this ability, but pineals of neonatal rats are capable of one cycle in culture.

Still other observations are: Species differences in gross and fine anatomy (Fig. 14.1) may be correlated with specific functions of the pineal in a given species: (1) the pineal may develop as a single organ (as in mammals) or as part of a complex of organs (as in lizards); (2) variation occurs in the degree to which pinealocytes are similar to retinal photoreceptor cells.

Nighttime synthesis of melatonin in adult pineals seems to be universal. Variation occurs in (1) the neural regulation of the process, which, for example, is dependent upon sympathetic signals in rats and is more independent in birds; (2) the extent to which extrapineal rhythmic melatonin synthesis occurs (ocular melatonin rhythms rival pineal in some birds); (3) the degree of sensitivity to light, especially in the rapid plummet response; (4) the modification by photoperiod, which takes one of two patterns: alteration of dark-time duration or phase.

The author views "time" relationships as crucial to pineal function. Pineal function depends on species, season, stage of life, and time of day. There is circadian clock involvement in all pineal functions; however, there is specialization in different animals: (1) the pineal is capable of self-generated oscillations in some birds and lower vertebrates; but this ability appears to be lost in mammals; (2) pineal light perception is confined to the birds and lower vertebrates and seems to be lost in adult mammals; (3) pineal involvement in reproductive function is developed in animals, especially in seasonal breeders, but the evidence for pineal involvement in avian reproduction is so far sparse; (4) melatonin control of circadian behavioral rhythms is found in birds and lizards but appears to be reduced in mammals; and (5) rapid skin color responses to melatonin are confined to lower vertebrates; changes in pelage coloration that may be influenced by the pineal are found in mammals that exhibit seasonal coat color changes.

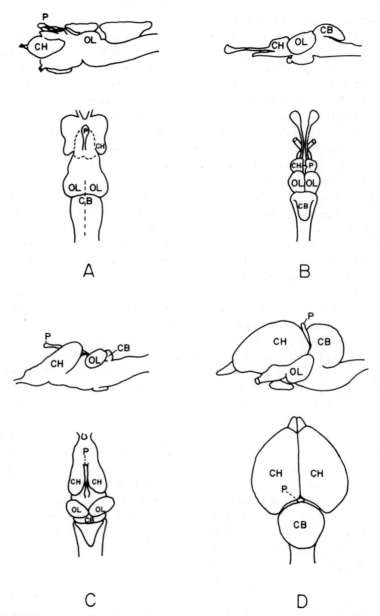

Figure 14.1 Diagrammatic representation of the gross anatomy of brains showing the location of the pineal in (A) lampreys, (B) teleost fish, (C) frogs, and (D) birds. CH = cerebral hemisphere; OL = optic lobe; CB = cerebellum; P = pineal. (After Reiter [51]; Romer [63]; and Vollrath [75].)

14.2 Mammals

The work with mammals has concentrated on rodents with some studies of humans, nonhuman primates, and ungulates. Most of the work falls into established patterns for the pineal. All mammals studied synthesize melatonin in the dark-time (see Table 10.1) irrespective of whether their behavior is nocturnal (hamsters, rats, mice) or diurnal (humans, monkeys, ground squirrels, sheep). (NAT activity, an indicator of melatonin synthesis, is shown for various species in Table 14.1.) Mammals, especially rats, were used to establish the neural pathway for pineal regulation by light and its relationship to the hypothalamus. Mammals, especially hamsters, were the group in which the pineal role in reproduction was established.

14.2.1 Humans

Most of the work with primates has been with humans (see Chapter 12) although there is some work with a variety of species of nonhuman primates.

The pineal was named for its pine-cone-like shape in humans. The human pineal can be a variety of colors (grey, white, yellow, red); there is a pineal recess in the third ventricle and the pineal is in the subarachnoid space and thus has access to cerebrospinal fluid (CSF) [75]. Human pinealocytes are polymorphic (different shapes with single, double, or more processes). The noteworthy aspect of human pineal anatomy has been the formation of concretions.

TABLE 14.1 N-acetyltransferase (NAT) activity comparisons (nmol/pineal/hr)

Organism	Light	Dark	Assay[a]
Human	3.9	4.3	S
Albino rat	0.2	2.8	S
Albino rat	0.2	22.8	T
Mexican Ground squirrel	0.5	2.7	S
Richardson's Ground squirrel	0.2	2.0	T
Eastern chipmunk	0.2	1.4	T
Guinea pig	0.7	1.0	T
Hamster	0.2	0.6	T
Gerbil	0.1	0.3	T
Chicken	1.8	47.0	S
Sparrow	0.2	3.8	S
Quail	0.3	6.1	S

Sources: Binkley [4] and Underwood et al. [72].
[a] S = serotonin substrate in the assay; T = trytamine substrate in the assay.

The human pineal contains the necessary substrates and enzymes for melatonin synthesis. Rhythmic melatonin production has been confirmed by the occurrence of melatonin at night in body fluids. There is evidence for regulation by light and dark—the rhythm is synchronized with environmental cycles. Light at night reduces melatonin but the light must be brighter than that required by some other species. Human serum sampled for melatonin at 20-minute intervals exhibited single high values up to 700 pg/ml which was taken as evidence for (1) episodic melatonin secretion in humans, and (2) melatonin half-life in humans of less than 30 minutes [78].

The evidence for human pineal function in reproduction is circumstantial. Precocious puberty associated with pineal tumors precipitated interest in the pineal in general in reproductive function.

14.2.2 Nonhuman primates

Pineals in nonhuman primates are not necessarily pine cone shaped, but are more elongated. Pineals of orangutans (*Pongo pygmaeus*) and rhesus monkeys (*Macaca macaca*) have relatively extensive contact with the CSF [75]. Pineals of some primates have NAT, hydroxyindole-O-methyltransferase (HIOMT), and melatonin. Daily profiles of serum melatonin in rhesus monkeys had dark-time levels three times the day levels [8]; however, the rhythms were apparent in only three of eight individual animals. In contrast, the serum prolactin rhythm (also two to three times higher at night) was present in all eight animals. Melatonin was high at night in rhesus monkey CSF [60].

Evidence for a pineal role in primate reproduction is scant. Unusually high melatonin (up to 410 pg/ml serum) was measured in a rhesus monkey that was anovulatory; melatonin of ovulating females' peaked at less than 150 pg/ml.

14.2.3 Sheep

Information on the physiological role of the pineal in large mammals is of particular interest because of potential use of the information in managing the reproductive capabilities of economically important species (sheep, goats, pigs, cows, etc.) [20]. Pineals from some of these species (particularly the cow) have been available in large quantities from slaughter houses and have been used in attempts to isolate putative pineal hormones or metabolites. While deer provide examples of more feral animals, sheep have been one of the most studied domestic animals. The sheep pineal is pea-like (4.5–7.5 mm; 69 mg) and is the proximal type with most of the gland found near the third ventricle [75].

Sheep pineal melatonin in different studies ranged from 0.8 to 4.0 ng/mg [20]. Because of the large blood volume of these animals, they

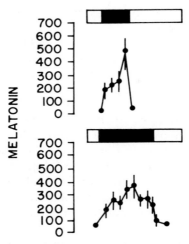

Figure 14.2 Melatonin profiles in the blood of sheep kept in long photoperiod (*top*) and short photoperiod (*bottom*). (After data in Bittman et al. [7].)

are particularly useful in studies where serial sampling of blood is a requirement. About 99.5% of circulating melatonin in the blood of sheep comes from the pineal, but there is also detectable melatonin in pinealectomized sheep. HIOMT has been detected in sheep pineal and was greatest in fetal pineals (dropping 5–6 days prior to parturition) and may vary with stage of estrous cycle.

Sheep pineal melatonin synthesis is responsive to light and dark. Sheep pineal NAT is higher at night (3.1 nmol/min/mg protein) than in the day (1.1 nmol/min/mg protein). Pineal HIOMT is 0.11–0.14 nmol/min/mg protein. Pineal 5-HT (serotonin) is 2.3 ng/mg wet weight in the day and 0.2 ng/mg wet weight in the night. Pineal melatonin is 1.2 ng/mg wet weight at night and 0.2 ng/mg wet weight in the day [34]. Plasma melatonin exhibits peak levels in the dark-time (100–300 pg/ml) and a nadir in the light-time (10–50 pg/ml). The rhythm persists in constant dark with increased amplitude (peaks up to about 450 pg/ml) and is attenuated in constant light (peaks less than 100 pg/ml) [62]. The duration of high melatonin in blood responds to light and dark (6 hours in LD 8:16; 14 hours in LD 16:8; see Fig. 14.2) [6, 7, 24]. One hour of light imposed in the late dark-time of LD 10:14 depresses circulating melatonin for the rest of the dark-time and damps the amplitude of the second cycle measured in DD [10].

Sheep are autumn breeders, and the ewes exhibit an estrous cycle that begins in the fall and recurs every 16 days until spring. The 16-day cycle is not altered by pinealectomy. There is a possible feedback relationship of the reproductive system and the pineal. The melatonin profile varies with phase of the estrous cycle [2]. Moreover, melatonin levels are three times normal in ewes 16 days after ovariectomy [1].

The onset of puberty in sheep was delayed by combined melatonin and constant light treatment, and prolactin was inhibited. Pinealectomy also inhibited puberty onset; puberty normally occurs at 44 weeks but with melatonin implants puberty occurred at 45 to more than 72 weeks of age [21].

Melatonin has been given to sheep by subcutaneous injections, in food, in continuous implants, and in infusions. Melatonin implants augmented plasma melatonin but did not alter the plasma melatonin rhythm; melatonin did not feed back to inhibit its own synthesis [23] but did lower plasma prolactin levels. Melatonin-fed ewes began cycling 78 to more than 103 days compared to control ewes that exhibited cycles of 65–88 days; thus melatonin delayed the onset of cyclicity [22].

Estradiol normally inhibits luteinizing hormone (LH) secretion in the ewe. Short photoperiods reduced the response to estradiol, but when ewes were pinealectomized, short days did not have the effect. When pinealectomized ewes were treated with melatonin infusions that mimicked long and short photoperiods, melatonin infusion with long duration (mimicking a long night) acted like the short days: the response to estradiol was decreased [6, 69]. Bittman et al. [7] have hypothesized that melatonin mediates daylength in the sheep by acting on an ensemble of neurons (in the hypothalamus) that control LH.

14.2.4 Deer

The pineal story is less easily developed in deer because several species have been subjects of study and the amount of information for each species is small.

White-tailed deer (*Odocoileus virginianus*) have seasonal changes that are cyclic and whose exact timing depends on latitude. For example, at 46°N, there are annual changes in antler development and shedding (mature by October–November; shed in December–February), testis size (small in March–June, largest in October), plasma testosterone levels (peak in October), male neck enlargement (peak in October–November), heat (November), fawning (June), coat color (molt to summer tan in June, molt to winter gray in September), metabolic rate (low in winter), blood volume (low in February–March), thyroxine (decreases in late winter), and heart rate (decreases in late winter) [44]. Some of the annual changes, such as antlers, are a consequence of changes in the reproductive hormones. The seasonal cycles in the physiology of deer respond to photoperiod, and they appear to have an endogenous component.

The effects of pinealectomy on antlerogenesis, neck swelling, body growth, and hormone levels were determined in red deer hinds, *Cervus elaphus* [77]. When deer were pinealectomized (March) they did not show a full fall neck growth or testis size increase. The annual plasma testosterone peak was delayed from November to March, antlerogenesis was delayed 2–3 months, peak body weight occurred in March instead of November, and winter coats were retained longer. Alterations of the seasonal cycles of LH and prolactin followed pinealectomy.

14.2.5 Laboratory rats

Pineals have been more extensively investigated in rodents than in any other group of vertebrates, probably because rodents include readily available laboratory species (rats, golden hamsters, gerbils) and wild species that can be maintained in the laboratory (mice, ground squirrels, Djungarian hamsters). Nocturnal (rats, hamsters, mice, gerbils) and diurnal (ground squirrels) species have been studied. The nocturnal albino laboratory rat (*Rattus norvegicus*) has been particularly useful for studying pineal biochemical responses to light and dark, pineal neural regulation, and the pineal melatonin generating system [5, 26].

The superficial pineal of rats (97.9–99.5% of the pineal) is club shaped with distal thickening (820–1950 μm; about 1.5 mg). Some (18%) rat pineals have a thin stalk to a small deep pineal (lamina intercalaris), but the stalk is missing in 6% of rats and interrupted in the remaining majority of rats. The structure extends from the third ventricle (deep) to just beneath the skull (superficial). Neonatal rat pinealocytes have structures that resemble pineal photoreceptors of lower vertebrates (i.e., with apical knobs and cilia-bearing bulges). Rat pinealocytes are arranged in cords, follicles, or rosettes [75].

The rat pineal melatonin-generating system is well characterized. Serotonin is high in the day and low at night; NAT, *N*-acetylserotonin (NAS), and melatonin peak in the dark-time; HIOMT is slightly higher at night. The indole changes can be explained by NAT and by the responses of NAT patterns to light and dark: entrainment of NAT rhythms to light-dark cycles, free-running rhythms of NAT in DD, attenuation of NAT rhythms by LL, refractory period for stimulation of NAT by dark in the early subjective day, and rapid plummet of NAT in response to light at night. Duration of high NAT depends on length of the dark-time. Phase advances occur in response to light pulses in the late subjective night; phase delays occur in response to light pulses in the early subjective night. The eyes are the photoreceptors for the light responses in adult rats; blinding abolishes the response to constant light and the rapid plummet.

Properties of pineal enzymes have been studied in rats. For example, properties of NAT—thermal instability, protection by acetyl CoA and cysteamine, inhibition by disulfides—were first established using rat pineal NAT. Rat retina has NAT and melatonin, but the rhythm in NAT is very small compared to the pineal gland. Removing the pineal from rats eliminates most, but not all, circulating melatonin.

The rat has been the animal model for the determination of the neural regulation of the pineal. In rats, light is perceived by the eyes. The information is transmitted to the suprachiasmatic nuclei (SCN) via a retinohypothalamic tract. The SCN is the source of circadian signals that are sent by a neural pathway to the superior cervical ganglia (SCG). The pineal is innervated by projections from the SCG. Norepineprine from the nerve terminals stimulates NAT and promotes melatonin production in the dark-time. There is evidence for β-adrenergic receptors (Section 6.3) and for cAMP acting as a second messenger (Section 6.4).

Adult rat pineals are not capable of generating a circadian rhythm in vitro; however, pineals of neonatal rats show one cycle of NAT or serotonin when they are placed in culture. Pinealectomy (removing the superficial pineal) does not abolish locomotor rhythms in rats. It produces only subtle changes in the locomotor rhythm of rats, more rapid phase adjustments to reversal of light-dark cycles. However, daily injections of melatonin (5 mg) synchronized the locomotor rhythm of rats with activity beginning near the time of the melatonin injection when melatonin would normally increase [49].

Elucidation of the role of the rat pineal in reproduction has been problematic. Laboratory rats are not markedly photoperiodic; that is, they are not strict seasonal breeders as are some other species of mammals. Therefore, it may not be unreasonable that pineal function in reproduction of rats is less well defined than in some other rodents. The sensitivity to pinealectomy can be increased in rats with factors that potentiate the retardation or regression of the reproductive system that occurs in blind rats: neonatal steroid treatment, anosmia, or food deprivation. Since pineal melatonin synthesis is normal in these situations, the potentiation may be due to increased sensitivity to pineal products [51].

Light deprivation slows growth and development of the reproductive systems of both sexes (e.g., testis, accessory organs, ventral prostate, ovary, uterus) and retards vaginal introitus. The inhibitory effect of blinding can be exacerbated by steroid hormone injections (e.g., 1 mg testosterone propionate at 5 days of age). The development in light-deprived rats was speeded by pinealectomy and mimicked by melatonin [61].

Once rats achieve adulthood, reproductive inhibition by blinding is small. However, the effects on the reproductive system can be magnified by several factors. First, potentiation by anosmia (olfactory bulb removal) occurs. Pinealectomy speeds reproductive development and inhibits regression in blind anosmic rats. Second, underfeeding together with blinding retards development of testes in rats; here again, pinealectomy overcomes the effects.

Melatonin effects on laboratory rat reproduction are less dramatic than its effects in some other species. Positive melatonin effects include delay of ovarian growth, decrease in incidence of estrous smears, decrease in LH in castrated male rats, decrease in follicle stimulating hormone (FSH), increase in prolactin, and depression of ovulation and LH in rats treated with pregnant mare's serum (PMS). Melatonin was more effective as an antigonadotropin in rats given one of the potentiating treatments such as food deprivation or anosmia.

In contrast to the results supporting an antigonadotropic hormone (e.g., melatonin) from the pineal, there is evidence that melatonin is counterantigonadotrophic in rats when subcutaneous implants of melatonin in beeswax are used.

14.2.6 Golden hamsters

The nocturnal golden hamster (*Mesocricetus auratus*, Syrian hamster) has been particularly useful for determining the pineal role in reproduction (see Section 7.4) [51]. The golden hamster has a deep pineal (80–280 μm, 3–12% of the pineal tissue) and a superficial pineal (600–820 μm). The two are connected by a long stalk (2700–3200 μm) that is not parenchymal but which consists of axons, blood vessels, and occasional clusters of pinealocyte-like cells.

Hamster pineal glands have serotonin, NAS, melatonin, NAT, and HIOMT. NAT and melatonin peak in the dark-time, and light exposure at night causes a rapid plummet. When the dark-time is lengthened, the duration of high NAT or melatonin does not change dramatically as in some other species; the decline in melatonin occurs just before lights-on. The hamster pineal is regulated by light and dark with the eyes acting as the photoreceptor.

The hamster reproductive system is exquisitely sensitive to photoperiod. The critical photoperiod is 12.5 hours in males. Male hamsters have large testes in long photoperiods. Female hamsters have 4-day estrous cycles (the cycles can be detected by observing elongated and oval nucleated cells in vaginal smears every 4 days); there is a surge in LH every fourth day (proestrous, preovulatory, afternoon). When light is reduced (via blinding, short photoperiod, or constant dark), the testes become small in the male, and estrous cycling is lost in the female (reduction of estrous smear incidence characteristic of anovulation). There is a LH and FSH surge every day even when the hamsters are ovariectomized, and prolactin levels drop 60–80%.

The testes of most pinealectomized male hamsters do not regress when the hamsters are deprived of light (via short days, constant dark, or blinding). Melatonin injections in the late light-time or late dark-time inhibited the testes; continuous melatonin administration with

Silastic capsules sometimes inhibited the testes; melatonin implants, however, were counterantigonadotrophic in some studies.

Pinealectomy prevents the pattern of reproductive inhibition seen in female hamsters that are deprived of light—estrous cycles persist. Injections of melatonin result in loss of the estrous cycle when the injections are in the late light-time (10 or 12 hours after lights-on, LD 14:10). Melatonin implants mimicked the effects of pinealectomy, a counterantigonadotrophic effect.

The neural regulatory pathway (eyes → SCN → SCG → pineal) proposed for rats is also supported in golden hamsters because bilateral ganglionectomy and lesions have the same effects on reproduction as pinealectomy [43]. However, β-adrenergic agents (isoproterenol injections, norepinephrine in organ culture) do not stimulate hamster pineal NAT [3] or melatonin, though blockers (propranolol) inhibit the pineal melatonin rhythm. It may be possible to explain the results and confirm the pathway (which do not agree with those in rats) because norepinephrine stimulates hamster pineal melatonin synthesis when it is combined with an MAO inhibitor such as desipramine [52].

Although most of the golden hamster work has concerned the pineal and reproduction, there are some other findings of interest. Hibernating golden hamsters have reduced plasma melatonin [73]. Melatonin injections increased eye weight [47]. Circadian rhythms of hamsters have not been markedly affected by pinealectomy or exogenous melatonin; however, lesions of the hypothalamus (SCN, paraventricular nuclei) altered locomotor rhythms in hamsters [43].

14.2.7 Djungarian hamsters

The nocturnal Djungarian hamster (*Phodopus sungorus sungorus*, Siberian, hairy-footed) exhibits seasonal changes (at 48°N latitude) in (1) testis weight (low in fall) and related androgen dependent parameters (spermatogenesis, accessory gland weight, abdominal marking gland weight); (2) body weight (30% less in winter with a 70% reduction in total body fat and an increase in brown fat); (3) pelage color (gray-brown in summer, whitish in winter); MSH (high in summer, low in winter); and daily torpor (in winter only). These seasonal physiological changes are responsive to photoperiod [33]. Body weight and pelage changes persist in castrated animals; photoperiod influences hamsters as early as 7–14 days of age, and short photoperiods delay reproductive development and molt to summer coat. The critical photoperiod is 13 hours, and 1 minute of light during the dark-time was sufficient to mimic long photoperiod.

NAT and melatonin patterns are affected by photoperiod in pineals of Djungarian hamsters. For example, the duration of high NAT was determined by the length of the dark (high 12 hours in LD 16:8; high

6 hours in LD 8:16) [14, 18]. One minute of light after 8 hours of dark in LD 8:16 reduced NAT, and NAT did not rise again, mimicking the long-day pattern. Hamsters have a cycle in pineal melatonin levels that is detectable as early as 15 days of age; at 60–75 days of age, day values are lower (50 pg/pineal) than night values (1200 pg/pineal) [68, 70]. The pineal melatonin rhythm free-runs: peak melatonin (1000 pg/pineal) occurred when free-running animals were active in constant dark, and nadir levels of melatonin (10 pg/pineal) occurred during hamster inactivity [84].

Pinealectomy retarded development of the testes, accessory glands, body weight, and change to summer pelage in long photoperiods. Pinealectomy also partially prevented the inhibitory effects of short days.

Melatonin implants delayed testicular development in young hamsters kept in long photoperiods and inhibited the size of adult gonads. However, when melatonin was implanted in early summer animals, it did not cause gonad regression, but it prevented the inhibitory effect of short photoperiods. Late in the summer, melatonin caused testicular regression. Pelage and weight were affected in parallel with the testis changes (late summer melatonin produced winter molt; winter melatonin retarded change to summer pelage). Thus it would appear that the effects of melatonin in Djungarian hamsters depend upon season of administration. Daily infusions (for 4–6 hours, with varied infusion onset time) of 10 ng melatonin per animal did not inhibit gonad development; melatonin infusion for 7–8 hours did, however, regress the testes [9, 14]. The timing of a melatonin infusion is important as is the duration. Short infusions inhibit the gonads when given during times that would augment the length of the endogenous melatonin peak [14]. Such duration is important even before the hamsters are born. When dams were infused with melatonin for 8 hours, the testes of the male offspring grew more than when the dams received 6-hour infusions at night; the offspring of pinealectomized dams had smaller testes [76].

14.2.8 Gerbils

The gerbil (*Meriones unguiculatus*) has an elongate (2.5–2.8 mm) pineal with superficial and deep parts connected by a parenchymal stalk to give a dumbell shape [75]. The deep pineal pinealocytes in the pineal recess are in contact with the CSF [80]. The pinealocytes are arranged in lobules separated by interstitial cells. Components of the cells exhibit changes with time of day [82, 83]. The gerbil pineal contains concretions (acervuli) composed of hydroxyapatite, like human pineal concretions. Gerbil concretions are spherical (10–65 μm) and are located in vacuoles. Human concretions have smaller, more condensed crystals; otherwise the acervuli of humans and gerbils are similar [27, 81]. The gerbil has thus provided an animal model in which to study pineal concretions.

The pineal NAT rhythm was measured in the gerbil; peak NAT in the dark-time (0.27 nmol/pineal/hr) was three times the daytime level [64]. NAT is quantitatively low in gerbils, and the day-night difference is small compared to other species. Norepinephrine levels did not exhibit a daily cycle, even though the gerbil pineal contains as much norepinephrine as the fivefold larger rat pineal [33]. It may be noteworthy that gerbil locomotor rhythms are not robust, implying that gerbils may have less well developed temporal organization in their physiology than other species of rodents.

Melatonin in beeswax implants lowered ovarian and uterine weight but did not reduce testis size (LD 14:10). Male gerbils were relatively unresponsive to photoperiod with only slight reductions in testis weight in LL and after blinding; pinealectomy had little effect [74].

Pineal concretions in gerbils increase with age as they do in humans. The concretions may be a result of secretory function because gerbil pineals did not have acervuli (nor pinealocyte vacuoles) following ganglionectomy [79, 81]). Long photoperiod and melatonin implants also reduced the number of concretions [79, 81].

Gerbils have been used to study convulsions as they are prone to seizures. Pinealectomy produces convulsions in over 90% of gerbils [41, 42] described by Philo and Reiter [41]:

> 30 minutes after pinealectomy a wild run began with brief, rapid tight circling (2 sec) followed by a linear running action rebounding off the cage walls for a total of 5–30 seconds. There was also hobbling, rear leg drumming, whisker twitching, and extremity twitching. The running phase was followed by a 5 second period where the trunk, limbs, and tail were extended. Death, more running, or cessation of the convulsions followed.

The convulsions (1) were greatest if pinealectomy was done at light onset, (2) were unaffected by photoperiod, (3) did not follow ganglionectomy, and (4) were not alleviated by melatonin, pineal extract, or serotoninergic drugs. Pinealectomy did reduce telecephalon norepinephrine levels; L-DOPA prevented the convulsions and blocked the norepinephrine reduction [40, 41, 42].

14.2.9 Ground squirrels and chipmunks

Ground squirrels and chipmunks (*Citellus mexicanus*, *Spermophilus mexicanus*, *Citellus tridecemlineatus*, and *Tamias striatus*) are of comparative interest; they are diurnal; some of them hibernate; and they are a nonlaboratory species. Ground squirrel pineals consist mainly of pinealocytes with nerve fibers and endings found in the pericapillary or intercellular spaces; synaptic ribbons were localized next to and perpendicular to the plasma membranes of the pineal-ocytes [32].

Ground squirrels have peak dark-time NAT (2.75 nmol/pineal/hr) that is five times day-time NAT [19, 54, 64, 67]. Serotonin peaks in the light-time; melatonin levels peak in the dark-time; and HIOMT levels are constant throughout the day. Rhythms in NAT, melatonin, and serotonin persisted in constant dark. The NAT and melatonin rhythms damped in constant light. Brighter light than for some other rodents is required to suppress NAT and melatonin in Richardson's ground squirrel and the Eastern chipmunk. Bright light extension did not prevent the dark-time rise in melatonin in chipmunks; however, as night progressed, sensitivity to light increased so that 7 hours after lights-out there was a rapid plummet in response to light. Raising squirrels in the laboratory increased the ability of light to depress NAT.

Isoproterenol stimulated pineal NAT and melatonin in Richard-son's ground squirrel. The α-blocker phentolamine partially blocked the dark-time rise; the β-blocker propranolol blocked the dark-time rise [19]. Propranolol did not block the rise of NAT in chipmunks but ganglionectomy eliminated the rhythm [32]. Retina and Harderian glands of Richardson's ground squirrel contained melatonin, but the amounts were small and not markedly rhythmic [53, 54, 55, 56, 57, 58, 59].

Pinealectomized ground squirrels exhibited the normal rhythm of hibernation, but melatonin increased the duration and incidence of hibernation [15, 35, 48, 66]. Pinealectomized golden-mantled ground squirrels (*Spermophilus lateralis*) had shorter annual rhythms of body weight (27 days shorter the first year, 58 days shorter the second year) [85].

14.2.10 White-footed mice

The white-footed mouse (*Peromyscus leucopus*) pineal is elongate and dumbell shaped. The staining properties of the pineal nuclei change in response to constant dark [45]. There is intraspecies variation in the occurrence of the stalk, which is continuous in only 31% of the mice examined. Pinealocytes were noted to contain a single myeloid-type body each (an array of flattened membranous cisternae) [65]. Old mice had decreases in the area of the Golgi apparatus and in dense core vesicles and increases in annulate lamellae-like structures [25].

Dark-time melatonin (85 pg/pineal) is higher than light-time mela-tonin (3 pg/pineal), and the duration of high melatonin lengthens with increased dark-time [37, 39].

The mice are photoperiodic [36]; mice raised in LD 8:16 had heavier testes (63 mg) than LD 16:8 controls (152 mg). Melatonin implants produced smaller testes (45 mg) in mice kept in LD 16:8 [11]. Short photoperiod and melatonin similarly reduced the testis size of adult mice and uterine weights of young mice [37, 38, 39]. Removing the superficial pineal resulted in larger testes (202 mg) in short photoperiod (LD 8:16) compared to sham-operated animals, whose testes regressed (to 97 mg). There was a daily rhythm of responsiveness to melatonin injections; afternoon injections in the SCN region reduced the female reproductive tract weight 66%, but morning injections had little effect on reproductive tract weight [12, 13]. Implants of melatonin into brain regions localized the site of action to the medial preoptic, suprachiasmatic, and retrochiasmatic areas [12, 13].

The effects of melatonin in the white-footed mouse are not limited to reproductive changes. Melatonin implants also cause a fall molt to occur and other changes characteristic of autumn's short days: hypertrophy of interscapular brown fat and increased basal metabolic rate [28]. Melatonin implants increased spontaneous daily torpor from 6 bouts to 13 bouts in the time period studied [31].

White-footed mice have a large enough geographical distribution to permit intraspecies comparisons. For example, when Georgia and Connecticut mice were compared, short days inhibited the reproductive system of the Connecticut but not the Georgia mice; pineals of both strains exhibited photoperiodic changes in their melatonin profiles. Likewise, melatonin injections had little effect on the Georgia mice [17, 29, 30].

REFERENCES

1. Arendt, J., C. Laud, A. Symons, and S. Pryde. 1983. Plasma melatonin in ewes after ovariectomy. *J. Reprod. Fert.* 68:213–218.
2. Arendt, J., A. Symons, and C. Laud. 1981. Pineal function in the sheep: Evidence for a possible mechanism mediating seasonal reproductive activity. *Experientia* 37:584–586.
3. Binkley, S. 1976. Comparative biochemistry of the pineal glands of birds and mammals. *Amer. Zool.* 16:57–65.
4. ———. 1981. Pineal biochemistry: Comparative aspects and circadian rhythms. In *The pineal gland I: Anatomy and biochemistry*, ed. R. Reiter, pp. 155–172. Boca Raton, Fla.: CRC Press.
5. ———. 1983. Circadian rhythms of pineal function in rats. *Endocrine Rev.* 4:255–270.
6. Bittman, E., R. Dempsey, and F. Karsch. 1983. Pineal melatonin secretion drives reproductive response to daylength in the ewe. *Endocrinology* 113:2276–2283.
7. Bittman, E., A. Kaynard, D. Olster, J. Robinson, S. Yellon, and F. Karsch. 1985. Pineal melatonin mediates photoperiodic control of pulsatile luteinizing hormone secretion in the ewe. *Neuroendocrinology* 40:409–418.

8. Brainard, G., R. Asch, and R. Reiter. 1981. Circadian rhythms of serum melatonin and prolactin in the rhesus monkey, *Macaca mulatta. Biomed. Res.* 2:291–297.

9. Carter, D., and B. Goldman. 1983. Antigonadal effects of timed melatonin infusion in pinealectomized male Djungarian hamsters (*Phodopus sungorus sungorus*): Duration is the critical parameter. *Endocrinology* 113:1261–1283.

10. Earl, C., M. D'Occhio, D. Kennaway, and R. Seamark. 1985. Serum melatonin profiles and endocrine responses of ewes exposed to a pulse of light late in the dark phase. *Endocrinology* 117:226–230.

11. Glass, J., and G. Lynch. 1981. The effect of superficial pinealectomy on reproduction and brown fat in the adult white-footed mouse, *Permomyscus leucopus. J. Comp. Physiol.* 144:145–152.

12. ———. 1982a. Melatonin: Identification of sites of antigonadal action in mouse brain. *Science* 214:821–823.

13. ———. 1982b. Diurnal rhythm of response to chronic intrahypothalamic melatonin injections in the white-footed mouse, *Peromyscus leucopus. Neuroendocrinology* 35:117–122.

14. Goldman, B., J. Darrow, and L. Yogev. 1984. Effects of timed melatonin infusions on reproductive development in the Djungarian hamster (*Phodopus sungorus*). *Endocrinology* 114:2074–2083.

15. Harlow, H., J. Phillips, and C. Ralph. 1981. Day-night rhythm in plasma melatonin in a mammal lacking a distinct pineal gland, the nine-banded armadillo. *Gen. Comp. Endocrinol.* 45:212–218.

16. Hartwig, H. 1984. Cyclic renewal of whole pineal photoreceptor outer segments. *Ophthalmic Res.* 16:102–106.

17. Heath, H., and G. Lynch. 1982. Intraspecific differences for melatonin-induced reproductive regression and the seasonal molt in *Peromyscus leucopus. Gen. Comp. Endocrinol.* 48:289–295.

18. Hoffman, K. 1981. Pineal involvement in the photoperiodic control of reproduction and other functions in the Djungarian hamster, *Phodopus sungorus.* In *The pineal gland II: Reproductive effects,* ed. R. Reiter, pp. 83–102. Boca Raton, Fla.: CRC Press.

19. Hurlbut, E., T. King, B. Richardson, and R. Reiter. 1982. The effects of the light:dark cycle and sympathetically-active drugs on pineal N-acetyltrans-ferase activity and melatonin content in the Richardson's ground squirrel, *Spermophilus Richardsonii.* In *The pineal and its hormones,* ed. R. Reiter, pp. 45–56. New York: Alan R. Liss.

20. Kennaway, D. 1984. Pineal function in ungulates. In *Pineal research reviews II,* ed. R. Reiter, pp. 113–140. New York: Alan R. Liss.

21. Kennaway, D., and T. Gilmore. 1984. Effects of melatonin implants in ewe lambs. *J. Reprod. Fert.* 70:39–45.

22. Kennaway, D., T. Gilmore, and R. Seamark. 1982a. Effect of melatonin feeding on serum prolactin and gonadotrophin levels and the onset of seasonal estrous cyclicity in sheep. *Endocrinology* 110:1766–1772.

23. ———. 1982b. Effects of melatonin implants on the circadian rhythm of plasma melatonin and prolactin in sheep. *Endocrinology* 110:2186–2188.

24. Kennaway, D., L. Sanford, G. Godfrey, and H. Friesen. 1983. Patterns of progesterone, melatonin, and prolactin secretion in ewes maintained in four different photoperiods. *J. Endocrinol.* 97:229–242.

REFERENCES   **237**

25. King, T., M. Karasek, L. Petterborg, J. Hansen, and R. Reiter. 1982. Effects of advancing age on the ultrastructure of pinealocytes in the male white-footed mouse (*Peromyscus leucopus*). *J. Exp. Zool.* 224:127–134.

26. Klein, D., and J. Weller. 1970. Indole metabolism in the pineal gland: A circadian rhythm in *N*-acetyltransferase. *Science* 169:1093–1095.

27. Krstić, R., and J. Golaz. 1977. Ultrastructural and X-ray microprobe comparison of gerbil and human pineal acervuli. *Experientia* 33:507–508.

28. Lynch, G., and A. Epstein. 1976. Melatonin induced changes in gonads, pelage, and thermogenic characters in the white-footed mouse, *Peromyscus leucopus*. *Comp. Biochem. Physiol.* 53C:67–68.

29. Lynch, G., H. Heath, and C. Johnston. 1981. Effect of geographical origin on the photoperiodic control of reproduction in the white-footed mouse, *Peromyscus leucopus*. *Biol. Reprod.* 25:475–480.

30. Lynch, G., J. Sullivan, H. Heath, and L. Tamarkin. 1982. Daily melatonin rhythms in photoperiod sensitive and insensitive white-footed mice. In *The pineal and its hormones*, ed. R. Reiter, pp. 67–73. New York: Alan R. Liss.

31. Lynch, G., S. White, R. Grundel, and M. Berger. 1978. Effects of photoperiod, melatonin administration, and thyroid block on spontaneous daily torpor and temperature regulation in the white-footed mouse, *Peromyscus leucopus*. *J. Comp. Physiol.* 125:157–163.

32. Matsushima, S., and R. Reiter. 1975. Fine structural features of adrenergic nerve fibers and endings in the pineal gland of the rat, ground squirrel, and chinchilla. *Amer. J. Anat.* 148:463–478.

33. Morgan, W., and R. Reiter. 1977. Pineal noradrenaline levels in the mongolian gerbil and in different strains of laboratory rats over a lighting regimen. *Life Sci.* 21:555–558.

34. Namboodiri, M., D. Sugden, D. Klein, L. Tamarkin, and I. Mefford. 1985. Serum melatonin and pineal indoleamine metabolism in a species with a small day/night *N*-acetyltransferase rhythm. *Comp. Biochem. Physiol.* 80B:731–736.

35. Palmer, D., and M. Riedesel. 1976. Responses of whole-animal and isolated hearts of ground squirrels, *Citellus lateralis*, to melatonin. *Comp. Biochem. Physiol.* 53C:69–72.

36. Petterborg, L., and R. Reiter. 1980. Effect of photoperiod and melatonin on testicular development in the white-footed mouse, *Peromyscus leucopus*. *J. Reprod. Fert.* 60:209–212.

37. ———. 1981. Effects of photoperiod and subcutaneous melatonin on the reproductive status of adult white-footed mice (*Peromyscus leucopus*). *J. Andrology* 2:222–224.

38. ———. 1982. Effect of photoperiod and pineal indoles on the reproductive system of young female white-footed mice. *J. Neural Trans.* 55:149–155.

39. Petterborg, L., B. Richardson, and R. Reiter. 1981. Effect of long or short photoperiod on pineal melatonin content in the white-footed mouse, *Peromyscus leucopus*. *Life Sci.* 29:1623–1627.

40. Philo, R. 1982. Catecholamines and pinealectomy-induced convulsions in the gerbil (*Meriones unguiculatus*). In *The pineal and its hormones*, ed. R. Reiter, pp. 233–241. New York: Alan R. Liss.

41. Philo, R., and R. Reiter. 1978. Characterization of pinealectomy-induced

convulsions in the Mongolian gerbil (*Meriones unguiculatus*). *Epilepsia* 19:485–492.

42. ———. 1981. The involvement of brain amines in pinealectomy-induced convulsions in the gerbil: Serotonin. *Behav. Brain Res.* 3:71–82.

43. Pickard, G., and F. Turek. 1983. The hypothalamic paraventricular nucleus mediates the photoperiodic control of reproduction but not the effects of light on the circadian rhythm of activity. *Neurosci. Lett.* 43:67–72.

44. Plotka, E., U. Seal, and J. Verme. 1982. Morphologic and metabolic consequences of pinealectomy in deer. In *The pineal gland III: Extra-reproductive effects*, ed. R. Reiter, pp. 153–169. Boca Raton, Fla.: CRC Press.

45. Quay, W. 1956. Volumetric and cytologic variation in the pineal body of *Peromyscus leucopus* (Rodentia) with respect to sex, captivity, and day-length. *J. Morph.* 98:471–495.

46. ———. 1980. Greater pineal volume at higher latitudes in rodentia: Exponential relationship and its biological interpretation. *Gen. Comp. Endocrinol.* 41:340–348.

47. ———. 1984. Increases in volume, fluid content, and lens weight of eyes following systemic administration of melatonin. *J. Pineal Res.* 1:3–13.

48. Ralph, C. 1984. Pineal bodies and thermoregulation. In *The pineal gland*, ed. R. Reiter, pp. 193–219. New York: Raven Press.

49. Redman, J., S. Armstrong, and K. Ng. 1983. Freerunning activity rhythms in the rat: Entrainment by melatonin. *Science* 219:1089–1091.

50. Reiter, R. 1981. The mammalian pineal gland: Structure and function. *Amer. J. Anat.* 162:287–313.

51. ———. 1982. Reproductive effects of the pineal gland and pineal indoles in the Syrian hamster and the albino rat. In *The pineal gland II: Reproductive effects*, ed. R. Reiter, pp. 45–81. Boca Raton, Fla.: CRC Press.

52. Reiter, R., and G. Vaughan. 1985. Personal communication.

53. Reiter, R., E. Hurlbut, G. Brainard, S. Steinlechner, and B. Richardson. 1983. Influence of light irradiance on HIOMT, NAT, and radioimmunoassayable melatonin levels in the pineal gland of the diurnally active Richardson's ground squirrel. *Brain Res.* 288:151–157.

54. Reiter, R., E. Hurlbut, A. Esquifino, T. Champney, and R. Steger. 1984. Changes in serotonin levels, *N*-acetyltransferase activity, hydroxyindole-O-methyltransferase activity, and melatonin levels in the pineal gland of the Richardson's ground squirrel in relation to the light-dark cycle. *Neuroendocrinology* 39:356–360.

55. Reiter, R., T. King, B. Richardson, and E. Hurlbut. 1982. Studies on pineal melatonin levels in a diurnal species, the Eastern chipmunk (*Tamias striatus*): Effects of light at night, propranolol administration or superior cervical ganglionectomy. *J. Neural Trans.* 54:275–284.

56. Reiter, R., T. King, B. Richardson, E. Hurlbut, M. Karasek, and J. Hansen. 1982. Failure of room light to inhibit pineal *N*-acetyltransferase activity and melatonin content in a diurnal species, the Eastern chipmunk (*Tamias striatus*). *Neuroendocrinol. Lett.* 4:1–6.

57. Reiter, R., and J. Peters. 1984. Non-suppressibility by room light of pineal *N*-acetyltransferase activity and melatonin levels in two diurnally active

rodents, the mexican ground squirrel (*Spermophilus mexicanus*) and the eastern chipmunk (*Tamias striatus*). *Endocrine Res.* 10:113–121.

58. Reiter, R., B. Richardson, and E. Hurlbut. 1981. Pineal, retinal and Harderian gland melatonin in a diurnal species, the Richardson's ground squirrel (*Spermophilus richardsonii*). *Neurosci. Lett.* 22:285–288.

59. Reiter, R., S. Steinlechner, B. Richardson, and T. King. 1983. Differential response of pineal melatonin levels to light at night in laboratory raised and wild-captured 13-lined ground squirrels (*Spermophilus tridecemlineatus*). *Life Sci.* 32:2625–2629.

60. Reppert, S., R. Chez, A. Anderson, and D. Klein. 1979. Maternal-fetal transfer of melatonin in the non-human primate. International Pediatric Research Foundation, Inc. pp. 788–791.

61. Rivest, R., U. Lang, M. Aubert, and P. Sizonenko. 1985. Daily administration of melatonin delays rat vaginal opening and disrupts the first estrous cycles: Evidence that these effects are synchronized by the onset of light. *Endocrinology* 116:779–787.

62. Rollag, M., and G. Niswender. 1976. Radioimmunoassay of serum concentrations of melatonin in sheep exposed to different lighting regimens. *Endocrinology* 98:482–489.

63. Romer, A. 1962. *The vertebrate body*, 3rd ed. Philadelphia: Saunders.

64. Rudeen, P., R. Reiter, and M. Vaughan. 1975. Pineal serotonin-N-acetyltransferase activity in four mammalian species. *Neurosci. Lett.* 1:225–229.

65. Samarasinghe, D., L. Petterborg, J. Zeigler, K. Tiang, and R. Reiter. 1983. On the occurrence of a myeloid body in pinealocytes of the white-footed mouse, *Peromycus leucopus*: An electron microscopic study. *Cell Tiss. Res.* 228:649–659.

66. Stanton, T., C. Craft, and R. Reiter. 1984. Decreases in pineal melatonin content during the hibernation bout in the golden-mantled ground squirrel (*Spermophilus lateralis*). *Life Sci.* 35:1461–1467.

67. Stephens, J., and S. Binkley. 1978. Daily change in pineal N-acetyltransferase in a diurnal mammal, the ground squirrel. *Experientia* 34:1523–1524.

68. Stetson, M. 1985. Personal communication.

69. Symons, A., and J. Arendt. 1982. Lack of effect of melatonin on the pituitary response to LH-RH in the ewe. *J. Reprod. Fert.* 64:103–106.

70. Tamarkin, L., S. Reppert, D. Orloff, D. Klein, S. Yellon, and B. Goldman. 1980. Ontogeny of the pineal melatonin rhythm in the Syrian (*Mesocricetus auratus*) and Siberian (*Phodopus sungorus*) hamsters and in the rat. *Endocrinology* 107:1061–1064.

71. Underwood, H. 1982. The pineal and circadian organization in fish, amphibians, and reptiles. In *The pineal gland III: Extra-reproductive effects*, ed. R. Reiter, pp. 1–25. Boca Raton, Fla.: CRC Press.

72. Underwood, H., S. Binkley, T. Siopes, and K. Mosher. 1984. Melatonin rhythms in the eyes, pineal bodies, and blood of Japanese quail (*Coturnix coturnix japonica*). *Gen. Comp. Endocrinol.* 56:70–81.

73. Vaněček, J., L. Jansky, H. Illnerová, and K. Hoffman. 1984. Pineal melatonin in hibernating and aroused golden hamsters. *Comp. Biochem. Physiol.* 77A:759–762.

74. Vaughan, M., G. Vaughan, D. Blask, and R. Reiter. 1976. Influence of

melatonin, constant light, or blinding on reproductive system of gerbils (*Meriones unguiculatus*). *Experientia* 32:9–10.

75. Vollrath, L. 1981. *The pineal organ.* Berlin: Springer-Verlag.

76. Weaver, D., and M. Reppert. 1986. Maternal melatonin communicates daylength to the fetus. Personal communication.

77. Webster, J., and G. Barrell. 1985. Advancement of reproductive activity, seasonal reduction in prolactin secretion and seasonal pelage changes in pubertal red deer hinds (*Cervus elaphus*) subjected to artificially shortened daily photoperiod or daily melatonin treatments. *J. Reprod. Fert.* 73:255–260.

78. Weitzman, E., U. Weinberg, R. D'Eletto, H. Lynch, R. Wurtman, C. Czeisler, and S. Erlich. 1978. Studies of the 24 hour rhythm of melatonin in man. *J. Neural Trans. Suppl.* 13:325–337.

79. Welsh, M. 1977. Effects of superior cervical ganglionectomy, constant light and blinding on the gerbil pineal gland: An ultrastructural analysis. *Anat. Rec.* 190:580.

80. ———. 1983. CSF-contacting pinealocytes in the pineal recess of the mongolian gerbil: A correlative scanning and transmission electron microscope study. *Amer. J. Anat.* 166:483–493.

81. ———. 1985. Pineal calcification: Structural and functional aspects. In *Pineal research reviews III,* ed. R. Reiter, pp. 41–68. New York: Alan R. Liss.

82. Welsh, M., I. Cameron, and R. Reiter. 1979. The pineal gland of the gerbil, *Meriones unguiculatus,* II: Morphometric analysis over a 24 h period. *Cell Tiss. Res.* 204:95–109.

83. Welsh, M., and R. Reiter. 1978. The pineal gland of the gerbil, *Meriones unguiculatus,* I: An ultrastructural study. *Cell Tiss. Res.* 193:323–336.

84. Yellon, S., L. Tamarkin, B. Pratt, and B. Goldman. 1982. Pineal melatonin in the Djungarian hamster: Photoperiodic regulation of a circadian rhythm. *Endocrinology* 111:488–492.

85. Zucker, I. 1985. Pineal gland influences period of circannual rhythms of ground squirrels. *Amer. J. Physiol.* 249:R111–R115.

15

Comparative Pineal Endocrinology: Birds, Reptiles, Amphibians, Fish, and Nonvertebrates

"Vertebrate pineal systems exhibit considerable morphological variability at both cellular and whole-organ levels of organization. The most striking anatomical feature of pineal systems is the presence in many lower vertebrates of a two-component system consisting of both the pineal organ proper (or epiphysis cerebri) and a second more superficial component generally termed the parapineal organ. Whereas the pineal organ is nearly universally present in vertebrates, the parapineal component is absent in birds and mammals. The pineal system has been implicated in a veritable host of functions including reproduction, thermoregulation, and circadian rhythmicity."

H. Underwood [97]

15.1 Introduction

As argued in Chapter 14, understanding the comparative function of the pineal is key to appreciating the physiology of the gland and to achieving an understanding of the obstacles that delayed the scientific unveiling of pineal function. In this chapter, the comparative physiology is discussed for birds and for lower vertebrates.

In discussing the pineal physiology of birds, it is possible to point to three species (chickens, quail, and sparrows) that have been extensively studied. In the reptiles, the most studied example is *Anolis carolinensis*. In the amphibians, not only particular species but also stage of development are important to pineal function. A variety of fishes each have contributed a small amount of information to our knowledge of the pineal. An uncharted area, but one that promises useful information, is that of possible melatonin synthesis and indole metabolism in invertebrate organisms.

15.2 Birds

Avian pineals are biochemically unique among vertebrates because they have particularly active enzymes and produce large amounts of melatonin. Moreover, the melatonin-synthesizing capacity of the pineal is matched by retinal melatonin synthesis in some birds. Birds are also the class in which pineal and retinal involvement in control of circadian behavior (locomotor activity) was established. The role of the pineal in avian reproduction is, however, less clear; generally, the pineal appears to be progonadal in developing birds and antigonadal in mature birds [83]. Many avian reproductive processes are unaffected by pinealectomy. In the weaver bird, however, pinealectomy produced early sexual maturation and stimulation by normally inhibitory short photoperiods [83]. In birds, β-adrenergic regulation of the pineal is not identical to that in mammals.

15.2.1 Domestic fowl

The chicken pineal (*Gallus domesticus*) has an enlarged distal portion lying just beneath the skull. The parenchymal stalk tapers and is not attached to the intercommissural region [108, 110]. The gland weighs 1.9 mg upon hatching and grows to 2.5 mg by the time the animals are 8 weeks old. Anatomically the gland develops with a primary follicle and rosettes of cells with central lumens and becomes compact in adults. Most investigators describe three cell types: receptor pinealocytes, glial cells, and a third kind in smaller numbers. The pinealocytes have cilia, inner-segment-like apical bulges, and there are lamellar bodies.

Chicken pineal biochemistry has been studied. The chicken pineal has a two-peaked serotonin rhythm (dark-time nadir, peaks at postdawn and predusk) [28]. The *N*-acetyltransferase (NAT) rhythm is especially well defined in chickens (in 3-week-old chicks, dark-time peak 30 nmol/pineal/hr, light-time nadir 2 nmol/pineal/hr). Hydroxyindole-O-methyltransferase (HIOMT) occurs in the gland and is affected by lighting (6.7–9.8 nmol/pineal/hr DD; 13.1–15.3 nmol/pineal/hr LL). Melatonin has rhythms whose patterns are similar to those of NAT (bioassay, 2 ng/pineal light-time nadir, 21 ng/pineal dark-time peak) [17, 25].

The chicken pineal is exquisitely sensitive to light and dark. The NAT rhythm persists in constant dark, damps in constant light, is refractory to stimulation by dark in the early light-time, plummets in response to light at night, and is phase-shifted by light and dark pulses [11, 14, 19, 20, 25]. The shape of the chick pineal NAT rhythm is modified by photoperiod [26]; constant light increases HIOMT, and constant dark decreases HIOMT [62, 85]. Pineal melatonin synthesis accounts for 80% of circulating melatonin [88].

Rhythms of NAT activity and melatonin content of the chicken retina quantitatively rival those in the pineal [15, 19, 49]. Retinal melatonin synthesis in the chick is regulated by light and dark in a manner similar to pineal. NAT exhibits a peak of activity in the dark time. The NAT rhythm persists in constant dark, and the rhythm is attenuated by constant light. There is a refractory period and rapid plummet [15, 22, 23]. Retinal melatonin synthesis accounts for most of the nonpineal circulating melatonin [88].

The chicken pineal gland is capable of generating circadian rhythms of cGMP, NAT, and melatonin in vitro [24, 91, 109]. Moreover, in keeping with the presence of photoreceptor-like pinealocytes, chick NAT is damped by constant light and amplified by light-dark cycles in vitro.

Blind chickens can detect light as measured by changes in pineal biochemical parameters: constant light induces an increase in HIOMT and damps the oscillations of NAT and melatonin; NAT and melatonin synchronize to light-dark cycles [63–85]. The locomotor activity of blinded chickens entrains to light-dark cycles [78].

Ganglionectomy results in disappearance of fluorescent amines from the pineal [83]. There is evidence for a neural control route from the eyes to the pineal. However, neural regulation of the pineal in chickens does not entirely follow the pattern established for rats. Isoproterenol inhibits (rather than stimulates) both chick retina and pineal NAT; ganglionectomy abolished the persistent NAT rhythm in DD but had no effect on the rhythm in LD [16, 18, 22, 23, 29, 85]. There is input to the pineal from the eyes because the rapid plummet response is slower in blinded chickens, and patching the eyes reduces (but does not eliminate) the pineal response to extended light [22, 23]. NAT is synthesized anew each night and continually throughout the night since cycloheximide reduces NAT whenever it is administered in the night [22, 23].

Both progonadal and antigonadal roles have been suggested for fowl pineal, and the possibility also exists that there is no pineal role in fowl reproduction. Early pinealectomy (during the first week after hatching) had little effect on ovarian weight but did delay sexual development of cockerels, implying a progonadal role for the pineal. In addition, melatonin stimulated testis and comb growth of juvenile fowl. In contrast, melatonin inhibited gonads of adult chickens [83].

Pinealectomy and ganglionectomy did not abolish circadian locomotor rhythms in fowl [69, 78]; however, blinding made two of five chickens arrhythmic in constant dark. In view of the discovery of substantive ocular melatonin synthesis in chickens, the possibility of a role for melatonin in behavioral rhythm regulation exists.

15.2.2 Quail

Quail (*Coturnix coturnix japonica*) pineal glands have receptor-type pinealocytes with abundant synaptic ribbons. The pineals lack nerve cell bodies seen in some avian pineals [108].

Quail pineals have daily cycles in melatonin (bioassay, light nadir 0.6 ng/pineal, dark peak 3.2 ng/pineal) [68]. The rhythms in melatonin, as expected, are similar to those in NAT (light nadir 0.2 nmol/pineal/hr, dark peak 6.2 nmol/pineal/hr) [3, 13, 30, 82]. The duration and amplitude of quail pineal melatonin responded to photoperiod (in much the same manner as described for chick pineal NAT) [30].

HIOMT activity was high in constant light and in the light-time and was low in darkness [1, 2, 79]. Quail retinas have NAT and melatonin cycles comparable to the quail pineal [13, 102] (Fig. 4.2). The melatonin peak in the pineal is synchronized with dark in blinded quail; the melatonin peak in the eye is synchronized with dark in pinealectomized quail [102]. Constant dark and LD 8:16 reduced HIOMT [1, 2]. Melatonin implants reduced HIOMT and NAT [83].

The effects of pinealectomy and/or blinding have been studied in quail. Arrhythmic locomotor activity is produced in two out of three quail by blinding, and in all quail by a combination of the blinding with pinealectomy; pinealectomy alone did not abolish rhythmicity [104].

When young quail were pinealectomized and placed in LD 16:8, their reproductive development was delayed—again, as in other birds, the pineal was progonadal. HIOMT declined during the period of rapid sexual development (25–52 days of age) [83, 89].

Quail exhibit photoperiodic reproductive responses that do not require the eyes. Pinealectomy has not affected the gonad response to photoperiod in blinded or intact quail; maturation occurs without either structure. Radioluminous paint implanted adjacent to the hypothalamus stimulated testis development in quail [83]. Ganglionectomy did not affect the rate of oviposition but did reduce pineal serotonin levels [83].

15.2.3 Sparrows

House sparrows (*Passer domesticus*) have saccular pineals with photoreceptor-like pinealocytes. The gland (0.3 mg) has an expanded top just below the skull and a long, thin parenchymal stalk. The sparrow pineal has nerve cell bodies (bipolar and unipolar) concentrated in the gland's center; nerve-like cells make contact (but not synapses) with hundreds of pinealocytes. Perivascular fiber bundles are found in the stalk; the fibers appear to merge with those of the habenular commissure. An antiserum to luteinizing hormone releasing hormone (LRH, a hormone of the hypothalamus) reacts with a bundle of fibers in the white-crowned sparrow; the fibers originate in the hypothalamus and enter the pineal stalk via a route through the habenula [27]. The pineals of juvenile sparrows are larger than those of sexually mature adults [108].

Sparrows have a pineal NAT cycle (light nadir 0.2 nmol/pineal/hr, dark peak 3.7 nmol/pineal/hr) [10]. As would be expected, there is a cycle of melatonin in the blood (light nadir 94 pg/ml, dark peak 840 pg/ml [Binkley and Mosher, unpublished data]. HIOMT activity is high compared to mammals (0.8 nmol/pineal/hr, 2.8 times the activity of the larger rat pineal). In one report, there was a dramatic seasonal cycle in HIOMT (high HIOMT September–April, low HIOMT May–August) that was the opposite of testis weight [7]. Isolated sparrow pineals are capable of generating melatonin cycles in vitro [90]. Sparrow retina has 0.1 nmol/retina/hr NAT in the light-time and 0.5 nmol/retina/hr NAT in the dark-time.

There is indirect evidence that sparrow pineals may be influenced by extraretinal and/or pineal photoreception. Blinded sparrows entrain their locomotor activity to light-dark cycles and exhibit photoperiodic reproductive responses [72, 73, 74]. Hartwig and van Veen [52] suggest that there may be "deep diencephalic photoreceptors" that account for the extraretinal light reception.

Pinealectomy abolishes circadian rhythms of locomotor activity and body temperature in sparrows [16, 39]. Melatonin injections lower body temperature in sparrows, reproducing normal 5° C daily excursion [9]. Transplantation of a pineal into the anterior chamber of the eye of a pinealectomized recipient sparrow restores circadian rhythmicity and timing characteristic of the donor bird [113]. Sparrow reproduction was unaffected by pinealectomy [74].

Attempts to demonstrate β-adrenergic control of the sparrow pineal through the superior cervical ganglia (SCG) have produced negative results. Neither 6-hydroxydopamine injections (meant as a chemical sympathectomy) nor pineal stalk deflection operations eliminated rhythmicity in the sparrows. However, lesions of the suprachiasmatic nuclei (SCN) produced arrhythmic birds [92, 112]. Isoproterenol injections did not stimulate NAT, nor did addition of norepinephrine to the culture medium [10].

Melatonin implants or oral administration alter sparrow circadian rhythms [12, 94]. Melatonin causes one of two effects: (1) shortening of the period of the free-running rhythm, or (2) arrhythmicity.

15.3 Reptiles

The possibility of pineal roles in reptiles is of particular comparative interest because of the presence of diverse pineal complexes [84, 94, 108]. Some reptiles (Crocodilia) lack an organized pineal gland; others have elaborate pineal complexes with an anterior parapineal organ (which may become a parietal eye) and a saccular posterior epiphysis cerebri.

Season of the year is an important consideration in reptile pineal physiology. The reptiles have distinct seasonal cycles in their biochemistry and some effects of pinealectomy and/or administration of melatonin are limited to certain seasons. For example, serotonin and melatonin have been measured throughout the year in tortoises (*Testudo hermanni Gmelin*) [105]. Both diurnal and seasonal changes were found. When rhythms were observed, serotonin peaked at the end of the light-time and melatonin peaked at middark. However, a large amplitude melatonin rhythm was found only in June–October; large amplitude serotonin cycles were found in April–September.

Third or parietal eyes are found in 60% of lizards. One suggestion was that the presence of a third eye was associated with an arboreal lifestyle, whereas the absence of the organ was associated with a burrowing behavior [41, 42]. A second idea was that latitude was correlated with parietal eye distribution, parietal eyes being present in species of lizards that live at higher latitudes (e.g., 48°–66°N latitude where there are large annual fluctuations in temperature and photoperiod) and absent nearer the equator [84]. The meaning of the apparently redundant third eye is yet a mystery though there have been many proposals for its use, such as detection of overhead predators, radiation dosimetry, and photoperiod detection. Investigations of the pineal in reptiles have produced data for photoperiodic control of reproduction, regulation of color change, biological clock function, indole metabolism, thermoregulation, and the impact of environmental temperature.

A species of lizard that has been widely studied is *Anolis carolinensis* (American chameleon, Florida chameleon). Anatomically, *A. carolinensis* has a parietal eye located under a transparent scale, a parietal nerve coursing from the "eye" to the habenular nucleus, and a pineal proper [81, 108]. Biochemically, pineals of *A. carolinensis* have substantive melatonin rhythms but melatonin rhythms were not

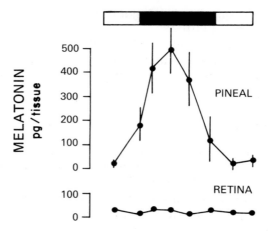

Figure 15.1 Melatonin peaks in the dark-time in pineals of *Anolis Carolinensis* but the eyes do not exhibit the same large change. (After data provided by Underwood [99].)

found in the lateral eyes (Fig. 15.1) [99]. Peak melatonin occurred in the dark-time in LD at 32° C. The duration of high melatonin was a function of the length of the dark-time. The lizards did not show the rapid plummet response to exposure to light at night. When a temperature cycle was given (32°/20° C) peak melatonin occurred at 20° C irrespective of the lighting.

Single pineals of *A. carolinensis* studied in organ culture exhibited persistent cycles at temperatures from 22° C to 37° C (up to 10 cycles were measured). The period length of the cycle was relatively unaffected by temperature (Q 10 = 1.135), a feature of circadian clocks that is called *temperature compensation* [75].

Pinealectomy produced arrhythmic locomotor activity in *A. carolinensis* in dim light or constant dark [98]. Entrainment was also abnormal with the daily onset advanced in pinealectomized lizards. Melatonin injections every 48 hours synchronized the activity to 24 hours [103].

Both temperature and photoperiod play roles in *A. carolinensis* reproduction. For example, long summer photoperiods maintain the testis, and shortening fall photoperiods produce testis regression. The restoration of spermatogenesis is temperature dependent [66]. There are seasonal differences in the way pinealectomy and melatonin affect reproduction in *A. carolinensis* [64, 95, 96, 101]. According to Underwood [101] "progonadal effects of pinealectomy are observed: (1) under both stimulatory and nonstimulatory photoperiods in the fall and (2) in winter when temperature, and not photoperiod is most important for gonadal development. Pinealectomy is without effect in the summer." In the lizards, melatonin was antigonadal (daily injections or Silastic® implants) in that it reversed the effects of pinealectomy. The results are consistent with a view that the pineal produces melatonin which acts in an antigonadal manner at some times of year. The stimulation of the testes by long photoperiods was blocked by covering the brain but not by blinding or parietalectomy, showing that the response can occur with extraretinal photoreceptors that are not located in the lateral or third eyes [94]. However, when the lizards were permitted to select environmental temperatures in an 18°–45° C thermal gradient in LD 13.5:10.5 (near the critical photoperiod), parietalectomy resulted in heavier testes; a parietal effect was not seen in lizards kept at 32° C [100]. In thermal gradients, *A carolinensis* selected warmer temperatures in the day and cooler ones at night and parietalectomized animals select about 2° C higher temperatures [98].

Body color is an area where the pineal and melatonin have been implicated (see Section 9.2.1). *A. carolinensis* exhibits a complex variety of color patterns in response to temperature, background, stress, time of day, and environmental lighting [6, 43]. In the light, the lizards turn brown when chilled (with ice) and green when heated (with a lamp), apparently irrespective of other conditions. The skin response to temperature can be obtained in vitro [43]. When the lizards are subjected to stress (handling), they turn green, a phenomenon called *excitement pallor*. This response is probably mediated by adrenergic stimulation. In vivo injections of epinephrine turn lizards green. *Anolis* skin responds to adrenergic agents in vitro: there is an α-adrenergic mechanism for aggregation and a β-adrenergic mechanism for dispersion of melanosomes. At normal temperatures, during the light of a light-dark cycle or in constant light, *Anolis* are green on a white background and dark on a black background, a phenomenon called *background adaptation*. The darkening response is due to melanophore stimulating hormone (MSH) from the pituitary gland and is controlled by the lateral eyes. The response is abolished by blinding or hypophysectomy. Further, *Anolis* skin is darkened by MSH or pituitary extract in vitro. Serotonin has been postulated to be an MSH releasing hormone; serotonin injections turned *Anolis* brown. In the dark of LD cycles or the subjective dark-time of constant dark, the lizards turn green. This response may be due to nocturnal pineal melatonin production. Other stimuli—background, stress, temperature—being absent, a pineal role seems likely for dark-time pallor. Melatonin implants (Silastic®, continuous) abolished the normal color rhythm and maintained the lizards in the green condition. Of lizards implanted with blank capsules, 83% were brown in the day on a natural background; 75% of the lizards were green in the day if they were implanted with capsules containing melatonin; all of the lizards were green at night [21]. In blind *Anolis* there are still color responses to light and dark. Skin color changes in *Anolis* have been attributed to movement of pigment in skin cells called *chromatophores*. Dispersion of melanin contained in organelles called *melanosomes* throughout cell processes produces darker skin; aggregation of the melanosomes to perinuclear regions produces light skin.

15.4 Amphibians

The work on pineals of amphibians has mainly involved studies of the anatomy, the function of the frontal organ, and of color change. A limitation for pinealectomy studies is posed by the fact that embryonic pinealectomy is often followed by regeneration of the pineal and frontal organ [5, 6, 36, 108].

Anatomically, amphibians may have a two-part pineal complex. The pineal portions of the complex of various amphibians have been described as saccular, tubular, containing septa, or relatively solid. In *Xenopus*, the pineal's dimensions are $450 \times 20 \times 40$ μm. The second portion of the amphibian pineal complex is called the *frontal organ* (Stirnorgan, brow spot). The organs have structures that seem like those in retinae; there are well-developed "photoreceptor-like cells" with apparent "outer segments" which seem to undergo "shedding." Both the frontal and pineal organs have supporting cells and intrapineal nerve cells. The interesting possibility that the outer segment-like structures have a spatial arrangement permitting detection of polarized light was raised [51, 52].

Electrical activity of amphibian frontal organs and the frontal nerve were measured and found to respond to light. Frontal organ electrical activity was inhibited by 355 nm and stimulated by 515 nm. The pineal was only inhibited. Evidence for photopigments with rhodopsin-like absorption maxima have been found in pineals and frontal organs [50]. A sudden drop of light intensity (which evokes locomotor activity bursts in *Xenopus*), provokes a burst of impulses and increased firing frequency from the "pineal eye" [38].

Attempts have been made to produce evidence that amphibian pineals have acute roles in behavior, including involvement in phototaxis and use in compass orientation [108]. For example, eyeless tiger salamanders previously trained to orient under the sun (take a particular compass direction) did not orient when their heads were covered or they were pinealectomized [93].

Biochemically, amphibian pineals contain serotonin, melatonin, and HIOMT and thus seem likely to be capable of melatonin synthesis. The retina of *Xenopus* contains HIOMT activity, and retinal cones contract in response to melatonin. *Xenopus* retinas are capable of rhythmic NAT cycles in vitro [8].

In reproduction, an antigonadal role for melatonin is supported by melatonin inhibition of gonad enlargement on a long photoperiod in

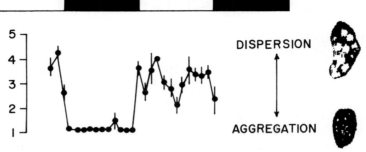

Figure 15.2 Daily cycle of melansome aggregation (night) and dispersion (day) in melanophores of 4-day-old tadpoles (*Xenopus laevus*). The horizontal bar over the record illustrates the LD 12:12 cycle to which the tadpoles were exposed. Units for dispersion indicate the Hogben melanophore indices. Image analyses (Bioquant) of patches of skin showing dispersion (light spots are dispersed melanophores) and aggregation (light dots are punctate melanophores) are shown to the right. (Data Courtesy of Binkley, Mosher, Rubin, and White).

December; however, there are negative studies where pinealectomy did little or pinealectomy inhibited spermatogenesis [108].

The melatonin bioassays (see Fig. 2.6) have been based on color changes that can be obtained with amphibian skins [5, 6, 40, 65, 86]. The assays were based on the fact that pineal extracts (from pig, beef, and man) contain melatonin and that extracts or melatonin aggregate melanosomes of dermal melanophores (e.g., in both larval and adult *Xenopus*, Fig. 15.2).

Xenopus exhibit a paling (blanching) reaction when placed in the dark. The reaction occurs in tadpoles from which the eyes, pituitary, or frontal organ is removed, but pinealectomized *Xenopus* do not show the reaction. Bagnara [4] suggested that absence of light causes the pineal to produce a melanosome-aggregating agent (melatonin) which caused paling. The paling response to darkness should be distinguished from the background adaptation response (which occurs in the light); background adaptation involves the eyes and MSH.

Color responses can be obtained with pieces of skin in vitro, which provides a system for study of possible melatonin receptors. A description of possible melatonin receptors based on their responses to various melatonin analogues (specificity, inhibition) has been developed using *Rana pipiens* skin in vitro [53] (see Sections 10.3.7 and 10.4.1).

15.5 Fish and Lampreys

Work with fish and lamprey pineals has produced detailed comparative anatomical information. For physiology of the pineal in fish, some information is available for roles in behavior, thermoregulation, color change, reproduction, carbohydrate metabolism, and circadian retino-motor movements.

Anatomically, fishes and lampreys have a pineal complex (pineal and parapineal) whose details are characterized by species variation [47, 70, 71, 97]. There may also be a circumventricular organ called the *paraphysis*. The pineal may be hollow or compact with variable quantities of the cell types. The pinealocytes appear to be sensory cells with outer and inner segments. The outer segments are not well developed as compared to retina; sloughing, phagocytosis, and renewal have been suggested. Synaptic ribbons in trout and goldfish pineals peak in number and size in the dark-time. There are other types of cells—supporting cells, nerve cells, macrophage-like cells. Many species have pineal glands with lumens that extend to the third ventricle so that pineal cells are in contact with cerebrospinal fluid.

Goldfish pineals exhibit daily changes in morphology with dark-time peaks in photoreceptor cell volume, inner segment volume, outer segment volume, nucleolar diameter, and vesicles per Golgi body. In goldfish kept in artificial environments simulating the photoperiod and temperature changes that occur in a year, peak sizes of cells, nuclei, nucleoli, mitochondria, endoplasmic reticulum, and Golgi bodies were found in the fall and winter months; reproductive activity (mature oocytes, spermatozoa) was present in April. Constant light and dark altered the morphology [70, 71].

The presence of photoreceptor-like pinealocytes in fish pineals suggests pineal light sensitivity. There is more direct evidence. First, the structure of the trout pineal was altered by environmental lighting and the effects were attributed to both light impinging directly on the pineal and to light information received by the lateral eyes [47]. Second, single pineal photoreceptors in isolated lamprey pineals hyperpolarized in response to light stimulation [77].

Biochemically, pineals of various fishes have serotonin (peak at the end of the light-time), melatonin, HIOMT, and a peptide similar to arginine vasotocin (AVT) [45, 48, 70, 71, 108]. The pineals and lateral eyes of ammocoetes exhibit seasonal variations (two cycles per year) in serotonin (Fig. 15.3) [106].

The pineal may function in fish locomotor activity and in behavioral thermoregulation. Pinealectomy did not alter phototactic responses in trout [46], but melatonin caused them to wobble, tilt, and lie on their sides [44]. Pinealectomized lake chub exhibited free-running and entrained locomotor activity. There were subtle effects of pinealectomy on the distribution of activity and period length. Blinded-pinealectomized lake chub increased activity in response to light and exhibited a rhythm of extraretinal sensitivity (more sensitivity in the light-time) in LD 12:12. Pinealectomized white suckers exhibited changes in period length, precision of circadian activity, and rhythm

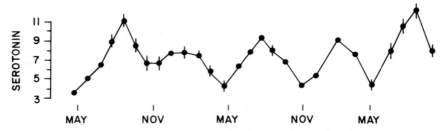

Figure 15.3 Pineal serotonin (5-HT) in ammocoetes showing five cycles (two cycles/yr). (After data in Vivien-Roels and Meinel [106].)

splitting. Pinealectomy increased circadian period length (from 22.1 to 23.4 hours) in winter and decreased it in summer (from 23.5 to 21.9 hours) [54, 55, 56, 57, 80]. In thermal gradients, some fish select higher temperatures in a rhythmic manner. Daily temperature preferences in the presence of endorphin by goldfish were eliminated by pinealectomy and pinealectomy increased body temperatures of control fish by 2°–4° C in thermal gradients [59, 60]. Shielding the pineal regions of white suckers caused them to reduce the time spent in dark by 25–30% [58].

In goldfish reproduction, the pineal may be both progonadal and antigonadal. Short photoperiods (LD 8:16, February–July) reduced gonad activity (based on ovary and testis histology); this effect was reversed by pinealectomy. Long photoperiods (LD 16:8 February–July) stimulated the gonads; pinealectomy blocked the effect [35].

Color changes occur in fish. Rhythms are present with dark-time pallor. Pinealectomy alone eliminated the color rhythm in juvenile lampreys [111]. Pinealectomy also eliminated the color change rhythm of killifish kept in constant light but did not alter the background response [61]. However, in trout the rhythm was reduced by blinding, unaffected by pinealectomy alone, and eliminated altogether by blinding together with pinealectomy [44]. Melatonin has not affected fish color in some studies; however, there are examples where it has been effective. In the pencilfish, there is a daily rhythm in day (black band) versus night (two spots) markings. Melatonin in the water (0.03 µg/ml or more) produced the night pattern [87].

The pineal may function in carbohydrate metabolism in fishes. In goldfish in LD 12:12, liver glycogen was high (about 2400 µg/mg protein) in October and reduced (to about 700–1000 µg/mg protein) in January and May. In May, the liver glycogen was increased by short photoperiods. Pinealectomy lowered liver glycogen in October or May; melatonin increased liver glycogen in constant light [33, 34]. Optic nerve section reduced liver glycogen in May and October [32].

15.6 Nonvertebrates

Pineals are not found in plants or in invertebrates (which do have circadian rhythms, photoperiodism, and color changes). However, some aspects of pineal physiology may be relevant to these other organisms.

The pathway for melatonin synthesis from serotonin is an indole pathway. One of the most studied plant hormones is auxin, which is indoleacetic acid. Moreover, auxin has a role in plant responses to light and dark. Plants have precise seasonal and daily rhythms. Plant enzyme activities are altered by photoperiod [67]. This line of reasoning leads to the possibility that indole or enzyme rhythms may play a role in plant rhythmicity as they do in vertebrates. Evidence for melatonin biosynthesis has been found in nonvertebrates. Melatonin was identified in the compound eyes of the locust (8–15 pg/eye) [107]. NAT (6–20 nmoles/brain/hr) was found in cockroaches and a melatonin rhythm was present. [Binkley, Mosher, Rollag, and Roberts, unpublished].

In the flatworm, planaria (*Dugesia dorotocephala*), two effects of melatonin have been noticed. First, melatonin, serotonin, and tryptamine contracted pigment cells 30–46% in planaria [31]. Second, melatonin suppressed the rate of "fissioning" of decapitated planarians (fissioning is an asexual form of reproduction in planarians that is sensitive to photoperiod) [76].

Fingerman [37] exposed fiddler crabs (*Uca pugilator*) to melatonin (2×10^{-3} and 2×10^{-4} M) and found no pigment-concentrating or dispersing effects; serotonin does change the crabs' color.

In plotting a course of study to find correlates of pineal physiology in nonvertebrate organisms, one would look for rhythms in indoles and enzymes, and one would seek responses (e.g., color) to indoles in pigment cells, especially in photoreceptor organs.

REFERENCES

1. Alexander, B., A. Dowd, and A. Wolfson. 1970a. Effect of continuous light and darkness on hydroxyindole-O-methyltransferase and 5-hydroxytryptophan decarboxylase activities in Japanese quail. *Endocrinology* 86:1441–1443.

2. ———. 1970b. Pineal hydroxyindole-O-methyltransferase (HIOMT) activity in female Japanese quail. *Neuroendocrinology* 6:236–246.

3. Bäckstrom, M., J. Hetta, G. Wahlstrom, and L. Wetterberg. 1972. Enzyme regulation of melatonin synthesis in the pineal gland of Japanese quail. *Life Sci.* 11:493–498.

4. Bagnara, J. 1960. Pineal regulation of the body lightening reaction in amphibian larvae. *Science* 132:1481–1483.

5. Bagnara, J., and M. Hadley. 1970. Endocrinology of the amphibian pineal. *Amer. Zool.* 10:201–216.

6. ———. 1973. *Chromatophores and color change.* Englewood Cliffs, N.J.: Prentice-Hall.

7. Barfuss, D., and L. Ellis. 1971. Seasonal cycles in melatonin synthesis by the pineal gland as related to testicular function in the house sparrow, *Passer domesticus. Gen. Comp. Endocrinol.* 17:183–193.

8. Besharse, J., and M. Iuvone. 1983. Circadian clock in *Xenopus* eye controlling retinal serotonin *N*-acetyltransferase. *Nature* 305:133–135.

9. Binkley, S. 1972. Pineal and melatonin: Circadian rhythms and body temperatures of sparrows. In *Chronobiology*, ed. L. Scheving, F. Halberg, and J. Pauly, pp. 581–585. Tokyo: Igaku Shoin.

10. ———. 1976. Comparative biochemistry of the pineal glands of birds and mammals. *Amer. Zool.* 16:57–65.

11. ———. 1983. Circadian rhythm in pineal *N*-acetyltransferase activity: Phase shifting by light pulses II. *J. Neurochem.* 41:273–276.

12. ———. 1985. Oral melatonin produces arrhythmia in sparrows. *Experientia* 41:1615–1617.

13. ———. 1986. Melatonin and *N*-acetyltransferase rhythms in pineal and retina. In *Pineal-retinal relationships*, ed. D. Klein and P. O'Brien, pp. 185–196. Elmsford, NY: Pergamon Press.

14. Binkley, S., and E. Geller. 1975. Pineal *N*-acetyltransferase in chickens: Rhythm persists in constant darkness. *J. Comp. Physiol.* 99:67–70.

15. Binkley, S., M. Hryshchyshyn, and K. Reilly. 1979. *N*-acetyltransferase activity responds to environmental lighting in the eye as well as in the pineal gland. *Nature* 281:479–481.

16. Binkley, S., E. Kluth, and M. Menaker. 1971. Pineal function in sparrows: Circadian rhythms and body temperature. *Science* 174:311–314.

17. Binkley, S., S. MacBride, D. Klein, and C. Ralph. 1973. Pineal enzymes: Regulation of avian melatonin synthesis. *Science* 181:273–275.

18. ———. 1975. Regulation of pineal rhythms in chickens: Refractory period and nonvisual light perception. *Endocrinology* 96:848–853.

19. Binkley, S., K. Mosher, and B. White. 1985. Circadian rhythm in pineal *N*-acetyltransferase activity: Phase shifting by dark pulses III. *J. Neurochem.* 45:875–878.

20. Binkley, S., G. Muller, and T. Hernandez. 1981. Circadian rhythm in pineal *N*-acetyltransferase activity: Phase shifting by light pulses I. *J. Neurochem.* 37:798–800.

21. Binkley, S., K. Reilly, V. Hermida, and K. Mosher. 1987. Circadian rhythm of color change in *Anolis carolinensis*: Reconsideration of regulation, especially the role of melatonin in dark-time pallor. In *Pineal research reviews* V, ed. R. Reiter. New York: Alan R. Liss. In press.

22. Binkley, S., K. Reilly, and T. Hernandez. 1980. *N*-acetyltransferase in the chick retina II: Interactions of the eyes and pineal gland in response to light. *J. Comp. Physiol.* 140:181–183.

23. Binkley, S., K. Reilly, and M. Hryshchyshyn. 1980. *N*-acetyltransferase in the chick retina I: Circadian rhythms controlled by environmental

lighting are similar to those in the pineal gland. *J. Comp. Physiol.* 139:103–108.

24. Binkley, S., J. Riebman, and K. Reilly. 1978a. "The pineal gland: A biological clock in vitro. *Science* 202:1198–1201.

25. ———. 1978b. Regulation of pineal rhythms in chickens: Inhibition of dark-time N-acetyltransferase activity. *Comp. Biochem. Physiol.* 59C:165–171.

26. Binkley, S., J. Stephens, J. Reibman, and K. Reilly. 1977. Regulation of pineal rhythms in chickens: Photoperiod and dark-time sensitivity. *Gen. Comp. Endocrinol.* 32:411–416.

27. Blahser, S., A. Oksche, and D. Farner. 1986. Projection of fibers immunoreactive to an antiserum against gonadoliberin (LHRH) into the pineal stalk of the white-crowned sparrow, *Zonotrichia leucophrys gambelii. Cell Tiss. Res.* 244:193–196.

28. Brammer, M., and S. Binkley. 1979. Daily rhythms of serotonin and N-acetyltransferase in chicks. *Comp. Biochem. Physiol.* 63C:305–307.

29. Cassone, V., and M. Menaker. 1983. Sympathetic regulation of chicken pineal rhythms. *Brain Res.* 272:311–317.

30. Cockrem, J., and B. Follett. 1985. Circadian rhythm of melatonin in the pineal gland of the Japanese quail (*Coturnix coturnix japonica*). *J. Endocrinol.* 107:317–324.

31. Csaba, G., J. Bierbauer, and Z. Feher. 1980. Influence of melatonin and its precursors on the pigment cells of planaria (*Dugesia lugubris*). *Comp. Biochem. Physiol.* 67C:207–209.

32. Delahunty, G., G. Bauer, M. Prack, and V. DeVlaming. 1978. Effects of pinealectomy and melatonin treatment on liver and plasma metabolites in the goldfish, *Carassius auratus*: Role of the pineal and retinal pathways. *Gen. Comp. Endocrinol.* 35:99–109.

33. Delahunty, G., J. Olcese, and V. de Vlaming. 1980. Photoperiod effects on carbohydrate metabolites in the goldfish, *Carassius auratus*: Role of the pineal and retinal pathways. *Rev. Can. Biol.* 39:173–180.

34. Delahunty, G., and M. Tomlinson. 1984. Hypoglycemic effects of melatonin in the goldfish, *Carassius auratus. Comp. Biochem. Physiol.* 78A:871–875.

35. De Vlaming, V., and M. Vodicinik. 1978. Seasonal effects of pinealectomy on gonadal activity in the goldfish, *Carassius auratus. Biol. Reprod.* 19:57–63.

36. Eichler, V. 1968. Pineal regeneration in the frog, *Rana pipiens*, following embryonic extirpation. *J. Morph.* 125:253–258.

37. Fingerman, M. 1984. Personal communication.

38. Foster, R., and A. Roberts. 1982. The pineal eye in *Xenopus laevis* embryos and larvae: A photoreceptor with a direct excitatory effect on behavior. *J. Comp. Physiol.* 145:413–419.

39. Gaston, S., and M. Menaker. 1968. Pineal function: The biological clock in the sparrow? *Science* 160:1125–1127.

40. Gern, W., T. Gorell, and D. Owens. 1981. Melatonin and pigment cell rhythmicity. In *Melatonin: Current status and perspectives*, ed. N. Birau and W. Schloot, pp. 223–233. Oxford: Pergamon Press.

41. Gundy, G., and C. Ralph. 1975. Parietal eyes in lizards: Zoogeographical correlates. *Science* 190:671–673.

42. Gundy, G., and G. Wurst. 1976. Parietal eye-pineal morphology in lizards and its physiological implications. *Anat. Rec.* 185:419–432.

43. Hadley, M., and J. Goldman. 1969. Physiological color changes in reptiles. *Amer. Zool.* 9:489–504.

44. Hafeez, M. 1970. Effect of melatonin on body coloration and spontaneous swimming activity in rainbow trout, *Salmo gairdneri*. *Comp. Biochem. Physiol.* 36:639–656.

45. Hafeez, M., and W. Quay. 1970a. Pineal acetylserotonin methyltransferase activity in the teleost fishes, *Hesperoleucus symmetricus* and *Salmo gairdneri*, with evidence for lack of effect of constant light and darkness. *Comp. Gen. Pharmacol.* 3:257–262.

46. ———. 1970b. The role of the pineal organ in the control of phototaxis in rainbow trout (*Salmo gairdneri, Richardson*). *Z. Vergl. Physiol.* 68:403–416.

47. ———. 1978. Mediation of light-induced changes in pineal receptor and supporting cell nuclei and nucleoli in steelhead trout (*Salmo gairdneri*). *Photochem. Photobiol.* 28:213–218.

48. Hafeez, M., and L. Zerihun. 1976. Autoradiographic localization of 3H-5-HTP and 3H-5-HT in the pineal organ and circumventricular areas in the rainbow trout, *Salmo gairdneri Richardson*. *Cell Tiss. Res.* 170:61–76.

49. Hamm, H., and M. Menaker. 1980. Retinal rhythms in chicks: Circadian variation in melatonin and serotonin N-acetyltransferase. *Proc. Natl. Acad. Sci. USA* 77:4998–5002.

50. Hartwig, H. 1984. Cyclic renewal of whole pineal photoreceptor outer segments. *Ophthalmic Res.* 16:102–106.

51. Hartwig, H., and H. Korf. 1978. The epiphysis cerebri of poikilothermic vertebrates: A photosensitive neuroendocrine circumventricular organ. In *Scanning electron microscopy II*, ed. R. Becker and O. Johari, pp. 163–168. Chicago, Ill.: Research Institute.

52. Hartwig, H., and T. van Veen. 1979. Spectral characteristics of visible radiation penetrating into the brain and stimulating extraretinal photoreceptors. *J. Comp. Physiol.* 130:277–282.

53. Heward, C., and M. Hadley. 1976. Structure-activity relationships of melatonin and related indoleamines. *Life Sci.* 17:1167–1178.

54. Kavaliers, M. 1980a. Pineal control of ultradian rhythms and short-term activity in a cyprinid fish, the lack chub, *Couesius plumbeus*. *Behav. Neural Biol.* 29:224–235.

55. ———. 1980b. Circadian locomotor activity rhythms of the burbot, *Lota lota*: Seasonal differences in period length and effect of pinealectomy. *J. Comp. Physiol.* 136:215–218.

56. ———. 1981a. Circadian rhythm of nonpineal extraretinal photosensitivity in a teleost fish, the lake chub, *Couesius plumbeus*. *J. Exp. Zool.* 216:7–11.

57. ———. 1981b. Circadian organization in white suckers *Catostomus commersoni*: The role of the pineal organ. *Comp. Biochem. Physiol.* 68A:127–129.

58. ———. 1982a. Effects of pineal shielding on the thermoregulatory behavior of the white sucker *Catostomus commersoni*. *Physiol. Zool.* 55:155–161.

59. ———. 1982b. Pinealectomy modifies the thermoregulatory effects of bombesin in goldfish. *Neuropharmacology* 21:1169–1982.

60. ———. 1982c. Pineal mediation of the thermoregulatory and behavioral activating effects of β-endorphin. *Peptides* 3:679–685.

61. Kavaliers, M., B. Firth, and C. Ralph. 1980. Pineal control of the circadian rhythm of colour change in the killifish (*Fundulus heteroclitus*). *Can. J. Zool.* 58:456–460.

62. Krstić, R., and J. Golaz. 1977. Ultrastructural and X-ray microprobe comparison of gerbil and human pineal acervuli. *Experientia* 33:507–508.

63. Lauber, J., J. Boyd, and J. Axelrod. 1968. Enzymatic synthesis of melatonin in avian pineal body: Extraretinal response to light. *Science* 161:489–490.

64. Levey, I. 1973. Effects of pinealectomy and melatonin injections at different seasons on ovarian activity in the lizard, *Anolis carolinensis. J. Exp. Zool.* 185:169–174.

65. Lerner, A., J. Case, Y. Takahashi, T. Lee, and W. Mori. 1958. Isolation of melatonin, the pineal gland factor that lightens melanophores. *J. Amer. Chem. Soc.* 80:2587.

66. Licht, P. 1971. Regulation of the annual testis cycle by photoperiod and temperature in the lizard, *Anolis carolinensis. Ecology* 52:240–252.

67. Lobban, C., M. Weidner, and K. Luning. 1981. Photoperiod affects enzyme activities in the kelp, *Laminaria hyperborea. Z. Pflanzenphysiol. Bd.* 105:81–83.

68. Lynch, H. 1971. Diurnal oscillations in pineal melatonin content. *Life Sci.* 10:791–795.

69. MacBride, S. 1973. Pineal biochemical rhythms of the chicken: Light cycle and locomotor activity correlation. Ph.D. Diss., Univ. of Pittsburgh.

70. McNulty, J. 1981. Synaptic ribbons in the pineal organ of the goldfish: Circadian rhythmicity and the effects of constant light and constant darkness. *Cell Tiss. Res.* 215:491–497.

71. ———. 1982. Morphologic evidence for seasonal changes in the pineal organ in the goldfish, *Carassius auratus*: A quantitative study. *Reprod. Nutr. Develop.* 22:1061–1072.

72. Menaker, M. 1968a. Light perception by extra-retinal receptors in the brain of the sparrow. *Proc. 76th Annual Convention APA*, pp. 299–300.

73. ———. 1968b. Extraretinal light perception in the sparrow II: Photoperiodic stimulation of testis growth. *Proc. Nat. Acad. Sci. USA* 60:146–151.

74. Menaker, M., R. Roberts, J. Elliott, and H. Underwood. 1970. Extraretinal light perception in the sparrow III: The eyes do not participate in photoperiodic photoreception. *Proc. Nat. Acad. Sci. USA* 67:320–325.

75. Menaker, M., and S. Wisner. 1983. Temperature-compensated circadian clock in the pineal of *Anolis. Proc. Nat. Acad. Sci. USA* 80:6119–6121.

76. Morita, M., and J. Best. 1984. Effects of photoperiods and melatonin on planarian asexual reproduction. *J. Exp. Zool.* 231:273–282.

77. Morita, Y., K. Segi, M. Samejima, and T. Nakamura. 1984. Intracellular dynamic response characteristics of pineal photoreceptors. *Ophthalmic Res.* 16:119–122.

78. Nyce, J., and S. Binkley. 1977. Extraretinal photoreception in chickens: Entrainment of the circadian locomotor activity rhythm. *Photochem. Photobiol.* 25:529–531.

79. Oishi, T., and J. Lauber. 1973. Effect of light and darkness on pineal hydroxyindole-O-methyltransferase (HIOMT) in Japanese quail. *Life Sci.* 13:1105–1116.

80. Olcese, J., T. Hall, H. Figueroa, and V. DeVlaming. 1981. Pinealectomy and melatonin effects on daily variations of the hypothalamic serotonergic system in the goldfish. *Comp. Biochem. Physiol.* 70A:69–72.

81. Ortman, R. 1960. Pariental eye and nerve in *Anolis carolinensis*. *Anat. Rec.* 137:386.

82. Pang, S., P. Chow, T. Wong, and E. Tso. 1983. Diurnal variations of melatonin and N-acetylserotonin in the tissues of quails (*Coturnix* sp.), pigeons (*Columbia livia*), and chickens (*Gallus domesticus*). *Gen. Comp. Endocrinol.* 51:1–7.

83. Ralph, C. 1981. The pineal and reproduction in birds. In *The Pineal gland II: Reproductive effects*, ed. R. Reiter, pp. 31–43. Boca Raton, Fla.: CRC Press.

84. ———. 1984. Pineal bodies and thermoregulation. In *The pineal gland*, ed. R. Reiter, pp. 193–219. New York: Raven Press.

85. Ralph, C., S. Binkley, S. MacBride, and D. Klein. 1975. Regulation of pineal rhythms in chickens: Effects of blinding, constant light, constant dark, and superior cervical ganglionectomy. *Endocrinology* 97:1373–1378.

86. Ralph, C., and H. Lynch. 1970. A quantitative melatonin bioassay. *Gen. Comp. Endocrinol.* 15:334–338.

87. Reed, B. 1968. The control of circadian pigment changes in the pencil fish: A proposed role for melatonin. *Life Sci.* 7:961–973.

88. Reppert, S., and S. Sagar. 1983. Characterization of the day-night variation of retinal melatonin content in the chick. *Invest. Ophthalmol. Vis. Sci.* 24:294–300.

89. Saylor, A., and A. Wolfson. 1967. Avian pineal gland: Progonadotropic response in the Japanese quail. *Science* 158:1478–1479.

90. Takahashi, J. 1981. Neural and endocrine regulation of avian circadian systems. Ph.D. diss., Univ. of Oregon.

91. Takahashi, J., H. Hamm, and M. Menaker. 1980. Circadian rhythms of melatonin release from individual superfused chicken pineal glands in vitro. *Proc. Natl. Acad. Sci. USA* 77:2319–2322.

92. Takahashi, J., and M. Menaker. 1982. Role of the suprachiasmatic nuclei in the circadian system of the house sparrow, *Passer domesticus*. *J. Neurosci.* 2:815–828.

93. Taylor, D., and K. Adler. 1978. The pineal body: Site of extraocular

perception of celestial cues for orientation in the tiger salamander (*Ambystoma tigrinum*). *J. Comp. Physiol.* 124:357–361.

94. Turek, F., J. McMillan, and M. Menaker. 1976. Melatonin: Effects on the circadian locomotor rhythm of sparrows. *Science* 194:1441–1443.

95. Underwood, H. 1980. Photoperiodic photoreception in the male lizard, *Anolis carolinensis*: The eyes are not involved. *Comp. Biochem. Physiol.* 67A:191–194.

96. ———. 1981. Effects of pinealectomy and melatonin on the photoperiodic gonadal response of the male lizard, *Anolis carolinensis. J. Exp. Zool.* 217:417–422.

97. ———. 1982. The pineal and circadian organization in fish, amphibians, and reptiles. In *The pineal gland III: Extra-reproductive effects*, ed. R. Reiter, pp. 1–25. Boca Raton, Fla.: CRC Press.

98. ———. 1983. Circadian organization in the lizard *Anolis carolinensis*: A multioscillator system. *J. Comp. Physiol.* 152:265–274.

99. ———. 1985a. Pineal melatonin rhythms in the lizard *Anolis carolinensis*: Effects of light and temperature cycles. *J. Comp. Physiol.* A 157:57–66.

100. ———. 1985b. Parietalectomy affects photoperiodic responsiveness in thermoregulating lizards (*Anolis carolinensis*). *Comp. Biochem. Physiol.* 80A:411–413.

101. ———. 1985c. Annual testicular cycle of the lizard, *Anolis carolinensis*: Effects of pinealectomy and melatonin. *J. Exp. Zool.* 233:235–242.

102. Underwood, H., S. Binkley, T. Siopes, and K. Mosher. 1984. Melatonin rhythms in the eyes, pineal bodies, and blood of Japanese quail (*Coturnix coturnix japonica*). *Gen. Comp. Endocrinol.* 56:70–81.

103. Underwood, H., and M. Harless. 1985. Entrainment of the circadian activity rhythm of a lizard to melatonin injections. *Physiol. Behav.* 35:267–270.

104. Underwood, H., and T. Siopes. 1984. Circadian organization in Japanese quail. *J. Exp. Zool.* 232:557–566.

105. Vivien-Roels, B., J. Arendt, and J. Bradtke. 1979. Circadian and circannual fluctuations of pineal indoleamines (serotonin and melatonin) in *Testudo hermanni Gmelin* (Reptilia, Chelonia). *Gen. Comp. Endocrinol.* 37:197–210.

106. Vivien-Roels, B., and A. Meinel. 1983. Seasonal variations of serotonin content in the pineal complex and the lateral eye of *Lampetra planeri* (Cyclostoma, Petromyzontidae). *Gen. Comp. Endocrinol.* 50:313–323.

107. Vivien-Roels, B., P. Pévet, O. Beck, and M. Fevre-Montange. 1984. Identification of melatonin in the compound eyes of an insect, the locust (*Locusta migratoria*) by radioimmunoassay and gas chromatography-mass spectrometry. *Neurosci. Lett.* 49:153–157.

108. Vollrath, L. 1981. *The pineal organ*. Berlin: Springer-Verlag.

109. Wainwright, S., and L. Wainwright. 1980. Diurnal cycles in serotonin acetyltransferase activity and cyclic GMP content of cultured chick pineal glands. *Nature* 285:478–480.

110. Wight, P. 1971. The pineal gland. In *Physiology and biochemistry of the domestic fowl I*, ed. D. Bell and B. Freeman, pp. 549–574. London: Academic Press.

111. Young, J. 1935. The photoreceptors of lampreys II: The functions of the pineal complex. *J. Exp. Biol. Med.* 12:254–270.

112. Zimmerman, N., and M. Menaker. 1975. Neural connections of sparrow pineal: Role in circadian control of activity. *Science* 190:477–479.

113. ———. 1979. The pineal gland: A pacemaker within the circadian system of the house sparrow. *Proc. Nat. Acad. Sci. USA* 76:999–1003.

16

Perspectives

"Tortoise pineal serotonin and melatonin levels show marked circadian and circannual rhythms in a natural environment. . . . In these reptiles, as in mammals and birds, serotonin is synthesized during the day, while melatonin is synthesized at night. Both the maximum concentration and the amplitude of circadian fluctuations are increased during the breeding season; circadian rhythms disappear completely during winter and hibernation."

B. Vivien-Roels, J. Arendt, and J. Bradtke [25]

16.1 Introduction

Various hypotheses have been proposed to explain pineal physiology and its relationship to time of day and season. As is the nature of science, the original hypotheses have changed as new information became available. There has been an "evolution" of ideas.

For the pineal, comparative physiology is important. That is, not only is it not necessary that the pineal work the same way in all species, but variation in pineal function is in fact required for adaptation by different species to the particular needs of their environments. Many questions remain, but a pattern has emerged for the

TABLE 16.1 Hypothesis for pineal function as a circadian biological clock

The pineal functions as a biological clock in one or both of two ways:
1. The pineal acts as "clockworks" generating periodic signals with a period near 24 hours (frequency = 1 cycle/24 hr).
2. The pineal relays periodic signals that originate in the supra-chiasmatic nuclei.

The pineal sends time information to other parts of the body via melatonin, which it produces in the dark-time of a daily environmental light-dark cycle.

TABLE 16.2 Hypothesis for pineal function in color change

The pineal functions in color change.
1. The pineal synthesizes a hormone, melatonin, in the dark-time.
2. Melatonin produces dark-time pallor in some lower vertebrates (fish, amphibians, and reptiles).

TABLE 16.3 Hypothesis for pineal function in reproduction

The pineal functions in reproduction.
1. The pineal functions in seasonal photoperiodism. The phase, amplitude, and duration of nightly melatonin production are consequences of photoperiod. The melatonin signal acts to mediate seasonal changes in reproductive function.
2. Melatonin may be progonadal or antigonadal depending on the developmental age, species, and time of year.

pineal functioning as a clock and/or calendar in behavioral rhythms, color change, and reproduction (Tables 16.1–16.3).

Consideration of some aspects of pineal physiology (e.g., rhythms associated with time of day or month of year; whether the melatonin is progonadal or antigonadal) leads to a complex view of the gland's function. However, there is a simple overriding idea that provides a framework for thinking about pineal function, to wit: melatonin is produced at night (by the eyes and/or the pineal); light and dark precisely determine the amount and timing of melatonin secretion; and melatonin acts on targets as a hormone that provides signals with time and/or lighting information [3, 4, 7, 10, 14, 18, 19, 20, 21, 24, 27].

Most of the model building concerning the pineal has centered around the manner in which it may mediate photoperiodically con-trolled reproduction.

16.2 The Pineal as a Photoreceptor

Photoreceptors are structures capable of detecting light. The idea that the pineal of some species is a photoreceptor derived from the anatomical presence of photoreceptor-like cells in the pineal. Evidence that some pineals are in fact themselves capable of light perception is unequivocal: pineal indole metabolism responds to light and dark in vitro, and the pineal exhibits electrical responses to light and dark. It is possible that direct pineal light detection parallels that for the eye; in other words, that there are photosensitive cells with a photopigment, probably rhodopsin.

Pineals—both those that are directly photosensitive and those that are not—receive light information from other sources (eyes, extraretinal light receptors), probably by neural means.

16.3 The Pineal as an Endocrine Gland

Endocrine glands are classically defined as ductless glands that secrete chemical products (hormones) into the blood. Examples of classic endocrine glands are the pituitary, thyroid, parathyroids, pancreas, adrenals, and gonads. The pineal appears to qualify as an endocrine gland by virtue of the fact that it synthesizes a hormone (or hormones) and secretes it into the blood. The evidence for this is that the pineal can synthesize melatonin and other products when it is isolated in culture; moreover, pinealectomy results in a lowering of circulating melatonin in a number of species.

16.4 The Pineal as a Neuroendocrine Transducer

A neuroendocrine transducer is a gland that receives information by neural signals from some part of the brain or nervous system and converts that signal to an endocrine signal. Three neuroendocrine transducers were described for vertebrates [30]:

1. The hypothalmic median eminence secretes its hormones into a portal circulation; they are then delivered selectively to the anterior pituitary gland where they influence the release of its tropic hormones (e.g., ACTH and the gonadotropins) into the general circulation.
2. The adrenal medulla responds to stimulation of its sympathetic nerves by releasing adrenaline directly into the venous blood.
3. The (mammalian) pineal gland's ... activity is controlled by nervous signals generated by environmental lighting and transmitted to the pineal by its sympathetic nerves. In response to absence of a light input, the mammalian pineal synthesizes its characteristic hormone, melatonin and releases this compound into the bloodstream.

Variations on the term *neuroendocrine transducer* can be imagined. *Photoneuroendocrine transducer* incorporates the pineal regulation by light from the eyes. Pineals that detect light directly and convert the information to a hormone signal might be termed *photoendocrine transducers*.

16.5 The Place of the Pineal in Endocrine Hierarchies

In placing pineals in relationships to other glands and photoreceptors, the concept of a hierarchy has often been used (Fig. 16.1A). There are several advantages of such hierarchies: (1) they permit coordination of information (e.g., from photoreceptors and clocks) into output (e.g., melatonin) of endocrine glands, and (2) they provide a means for amplification of a signal. For the stimulation of the adrenal by the pituitary, for example, 56,000-fold amplification was estimated (Fig. 16.1B) [2]; each molecule that acts on a target causes production of many molecules by the target, and a series of such sequences produced amplification.

Many endocrinologists view the endocrine and neuroendocrine systems as comprised of a complex set of interactions. The models involve feedback (usually negative). This view of the pineal role in endocrine and neuroendocrine function has also been taken. One such model (Fig 16.2) was drawn by Quay [16] who pointed to the brain as the central focus of pineal function:

> The diversity, physiological relations, and variability of the pineal's peripheral effects, and the constancy, rapidity, and homeostatic nature of its central and behavioral effects are consistent with the view that the pineal's primary action is on brain tissue. It remains probably that on a seasonal basis, the pineal's vegetative and homeostatic effects may contribute to the adaptive physiological changes in particular mammalian species under the influence of changes in photoperiod and possibly other environmental factors [17].

16.6 The Role of the Pineal in Clocks

The clock role of the pineal is species dependent. There is evidence that four vertebrate structures may be biological pacemakers: in vitro oscillatory capability is evidence for clock function in pineal, retina, and adrenal; rhythmic electrical activity in isolated hypothalmic islands is evidence for clock function in the suprachiasmatic nuclei. Loss of rhythmicity after ablation of the structures is evidence that they may function as pacemakers that provoke rhythms in other structures or synchronize rhythms of other structures. The pineal may act as its own photoreceptor for circadian synchronization, detecting

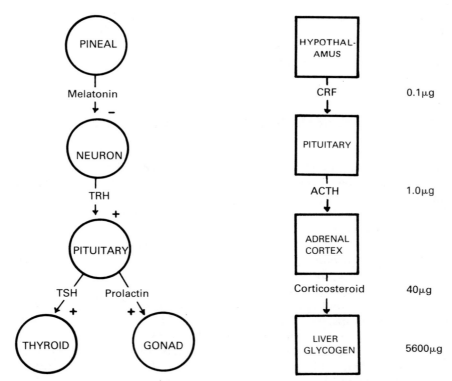

Figure 16.1 Models of endocrine hierarchies showing (*A*) pineal involvement (TRH hypothesis of pineal function), and (*B*) signal amplification. In *A*, the pineal secretes melatonin, which inhibits neurons in the hypothalamus that secrete TRH (thyroid stimulating hormone releasing hormone). When TRH secretion is not inhibited by melatonin, it stimulates the pituitary to secrete TSH (thyroid stimulating hormone), which in turn stimulates the thyroid to secrete thyroid hormones; TRH also stimulates prolactin secretion by the pituitary which in turn stimulates reproduction. (After Vriend [23].)

In *B*, 0.1 μg of CRF (corticotropin releasing hormone) secreted from the median eminence of the hypothalamus releases 1.0 μg of ACTH (adrenocorticotropin) from the pituitary. The ACTH stimulates the adrenal cortex to produce 40 μg of corticosteroid, which in turn causes deposit of 5600 μg of glycogen in the liver. The amplification is 56,000 times (10 × 40 × 140). (After Bentley [2].)

light with mechanisms within its own cells. On the other hand, the pineal may act as a slave driven by a clock that is located elsewhere and receives light information from retinal and nonretinal receptors.

16.6.1 The pineal as a pacemaker

The pineal is a circadian biological clock in some species; however, in those species it is not the only clock, but one of several. The

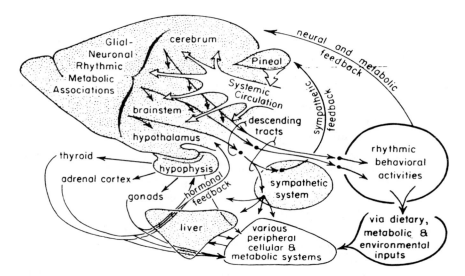

Figure 16.2 Representation of the interaction between the pineal, its targets, and factors that influence the pineal. (From Quay [16] with permission of *American Zoologist*).

melatonin-generating system is likely a means of conveying time information from the pineal. Ablation of the pineal produces arrhythmicity in some species. Moreover, removing the eyes (and their melatonin-generating system) renders yet other species arrhythmic. The evidence is thus strong that nightly melatonin synthesis can provide a periodic time signal. The simple idea is that nightly melatonin production is somehow responsible for rest in diurnal organisms and for activity in nocturnal organisms.

Components of the oscillating system have been considered in the pineal; in particular, the question has been asked, Is there a population of oscillators in the pineal? The pineal has clock capabilities in culture: rhythms persist in DD, entrain to LD, and damp in LL; the glands exhibit timekeeping; the glands exhibit a rapid plummet. For the pineal there is evidence that the clock may reside in a single cell type (possibly the pinealocyte) because cells isolated in culture exhibit persistent rhythms [9]. Moreover, when pineals are cut into smaller and smaller pieces, the pieces exhibit rhythms [23]. Single-celled organisms exhibit circadian rhythms so the possibility of the circadian clock mechanism, and even the photoreceptive component, residing in single cells in not outrageous. Even in those species whose pineals are capable of independent melatonin rhythm generation in vitro, however, there is evidence of neural input, providing means of entering extrapineal data from the organism into the pineal clock.

There is a virtual clockshop of models for possible circadian rhythm generation by cells, and these models include most of the available cell parts (the nucleus, the mitochondria, the cell membrane, etc.) as possible "wheels" and "mainsprings." An "enzyme clock" model was proposed for the pineal clock based on the properties of N-acetyltransferase (NAT) [5]. In the enzyme model, high melatonin is produced by continous production of new NAT molecules in the dark for a period of time specified by a "program" that is generated in the prior light-time. The amount of the NAT synthesized, the exact molecular form of NAT synthesized, and the duration of NAT production are programmed. Cessation of NAT synthesis is accomplished two ways. First, NAT declines when the programmed sequence ends; this occurs in DD. Second, light has two effects: (1) it causes a rapid plummet; and (2) it begins to reprogram the phase (rise time), amplitude, and duration of the next cycle. If the light is brief (a pulse) and the program was not completed, NAT reinitation occurs when dark is reimposed.

The properties of the NAT rhythm (and melatonin output) correlate with behavioral changes in rhythms including entrainment, free-run in DD, suppression by light, photoperiod compression and decompression of activity and rest times, and phase shifting. Most interesting, it is possible to explain phase responses (phase changes of the rhythm following a perturbation).

A property of the NAT system is the presence of a sensitive time (when NAT can be stimulated by dark) beginning in the late subjective day and continuing into the early subjective night. A shift to an insensitive refractory state occurs in the night so that the system is insensitive in the late subjective night and early subjective day. A shift from delays to advances occurs in the mid-subjective night in response to light pulses imposed in dark. The shift may be due to the change from sensitive to refractory status. That is, if light is imposed while the system is sensitive, most of the NAT cycle is completed upon restoration of dark, a subjective day of roughly fixed duration passes, and the subsequent cycle is delayed a bit by the duration of the pulse. If light is imposed while the system is refractory, NAT does not rise, the passage of the subjective day is begun, and the next cycle is advanced. A dark pulse in the sensitive time permits initiation of a cycle; return to light begins the passage of the subjective day, and the subsequent cycle is advanced. A dark pulse in the refractory portion has little effect on the cycle because NAT cannot initiate.

The fact that the NAT rhythm and other circadian rhythms have similar properties (e.g., locomotor activity) could derive from (1) the NAT cycle being part of a clock, or (2) NAT and the other rhythms both being driven by the same clock. The evidence that the NAT rhythm may be part of the clock mechanism comes from its persistence in vitro and the fact that rhythms in NAT respond at once to the lighting changes, which would be expected if they in turn drive other rhythms.

Moreover, the properties of NAT provide a rationale for measurement of the dark period (Section 16.7.2).

16.6.2 The Pineal as one of several oscillators

Since the eyes may also produce rhythmic melatonin, the pineal may be one of several oscillators (at least three, two eyes and one pineal) providing time information via melatonin production. Ablation of either structure may cause arrhythmia, or it may be necessary to ablate both structures. In an intact individual, with several oscillators, synchronization among the oscillators would be the normal physiological state.

In a multicellular organism, even if all its cells possess clock capability, there is the added problem of synchronizing the oscillations. The solution to this problem may be that the components are arranged in hierarchies of oscillators [11] (see Fig 16.3). In such a hierarchy (1) photoreceptors, which may not be oscillators themselves, are at the pinnacle: (2) the photoreceptors inform the independent oscillators (pacemakers, driving oscillators) about environmental light and dark so that the oscillators synchronize with light-dark cycles; (3) where several independent oscillators are present, one dominates by synchronizing the others (driven or slave oscillators); and (4) signals from slave oscillators in turn drive yet other rhythms in structures that do not have oscillatory capability themselves. The pineal may fit into hierarchical schemes in different positions depending upon the species.

One model, the "neuroendocrine loop" model, in which the pineal is one of several oscillators is that proposed by Cassone and Menaker [8] for birds in which there are oscillators in the eye, suprachiasmatic nuclei (SCN), and pineal (Fig. 16.4). Their proposition is: "The avian circadian system has as its core the mutual interactions of the pineal, retinae, and SCN. . . . these three components contain multiple circadian oscillators." They go on to describe details:

> The pineal actively secretes melatonin during subjective night into the blood. This melatonin is concentrated by the hypothalamus where it inhibits SCN activity, possibly via the activation of inhibitory 5-HT pathways. As melatonin levels fall with the approach of dawn, the SCN is disinhibited and its cells activate in synchrony, increasing metabolic and electrical activity and output. This output, through the sympathetic SCG, inhibits the production of melatonin during the subjective day through the secretion of inhibitory norepinephrine within the pineal. [8]

16.6.3 Redundancy

In the regulation of circadian rhythms as it relates to the pineal there appear to be three kinds of redundancy: (1) photoreceptors for

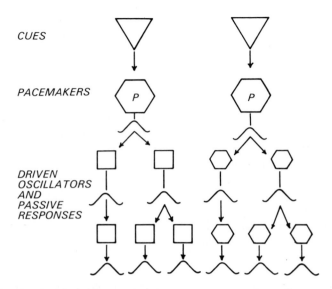

CUES

PACEMAKERS

DRIVEN
OSCILLATORS
AND
PASSIVE
RESPONSES

Figure 16.3 Models of hierarchical organizations of oscillators. Triangles represent receptors of external time cues (e.g., light and dark in the environment), which are at the apex of the hierarchy. Hexagons represent oscillators (e.g., a cell or group of cells with the ability to generate a circadian rhythm with a specific period). Hexagons with a P represent pacemakers (driving oscillators). Squares represent cells that respond passively. Sinusoidal lines represent oscillations in measurable parameters. The arrows represent the flow of information. The model to the left has a single pacemaker and the model on the right is a multioscillator model. (After Moore-Ede et al. [15].)

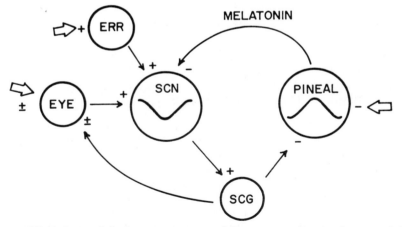

Figure 16.4 A simplified representation of the neuroendocrine loop model in which the suprachiasmatic nuclei (SCN) oscillator influences the pineal oscillator via the superior cervical ganglia (SCG), and the pineal oscillator feeds back on the rhythm in the SCN via melatonin. A possible third oscillation is in the eyes (not shown); melatonin may act within the eye. Light (*open arrows*) is perceived by the eyes and by extraretinal receptors (ERR). (After Cassone and Menaker [8].)

circadian rhythms include the eyes, pineal, and other extraretinal receptors; (2) in vertebrates, clocks include the pineal, eyes, SCN, and adrenal; and (3) there are multiple sites of melatonin synthesis. Each species may have formed its own hierarchy to suit its own requirements capitalizing on some of the components here while reducing others there. For example, in the mammalian system, photoreception has been reduced to the eyes, the pacemaker is localized in the SCN, and the pineal is driven by neural signals.

16.7 The Pineal as a Calendar

The seasonal and photoperiodic roles of the pineal [22] invite consideration of how the pineal might function in a calendar for yearly events. There are a number of hypotheses for how melatonin might mediate photoperiodic events (Fig. 16.5). Many of the hypotheses might be true simultaneously if different animals have exploited different aspects of pineal physiology to achieve photoperiodic time measurement each to suit its own needs.

16.7.1 Season analog model

The simplest idea is that the pineal converts changes in night (and day) length to a hormone signal, a "season analog" model. In such a model, circadian rhythmicity, an endogenous clock, is not necessary. The pineal could change the overall level of some parameter with season.

Initial attempts to find evidence for a seasonal model have focussed on hydroxyindole-O-methyltransferase (HIOMT; Fig. 16.5A). A relatively simple correlation between HIOMT and season (natural photoperiods) that is the reverse of the testes cycle has been reported for sparrows and ground squirrels [1]. Laboratory evidence was sought and found in some experiments where HIOMT was measured in different photoperiods, in constant light, and in constant dark.

16.7.2 Nightlength measurement using duration

A number of descriptions and models exist that are based on pineal measurement of nightlength (Fig. 16.5B). A biochemical event that tracked day- or nightlength by accumulation of some substance would provide a means for photoperiod or scotoperiod measurement. This view of the author's was stated as a "duration" model [11]:

> The large changes in indole metabolism that occur in the pineal gland during the course of the day provide a means of turning environmental light signals into biochemical messages that are measurements of the *duration* of the dark and light periods. Long dark periods would allow

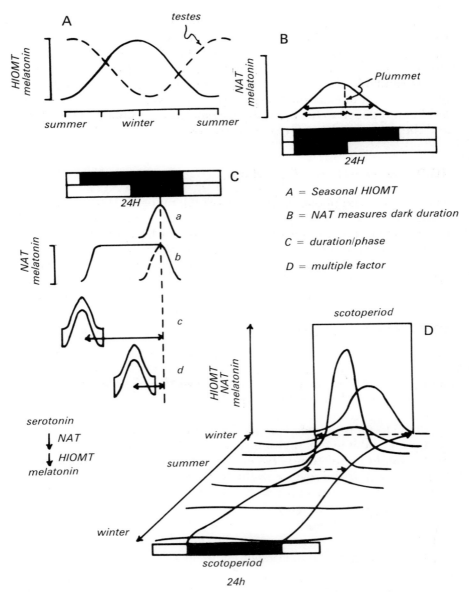

Figure 16.5 Models for pineal function as a calendar. *A* shows the simplest idea, that a pineal parameter (HIOMT) might simply fluctuate on a seasonal basis. Melatonin in turn would fluctuate, and, through antigonadal action, would produce a cycle of reproduction (testis size).

B shows the idea that the pineal can keep track of the length of the dark-time. When the dark is long, NAT and melatonin are produced for a long time (e.g., 12 hours); when the dark is short, NAT and melatonin are high for a shorter period of time (e.g., 8 hours in LD 16:8). NAT and melatonin can only rise when permitted by the circadian clock to do so, when the system is not refractory, during the subjective night. (After Binkley [3, 4]).

longer periods of high melatonin and N-acetylserotonin production to occur, and these would presumably result in periods during which blood levels of these compounds would be elevated.

Experimentally, NAT duration was shown to be lengthened in a long night (lower amplitude) and shortened in a short night (higher amplitude) in chickens [7]. The finding that melatonin duration is important in some species, coupled with the way NAT duration responded to nightlength provided a basis for consideration of the possibility that NAT's map of the nightlength is used as a timestick to measure nightlength and convert it to a melatonin signal. Goldman and Darrow [10] stated the duration hypothesis for photoperiodism in the Djungarian hamster:

> The duration of the nocturnal peak of melatonin is inversely related to daylength. The reproductive system appears to receive daylength information "coded" in the form of a nocturnal melatonin peak of variable duration; long duration peaks (i.e., 8–12 h) signal short days, while short duration peaks (i.e., 4–6 h) signal long days. In the context of this hypothesis, pinealectomy must be viewed as an operation which prevents the reproductive system from receiving daylength information. The hypothesis . . . leads to the prediction that pinealectomy would prevent the appearance of differential reproductive responses under different photoperiods.

For many photoperiodic systems, light-break and resonance experiments demonstrate a circadian component (the Bünning hypothesis: *when* light is imposed is important, not just *how much* light there is). Short light periods that interrupt the subjective night can mimic results characteristic of short nights (long days). Models must explain this phenomenon. The enzyme model (Figs. 16.6–16.8) is consistent with the Bünning hypothesis. The properties of NAT (and serotonin and melatonin via NAT action) can explain light-break experiments. In the model, there is a "window" of time, a sensitive period (late subjective day, early subjective night) preprogrammed by the light

---

C shows the possibility that phases of two oscillators—one set by dawn (*line*), the other set by dusk (*open*)—are changed by photoperiod. The phase of the dawn-set oscillation (*a*) is indicated by the vertical dashed line. In a short photoperiod (*c*), the phase difference is larger than in a long photoperiod (*d*). The fact that the same thing can be achieved by duration is shown in (*b*) where the relevant parameter is the drop in NAT or melatonin that occurs at the end of the night.

D shows a seasonal model represented in three dimensions. In this presentation, the changing dark period (scotoperiod) is accompanied by changes in the amplitude and duration of melatonin, which together produce a dramatic signal for the change of season. (Based on data for the tortoise provided by Vivien-Roels, Arendt, and Bradtke [25].)

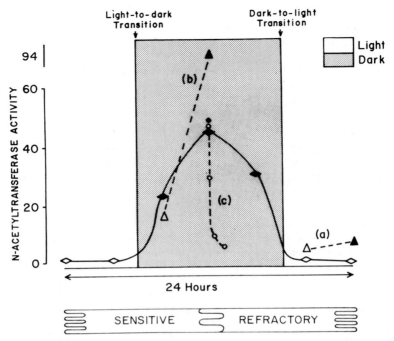

Figure 16.6 The enzyme clock model is based on the properties of the rhythm in *N*-acetyltransferase (NAT). The NAT cycle in LD 12:12 is shown by the solid line with diamonds. The triangles show that in the early subjective day, NAT does not rise much in response to imposition of dark (*a*); in the subjective night, however, NAT ascends if dark is imposed (*b*). The unfilled circles show how once NAT has risen, light imposition causes a rapid plummet (*c*). The response to dark has been mapped to divide the cycle into two portions: (1) a sensitive portion encompassing the late subjective day, the expected lights-off time, and the early subjective night, and (2) a refractory portion encompassing the late subjective night (shaded area), expected lights-on transition, and the early subjective day. The durations of the refractory and sensitive portions may be programmed by the prior light-dark cycle. (After Binkley [3, 4].)

when dark can stimulate NAT; there is a refractory period when NAT cannot be stimulated (late subjective night through early subjective day); that is, there is a circadian rhythm of pineal sensitivity to stimulation in dark [5, 6, 7]. Once NAT has risen in dark, its activity can be rapidly reduced by light (rapid plummet) [12]. So NAT provides a record of nightlength [3,4] and the interpretation of a light-pulsed night as a "short" night can be explained by the NAT refractory period.

The manner in which prior light "programs" the course (amplitude, duration) of the subsequent night's NAT activity (and thus melatonin profile) has been considered in the enzyme clock model [5]. Requiring explanation is the fixed NAT pattern [13]. This author has

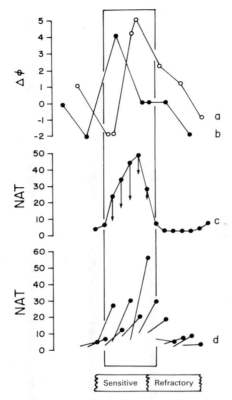

Figure 16.7 Representation of the relationship between phase-shifting the NAT rhythm (*a*, *b*), sensitivity of NAT to light in the dark-time (*c*), and refractoriness of NAT to stimulation by dark in the light-time (*d*) in the pineal NAT system using data derived from chicks. (*a*) Phase response curve derived for chick NAT using 4-hour light pulses. (*b*) Opposing phase response curve for chick NAT using 4-hour dark pulses. (*c*) Rapid plummets (*arrows*) which occur when chicks are exposed to 10 minutes of light in the dark-time (*closed circles* = NAT in the dark). (*d*) Points represent NAT levels reached after 4 hours of dark (lines extend back 4 hours to starting NAT values in the subjective first night of constant light) and show that NAT can be stimulated by dark only during the chick's expected, or subjective, night. The author contends that the middark changes from delay to advance phase shifts (*a*), from advance to delay phase shifts (*b*), from more to less sensitive to light (*c*), and from more to less refractory to dark (*d*) are caused by a common mechanism in the pineal gland deriving from the properties of NAT and the preprogramming of the course of NAT in the prior light period. (Unpublished synthesis by Binkley).

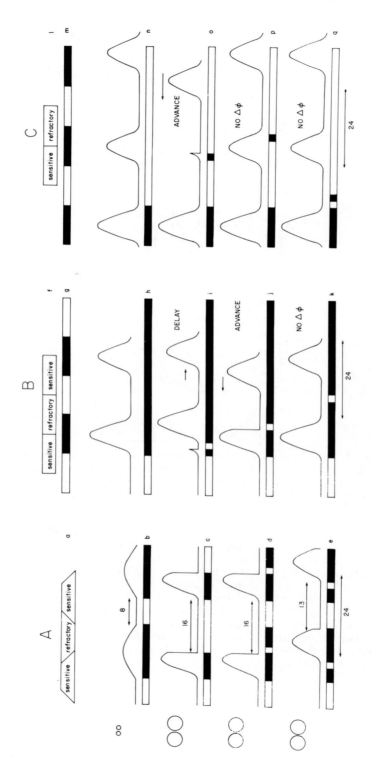

Figure 16.8

proposed that a nighttime pattern is a consequence of events that occur in the prior subjective day under the influence of light. Prior light exposure altered the response to dark of chick pineal glands in vivo [5] and of rat pineals to adrenergic stimulation [32]. It seems logical to consider the possibility that the biochemical basis for the responses might include events upon which NAT synthesis depends. One event might be the synthesis of the RNA which is used for NAT production; NAT appears to depend on early night production of RNA, though rat pineal RNA levels peak after 5 hours of light [5, 31, 32]. Interestingly, the initial induction of NAT requires RNA synthesis, but reinduction does not [31, 32]; Zatz has suggested the "cir-

---

Figure 16.8 Diagrammatic representation of the way the enzyme model with the shift from "sensitive" (dark stimulates NAT) to "insensitive" (dark does not stimulate NAT) explains (A) the way photoperiod is mimicked in light-break experiments, (B) phase shifts produced by light pulses, and (C) phase shifts produced by dark pulses. The model is drawn for a species whose NAT peak is lengthened in short photoperiod and shortened in long photoperiod. The horizontal bar over each figure (a, f, l) represents alternating 12-hour sensitive and refractory periods. Slanted lines in this bar in a represent the idea that the sensitive and refractory periods are malleable and are a function of photoperiod. The phase relationship of the sensitive-refractory cycle to light-dark cycles is represented in the horizontal bars, g and m. The graphs illustrate the time course of NAT and melatonin under the conditions shown in the horizontal bars below them (c—e, h—k, and n—q).

A, in short photoperiod (b, LD 8:16), the NAT cycle lengthens and damps, the testes (circles on left) are small. In long photoperiod (c, LD 16:8) the NAT cycle is shorter and of high amplitude; the testes are large. In a light-dark cycle with a late night light break (d, LDLD 8:8:2:6), the duration of NAT is short; the testes are large. In a light-dark cycle with an early night light break (e, LDLD 8:2:2:12), the duration of NAT is short; the testes are large. The amplitude of the NAT has not been measured for the light-break cycles shown in d and e.

B, the rhythm in NAT persists in DD (h) with reduced amplitude. If a single light pulse is imposed in the early subjective night (i), NAT plummets in the light and rises in the dark to "complete" its cycle because the system is still "sensitive." When NAT finally drops (later than usual), a new "day" is begun. The subsequent cycle is delayed. If a single light pulse is imposed in the late subjective night (j), NAT plummets in the light and does not reinitiate because the refractory period has been entered. The new "day" begins early. The subsequent cycle is advanced.

C, the rhythm in NAT persists in dim LL (n) although the peak time is delayed and the amplitude is altered. When a dark pulse is imposed in the early subjective night (o, during the sensitive period) it provokes an early peak in NAT. Abruptly a new "day" is begun and the subsequent cycle is advanced. If a dark pulse is imposed in the late subjective night (p), NAT is already up; the additional dark may provoke an increase in the NAT to higher levels because it removes the suppressive effect of light. However, because NAT has already increased, the effect on the subsequent cycle is negligible. When the dark pulse is imposed during the early subjective day (when the system is refractory), it has no effect (q).

cadian rhythm in presumptive messenger RNA parallels that of serotonin *N*-acetyltransferase" [31]. Wainwright and Wainwright [28] pushed the molecular events back yet another level by proposing that NAT was dependent upon excision repair of DNA. Alternatively, Klein and Weller [13] suggested explanations that involved nighttime events—the possibility that NAT fell in rat pineal cultures after 12 hours of norepinephrine (NE) stimulation because an "endogenous inhibitor" was formed or because a compound that stabilized NAT was gradually consumed.

16.7.3 Clock-gate model

Lewy [14] coined the term *clock-gate model* to describe the previously found [4] interaction of the circadian clock and dark in promoting melatonin synthesis. For melatonin synthesis to occur a "clock" (e.g., a circadian sensitive period for NAT stimulation) must be "on" and a "gate" (e.g., dark) must be "open." Lewy raised the possibility that light suppression of melatonin and generation of the dark-time rise by a clock may involve separate mechanisms:

> Because of the suppressant effect of light, darkness acts as a "gate" that must be open in order for melatonin production to be expressed, providing that it coincides with the proper circadian phase (as set by the endogenous "clock" or pacemaker, the SCN). Light also entrains the endogenous pacemaker in a relationship described by a PRC [phase response curve]. In other words, light entrains the clock (the endogenous pacemaker for melatonin production), but light can also suppress the "hand of the clock" (melatonin production per se) . . . . these two effects of light appear to be different and the pathways mediating the suppressant and the entrainment effects of light may not be the same. [14]

16.7.4 Interval and circadian timers

Silver and Bittman [21] discussed "two-timer" models for reproductive events. In the models there are (1) 24-hour oscillators and (2) shorter-interval nonoscillatory timers. The interval timer accumulates information until some threshold is reached. Once the interval timer has stored enough information, it awaits the appropriate phase for activation of the circadian effector system: "The photoperiodic system which measures nightlength requires a melatonin stimulus that is nearly continuous over a critical duration that corresponds to the threshold nightlength" [21].

16.7.5 Coordinating signal

Tamarkin, Baird, and Almeida [24] pondered the dichotomy in the patterns of melatonin response to photoperiod: (1) "tailoring" the melatonin profile by photoperiod (alteration of the duration of high melatonin), versus (2) confinement of melatonin to the late dark-time (phase-locking it to dawn) with relatively little effect of photoperiod on duration.

> The mammalian pineal generates a daily melatonin signal that can be altered by light in its duration, phase, and amplitude. A signal that can be modulated in these ways has the potential for synchronizing complex physiological processes in which temporal coordination is crucial. [24]

It is not necessary for determination of nightlength to have a parameter that is actually of long or short duration. Another way to accomplish the same thing is to have two oscillations—the first rhythm must set its phase with dusk (light-to-dark transition), and the second rhythm must set its phase with dawn (dark-to-light transition). The effect of such a system is that the two oscillators change their relative positions as photoperiod increases and diminishes (Fig. 16.5C). This type of thinking helps explain the case in the golden hamster where the duration of the NAT rhythm is little modified by nightlength, but the decline in NAT is phase-locked to dawn. The duration and two-oscillator ideas are not mutually exclusive. The phase of an event coupled to dawn (e.g., fall in NAT) relative to an event whose phase is set with dusk can also be accomplished by changing the durations of one or both parameters. The melatonin secretion rhythm of the pineal is an obvious candidate for one of the oscillations (probably the one phase locked to dawn). A rhythm of sensitivity in a target (e.g., receptor sensitivity) could provide the second oscillation.

16.7.6 Down regulation

In one model, the receptor sensitivity rhythm is attributed to melatonin itself. Attempting to explain the effect of timed injections and continuous melatonin administration (which blocked the timed injection effects) in golden hamsters, Reiter [20] proposed a "down regulation" receptor model:

> Melatonin administered daily in the afternoon inhibits reproduction whereas in the morning it is without effect. Endogenously produced melatonin is normally secreted late during the dark phase. After melatonin acts on its receptors, it may render them temporarily insensitive (increased threshold) to additional melatonin, i.e., the receptor may become transiently refractory. Hence, early in the light phase the receptors are in a desensitized state and cannot respond to exogenously injected melatonin. By late afternoon the sensitivity of the receptors is reestablished. Thus, an injection of melatonin at this time is capable of acting, and reproductive atrophy ensues.

This model must yet explain the sensitivity to melatonin that occurs near dawn and the rhythmic sensitivity to melatonin in pinealectomized hamsters.

16.7.7 Mechanistic model

Ralph [18] proposed a "mechanistic model for the diurnal melatonin cycle serving as a determinant of seasonal adaptations." The model involves an interaction between a neural clock of fixed interval and melatonin duration. In the model, the phase of the onset of the neural clock is locked to the rise in melatonin.

> The rising titre of melatonin, after the onset of darkness, reaches threshold for starting a fixed-interval, neural clock. If time expires daily for the clock while still within the envelope of high melatonin titre, as during long nights, the winter program of adaptations is invoked (or maintained). During short nights, the fixed-interval clock advances through the shortened melatonin envelope, permitting the summer program of adaptations to be invoked. [18]

16.7.8 Rhythm of sensitivity model

Watson-Whitmyre [29] proposed a model for photoperiodic time measurement in hamsters that incorporated aspects of both external and internal coincidence. In the model the phase relationship of the melatonin rhythm and a rhythm of sensitivity to melatonin is recognized. The model was generated because pinealectomized hamsters exhibited a rhythm of sensitivity to melatonin injections (peak in early dark-time) whose phase differed from the endogenous rhythm in pineal melatonin (peak in late dark-time).

> The model recognizes that light entrains the circadian clock (the SCN) through a receptor, known to be the retina. The circadian clock is responsible for phasing the pineal melatonin rhythm, resulting in a longer duration of melatonin production as the dark period is increased. The circadian clock is also presumably responsible for phasing the rhythm of sensitivity to melatonin, which is likely located within the hypothalamus. Sensitivity to melatonin is maximal at CT 12 to CT 19 on short days. However, the rhythm of sensitivity to melatonin is not present on long days; it is induced only by short days. It is this feature which distinguishes the proposed model from either external or internal coincidence. Discrimination of daylength depends on the interaction between the rhythm of sensitivity to melatonin and the melatonin rhythm itself, as in internal coincidence. This interaction, probably receptor mediated, results in modulation of neurohormone secretion within the hypothalamus. [29]

16.7.9 Amplitude, phase, and duration

Seasonal changes in melatonin profiles have been measured in some species (e.g., tortoise [25]) and found to exhibit changes in amplitude and duration (Fig. 16.5*D*). Thus, the pineals of some species may exploit several of the possible strategies (amplitude, phase, duration) to convert seasonal changes in photoperiod into precise endocrine signals.

Alteration of the amplitude and duration of melatonin can be explained several ways:

1. There may be a seasonal shift in the rate-limiting enzyme. The nightlength may be measured by NAT and NAT may be the rate-limiting enzyme for the daily cycle of melatonin production when HIOMT is high. Low HIOMT during some seasons might render HIOMT the rate-limiting enzyme reducing melatonin production. Evidence for this kind of complex seasonal modulation of melatonin has been observed [25].

2. Alteration in the amplitude of the melatonin cycle may be accomplished or augmented by changing the average level achieved by NAT. Long dark (LD 8:16) lowered average chick pineal NAT amplitude by 35% compared to the excursion in short dark (LD 16:8). The duration of chick pineal NAT in short dark was compressed to as little as 8 hours; in long dark NAT stayed up 12 hours or more [7].

3. Changes in circulating melatonin amplitude could be a function of secretion rather than of synthesis. Pulsatile melatonin release (as is claimed for sheep, humans, and ponies) would permit variation in circulating duration/amplitude by pulse frequency and pulse height.

16.7.10 Lengthening or shortening

Measurement of photoperiod may not be enough. Since all photoperiods occur twice a year, an organism must detect the direction of change of the photoperiod—whether it is lengthening or shortening. In order to make the discrimination, some mechanism for "remembering" the prior photoperiod is prerequisite. As indicated, the time courses of the pineal enzymes under the influence of light and dark provide prior day's length information and could thus participate in the "memory" mechanism.

REFERENCES

1. Barfuss, D., and L. Ellis. 1971. Seasonal cycles in melatonin synthesis by the pineal gland as related to testicular function in the house sparrow (*Passer domesticus*) *Gen. Comp. Endocrinol.* 17:183–193.

2. Bentley, P. 1976. *Comparative vertebrate endocrinology.* Cambridge, England: Cambridge Univ. Press.

3. Binkley, S. 1976a. Comparative biochemistry of the pineal glands of birds and mammals. *Amer. Zool.* 16:57–65.

4. ———. 1976b. Pineal gland biorhythms: *N*-acetyltransferase in chickens and rats. *Fed. Proc.* 35:2347–2352.

5. ———. 1983. Rhythms in ocular and pineal *N*-acetyltransferase: A portrait of an enzyme clock. *Comp. Biochem. Physiol.* 75A:123–129.

6. Binkley, S., D. Klein, and J. Weller. 1973. Dark-induced increase in pineal serotonin *N*-acetyltransferase activity: A refractory period. *Experientia* 29:1339–1340.

7. Binkley, S., J. Stephens, J. Riebman, and K. Reilly. 1977. Regulation of pineal rhythms in chickens: Photoperiod and dark-time sensitivity. *Gen. Comp. Endocrinol.* 32:411–416.

8. Cassone, V., and M. Menaker. 1984. Is the avian circadian system a neuroendocrine loop? *J. Exp. Zool.* 232:539–549.

9. Deguchi, T. 1979. A circadian oscillator in cultured cells of chicken pineal gland. *Nature* 282:94–96.

10. Goldman, B., and J. Darrow. 1983. The pineal gland and mammalian photoperiodism. *Neuroendocrinology* 37:386–396.

11. Klein, D. 1974. Circadian rhythms in indole metabolism in the rat pineal gland. In *The neurosciences*, 3rd study program, ed. F. O. Schmitt and F. Worden, pp. 509–515. Cambridge, Mass.: MIT Press.

12. Klein, D., and J. Weller. 1972. Rapid light-induced decrease in pineal serotonin *N*-acetyltransferase activity. *Science* 177:532–533.

13. ———. 1973. Adrenergic-adenosine 3′,5′-monophosphate regulation of serotonin *N*-acetyltransferase activity and the temporal relationship of serotonin *N*-acetyltransferase activity to synthesis of 3H-N-acetylserotonin and 3H-melatonin in the cultured rat pineal gland. *J. Pharm. Exp. Therap.* 186:516–527.

14. Lewy, A. 1983. Biochemistry and regulation of mammalian melatonin reproduction. In *The pineal gland*, ed. R. Relkin, pp. 77–128. New York: Elsevier.

15. Moore-Ede, M., W. Schmelzer, D. Kass, and J. Herd. 1976. Internal organization of the circadian timing system in multicellular animals. *Fed. Proc.* 35:2333–2338.

16. Quay, W. 1955. Rhythmic and light-induced changes in levels of 5-hydroxyindoles in the pigeon (*Columba livia*). *Gen. Comp. Endocrinol.* 6:371–377.

17. ———. 1970. Endocrine effects of the mammalian pineal. *Amer. Zool.* 10:237–246.

18. Ralph, C. 1983. Evolution of pineal control of endocrine function in lower vertebrates. *Amer. Zool.* 23:597–605.

19. Reiter, R. 1972. The role of the pineal in reproduction. In *Reproductive biology*, ed. H. Balin and S. Glasser, pp. 71–114. Amsterdam: Excerpta Medica Monograph.

20. ———. 1980. The pineal and its hormones in the control of reproduction in mammals. *Endocrine Rev.* 1:109–131.

21. Silver, R., and E. Bittman. 1983. Reproductive mechanisms: Interaction of circadian and interval timing. *Ann. N.Y. Acad. Sci.* 423:488–514.

22. Stetson, M., and M. Watson-Whitmyre. 1984. Physiology of the pineal and

its hormone melatonin in annual reproduction in rodents. In *The pineal gland*, ed. R. Reiter, pp. 109–153. New York: Raven Press.

23. Takahashi, J., and M. Menaker. 1984. Multiple redundant circadian oscillators within the isolated avian pineal gland. *J. Comp. Physiol.* 154:435–440.

24. Tamarkin, L., C. Baird, and O. Almeida. 1985. Melatonin: A coordinating signal for mammalian reproduction. *Science* 227:714–720.

25. Vivien-Roels, B., J. Arendt, and J. Bradke. 1979. Circadian and circannual fluctuations of pineal indoleamines (serotonin and melatonin) in *Testudo hermanni Gmelin* (Reptilia, Chelonia). *Gen. Comp. Endocrinol.* 37:197–210.

26. Vriend, J. 1983. Pineal-thyroid interactions. In *Pineal Research Reviews I*, ed. R. Reiter, pp. 183–206. New York: Alan R. Liss.

27. Wainwright, S. 1982. Some answers to a 2000-year-old question: The role(s) of the pineal gland. *Rev. Pure Appl. Pharmacol. Sci.* 3:185–262.

28. Wainwright, S., and L. Wainwright. 1986. Effects of some inhibitors of DNA synthesis and repair upon the cycle of serotonin N-acetyltransferase activity in cultured chick pineal glands. *Biochem.* Cell Biol. 64:344–355.

29. Watson-Whitmyre, M. 1985. Photoperiodism in the golden hamster: Dependence on rhythmic sensitivity to melatonin. Ph.D. diss., Univ. of Delaware.

30. Wurtman, R., J. Axelrod, and D. Kelly. 1968. *The pineal*. New York: Academic Press.

31. Zatz, M. 1981. Pharmacology of the rat pineal gland. In *The pineal gland I: Anatomy and biochemistry*, ed. R. Reiter, pp. 229–242. Boca Raton, Fla.: CRC Press.

32. Zatz, M., J. Romero, and J. Axelrod. 1976. Diurnal variation in the requirement for RNA synthesis in the induction of pineal N-acetyltransferase. *Biochem. Pharmacol.* 25:903–906.

17

Epilogue

"Pineal (pīn´ ēal, pin´ ē ăl) n: a small gland located centrally in the brains of most vertebrates which functions in photoreception, seasonal reproduction, circadian rhythms, and integument color via production of a hormone, melatonin, and/or other hormones—also called *epiphysis cerebri*. adj: pertaining to the pineal."

Binkley

17.1 Introduction

It is the purpose of this chapter to provide a status report on pineal researches and the place they have earned for the gland in physiology. Pineal function—in reproduction and in rhythms—is now well established, whereas "Prior to 1950 one could confidently say that we were effectively ignorant of the influence of the pineal gland on the endocrine and reproductive systems" [14].

Thus, although pineal functions may yet be sought, the direction of research effort has shifted to how the pineal achieves its effects. As is generally the case in science, new findings have led to new questions.

As pointed out in Chapter 1, the author views the daily rhythms in the pineal and regulation of the pineal by environmental lighting as the first key to understanding pineal physiology. A second key that has opened doors to comprehension of pineal function has been the comparative approach, that is, the appreciation that pineal function is part and parcel of the adaptations of a species to its external environment. Based on our understanding of the pineal's rhythmic properties in animals and the recent advances in our ability to measure melatonin in human blood, it has become possible to consider how melatonin may function in humans.

At the time of this writing, the details of pineal anatomy, physiology, biochemistry, and regulation by light and dark comprise the most comprehensive description of a circadian biochemical system. As such, the body of knowledge about the pineal stands as a model for seeking circadian systems in invertebrates (which lack a pineal glad) and for understanding the role of natural rhythms in other endocrine glands.

17.2 Anatomical Relationships

Descriptions of slices of pineals from a variety of species with various techniques have been the basis of most of the extant anatomical work. New technology should permit more three-dimensional descriptions, which may be particularly interesting for pineals that have a stalk, a rosette arrangement of cells, and photoreceptor-like structures. Three-dimensional analyses may also prove that pineal cells and their contents have nonrandom orientations that are of physiological importance.

Histochemistry and autoradiography should enable us to continue assignment of pineal biochemical mechanisms to pineal cells and cell parts. In addition, it should be possible to make functional and anatomical distinctions (or to prove the lack of them) among putative pineal cell "types" using cloning methodology and cell cultures. The groundwork has been established in the finding that it is possible to grow pineal cells in culture, to stimulate their melatonin-synthesizing machinery with norepinephrine, and to obtain rhythms.

Most past work regarding the neural regulation of the pineal has focussed on the sympathetic innervation the pineal receives from the superior cervical ganglion (see Chapter 6). The β-regulation has not only been of interest to pinealogists, but because of the in vivo and in vitro responsiveness to β-adrenergic agents, the rat pineal has provided a model system for such regulation in general.

Always in the background and less understood has been the possibility of other neural connections between the pineal and the brain. For example, in the Djungarian hamster, immunocytochemistry has been used to trace the neural projections of pinealocytes [9]. The investigators used an antiserum to bovine retinal S-antigen and found that neural processes from pinealocytes of the deep pineal extended into the medial habenular nucleus and the posterior commissure of the brain. Based on this finding, the authors suggest that the cells are "derivatives of photoreceptor cells of the pineal complex of lower vertebrates that transmit signals to the brain by neural projections" [9].

17.3 Biochemistry

Probably the most significant biochemical advances attached to the pineal have been the realization first that hydroxyindole-O-methyltransferase (HIOMT), and second that N-acetyltransferase (NAT), had activities that were a consequence of environmental lighting. The changes in the enzymes that are brought about with lighting, especially the responses of NAT, explain the changes in pineal serotonin and in pineal melatonin production. Not only have the seasonal rhythms in the enzymes and their substrates provided a basis for explanation of pineal physiology, they have also been provocative of searches for other such rhythmic and environmental lighting control throughout the endocrine system [13].

The rhythmic responses of serotonin found explanation in the rhythmic and light-regulated properties of NAT (see Chapter 5). The details of NAT responses (e.g., dark-time peak whose amplitude and duration are a consequence of photoperiod and rapid plummet response to light) have been echoed in the determinations of pineal melatonin. The studies of NAT, which were all initially done in rodents and birds, have provided paradigms with which to study melatonin in pineals and body fluids of humans.

The properties of the pineal melatonin-generating system, particularly modification of phase, duration, and amplitude of NAT and melatonin by changing the spans of light and dark times, have provided a biochemical basis for photoperiodic time measurement [5]. It is the author's expectation that species-by-species elucidation of the seasonal changes in pineal biochemical rhythms will correlate in a meaningful way with species-by-species seasonal physiology.

The finding that eyes, as well as pineals, of some species are capable of rhythmic melatonin synthesis and responses to light and dark (Section 8.4) has required reconsideration of negative studies where pinealectomy had no effect [3]. A broader role of melatonin, including melatonin function in the eye, is a probable consequence of future research in this area.

Always possible, but elusive, is the potential for discovery of unsuspected other important biochemical products of any endocrine gland. The pineal, like other tissues, has this potential and papers appear daily noting the detection of additional biochemicals in the pineal. It remains for such studies to arrive at the detailed understanding that has been achieved for the melatonin-generating system.

We have reason to expect that investigators in the next few years will be able to provide fine descriptions of the characteristics of the pineal enzymes, especially NAT. Moreover, we can hope that the enzymes' properties can be compared for a variety of species, so that, for example, it may be possible to describe two forms of NAT in chick pineals as proposed by Wainwright and Wainwright [16] based on physiological evidence. Their proposal is that there is a "photostable" NAT molecule that accounts for the intermediate NAT levels seen in constant light during the projected subjective night; this NAT is not inhibited by light and does not respond with a rapid plummet. To account for the very high values of NAT seen in dark and the rapid plummet, the Wainwrights proposed a "photolabile" NAT, a molecule that is inhibited by light. NAT in pineal homogenates is not inhibited by light, so photolability must be indirectly regulated and is likely to be dependent upon intact cells. Moreover, it is possible that the daytime low (but nevertheless detectable) NAT can be attributed to still a third molecule. Characterizations of NAT molecules [12], which have been impeded by instability of the enzyme(s), should provide information as to the form(s) of the enzyme and their relationship to each other, as well as the meaning of disulfide inhibition and the rationale for cysteamine protection of NAT [4]. It is the author's further expectation that detailed examination of the forms of NAT produced following different photoperiods will provide clues to explanation of the observed duration-amplitude-phase consequences of photoperiod on NAT.

17.4 Regulation

For over a decade, work on the neural regulation of the pineal focussed on the β-adrenergic responses and the neural input the pineal receives via the superior cervical ganglia (Chapter 6). However, roles of other possible regulating agents have been considered. For example, Klein, Sugden, and Weller [11] have entered the idea that while "β-activiation is an absolute requirement, an α-adrenergic receptor mechanism potentiates β-adrenergic activation." The evidence for this is pharmacological—that phenylephrine (an α-agonist) potentiated NAT stimulation by isoproterenol and prazosin (an α-blocking agent) potentiated propranolol (a β-blocker) in blocking norepinephrine stimulation of melatonin synthesis.

In the "central dogma" of pineal regulation the β-adrenergic system triggers the NAT increase via cyclic AMP (Fig. 6.1). However, a mechanism has been proposed and dubbed *seesaw signal processing* [10] whereby norepinephrine also stimulates the production of cyclic GMP as well. By producing differential effects on the two cyclic nucleotides (termed homologous desensitization of cyclic AMP and homologous sensitization of cyclic GMP responses), a single norepinephrine input signal could provide two output messages.

17.5 Clock Function

Pineals of some species (lizards, chicks, sparrows) are of particular interest for their ability to generate circadian rhythms in NAT and/or melatonin production (see Chapters 6 and 15). Questions of how pineals generate the cycles are not only of interest to endocrinologists, but are of major importance to the field of circadian rhythms where the nature of circadian "clock" mechanism(s) is a primary concern.

An enzyme clock model for endogenous pineal generation of circadian cycles has been proposed [1, 2]:

> I will suggest an hypothesis for an enzyme clock based upon the properties of NAT in the chick pineal gland. The salient features of the clock include: enzyme synthesis and degradation; buildup of fixed amounts of an enzyme initiator; a rapid disulfide inactivation; and two forms of the enzyme, one photostable, one photolabile [2].

The enzyme clock model suggests a mechanism for determining the peak in NAT and its modification by lighting. The consequence is the ability to explain photoperiodism and resetting. The daily NAT peak's amplitude, phase, and duration are subject to modification by photoperiod and can provide a signal via melatonin for photoperiod-dependent events such as seasonal changes in reproductive function. Moreover, the changes between sensitive and refractory periods correlate with and can explain circadian resetting responses (see Chapter 16). There is evidence for a daytime event (the "initiator") that precedes and programs the subsequent night's NAT. At this point, that daytime event is unknown; RNA synthesis or DNA synthesis are candidates [2, 17, 18].

In seeking further details of the pineal clockworks, it would appear that pharmacological tools will provide an avenue of investigation. Using the rhythms of pineals in culture, drugs may be tested for their ability to (1) change the period length of the NAT/melatonin rhythm, or (2) reset or phase-shift the phase of the NAT-melatonin rhythm. This in vitro type of investigation may produce some information that can be correlated with properties of NAT or pineal physiology in some meaningful way. The potential difficulty is that some of the pharmacological successes may lack physiological meaning.

It seems unlikely, a priori, that pinealologists have happened on the single circadian clock mechanism in the elucidation of the properties of NAT. But there are two lines of research that should be pursued. First, the fate, possible rhythms, and regulation of serotonin (or other parts of melatonin-generating system) can be investigated in other circadian oscillators (the eye of *Aplysia*, the optic lobe of the cockroach). Lower vertebrates and some invertebrates do possess serotonin, melatonin, and HIOMT [15]. Some success has already been had in the finding that serotonin phase-shifts the rhythm of the *Aplysia* eye [7]. Second, other enzymes that have rhythms invite comparisons to search for similarities in regulation to those found in NAT [2, 8]. Accessible for study, for example, is the dinoflagellate, *Gonyaulax polyedra*, which has dark-time peaks in the activity of luciferase and total proteins [6]. The rhythms of this species are phase-shifted by protein synthesis inhibitors (e.g., anisomycin).

17.6 Calendar Function

As described throughout this book, the pineal has the capacity to respond to photoperiod. The principal response to lengths of light and dark that influences the output of the pineal is that of melatonin whose duration, amplitude, and phase are a consequence of NAT, whose duration, phase, and amplitude all respond to changing photoperiod. Moreover, it is possible that HIOMT, which also responds to photoperiod, provides an additional seasonal modulation of the melatonin output. In order to measure photoperiod, it does not seem that such a finely modulated signal would be required by all species—the phase or duration might be sufficient in some species. However, the potential exists for dramatic seasonal changes in the phase, amplitude, and duration of nightly melatonin secretion, which would provide an accurate conversion of the external lighting signal of season (photoperiod and scotoperiod) into an internal signal (daily melatonin pattern). (See Section 16.7.)

17.7 Output Signal and Targets

Melatonin has emerged as the primary candidate for a pineal secretory product. Identification of melatonin targets and receptors has not readily yielded the clear-cut mechanism whereby a hormone signal is recognized specifically and produces amplification that is the ideal in endocrinology. Hopefully, solutions will be found for target and receptor problems in the next decade. At this time, there is evidence for targets in the brain and in the skins of lower vertebrates (chromatophores). Pursuit of the manner in which known targets (e.g., chromatophores in amphibian skin) respond to melatonin may provide clues that will be useful in the search for other target cells. Identification of the targets and the receptor mechanism(s) within them is required for an understanding of how melatonin exerts its physiological effects.

REFERENCES

1. Binkley, S. 1979. A timekeeping enzyme in the pineal gland. *Sci. Amer.* 240:66–71.

2. ———. 1983. Rhythms in ocular and pineal *N*-acetyltransferase: A portrait of an enzyme clock. *Comp. Biochem. Physiol.* 75A:123–129.

3. Binkley, S., M. Hryshchyshyn, and K. Reilly. 1979. *N*-acetyltransferase activity responds to environmental lighting in the eye as well as in the pineal gland. *Nature* 281:479–481.

4. Binkley, S., D. Klein, and J. Weller. 1976. Pineal serotonin *N*-acetyltransferase activity: Protection of stimulated activity by acetyl-CoA and related compounds. *J. Neurochem.* 26:51–55.

5. Binkley, S., J. Stephens, J. Riebman, and K. Reilly. 1977. Regulation of pineal rhythms in chickens: Photoperiod and dark-time sensitivity. *Gen. Comp. Endocrinol.* 32:411–416.

6. Cornelius G., A. Schroeder-Lorenz, and L. Rensing. 1985. Circadian-clock control of protein synthesis and degradation in *Gonyaulax polyedra*. *Planta* 166:365–370.

7. Corrent, G., and A. Eskin. 1982. Transmitter-like action of serotonin phase shifting a rhythm from the *Aplysia* eye. *Amer. J. Physiol.* 242:R333–R338.

8. Johnson, C. H., and J. Hastings. 1986. The elusive mechanism of the circadian clock. *Amer. Sci.* 74:29–36.

9. Korf, H., A. Oksche, P. Ekstrom, I. Gery, J. Zigler, and D. Klein. 1986. Pinealocyte projections into the mammalian brain revealed with S-antigen antiserum. *Science* 231:735–737.

10. Klein, D., D. Auerbach, and J. Weller. 1981. Seesaw signal processing in pineal cells: Homologous sensitization of adrenergic stimulation of cyclic GMP accompanies homologous desensitization of β-adrenergic stimulation of cyclic AMP. *Proc. Nat. Acad. Sci. USA* 78:4625–4629.

11. Klein, D., D. Sugden, and J. Weller. 1983. Postsynaptic α-adrenergic receptors potentiate the β-adrenergic stimulation of pineal serotonin *N*-acetyltransferase. *Proc. Nat. Acad. Sci. USA* 80:599–603.

12. Klein, D., P. Voisin, and M. Namboodiri. 1986. The pineal family of aromatic amine *N*-acetyltransferases. *BioEssays* 3:217–220.

13. Krieger, D., ed. 1979. *Endocrine rhythms*. New York: Raven Press.

14. Reiter, R. 1972. The role of the pineal in reproduction. In *Reproductive biology*, ed. H. Balin and S. Glasser, pp. 71–114. Amsterdam: Excerpta Medica Monograph.

15. Takeda, M., Y. Endo, H. Saito, M. Nishimura, and J. Nishiitsutsuji-Uwo. 1985. Neuropeptide and monoamine immunoreactivity of the circadian pacemaker in *Periplaneta*. *Biomed. Res.* 6:395–406.

16. Wainwright, S., and L. Wainwright. 1981. Regulation of chick pineal serotonin *N*-acetyltransferase. In *Pineal function*, ed. C. D. Matthews and R. F. Seamark, pp. 199–210. Amsterdam: Elsevier/North-Holland.

17. ———. 1986. Effects of some inhibitors of DNA synthesis and repair upon the cycle of serotonin *N*-acetyltransferase activity in cultured chick pineal glands. *Biochem. Cell Biol.* 64:344–355.

18. Zatz, M. 1981. Pharmacology of the rat pineal gland. In *The pineal gland I: Anatomy and biochemistry*, ed. R. Reiter, pp. 229–242. Boca Raton, Fla.: CRC Press.

Glossary

amplitude The maximum minus the minimum value of a rhythm or oscillation.

antigonadal Inhibitory to the reproductive system; causing the testes and/or ovaries to decrease in size or weight or to become atrophic.

arrhythmic Lacking a discernible rhythm, a condition that sometimes results from pinealectomy or constant light.

atrophy A condition of wasting away or decline in functional ability.

AVT Arginine vasotocin, a nonapeptide that may be a hormone of the pineal.

β-receptor A theoretical membrane receptor for catecholamines (e.g., norepinephrine) that is defined pharmacologically (based on responses to stimulating and blocking agents).

biological clock A mechanism within an organism that is capable of generating repeated cycles (oscillations, rhythms) whose period is relatively insensitive to temperature, and which can be synchronized by environmental stimuli.

blood-brain barrier A term used to describe the inability of certain substances of the blood to be taken up by the brain. The pineal is commonly thought to be outside the blood-brain barrier for some substances.

cAMP Cyclic adenosine 3′, 5′ monophosphate; also abbreviated as cyclic AMP.

choroid plexus A vascular membrane located near the nether end of the pineal stalk, sometimes extirpated with the pineal. This structure is barely mentioned in association with the pineal despite its proximity to the gland (one investigator suggested that it concentrates melatonin and then secretes the melatonin into the CSF).

circadian rhythm A rhythm with a period of about 24 hours.

compensatory hypertrophy An endocrine phenomenon in which compensation for loss of a structure occurs. For example, when an ovary is removed, the remaining ovary compensates by increasing its function.

COMT Catecholamine-O-methyltransferase; catecholamine-O-methyltransferase activity.

critical photoperiod The duration of light in excess of which a photoperiodic reponse is that of a "long" day.

CT Circadian time; time from the organism's point of view in which the organism's circadian cycle is set "equal" to 24 and each $\frac{1}{24}$ of the cycle is considered to be an "hour." By convention CT 0 = onset of activity for diurnal animals and CT 12 = onset of activity for nocturnal animals.

diurnal Active in the daytime.

endocrine gland A ductless gland that secretes chemicals (hormones) into the blood.

entrainment Synchronization of a rhythm by a repetitive signal (e.g., the recurring light-dark cycle).

epiphysis cerebri Pineal.

free run Repetitive cycles of a rhythm in the absence of a synchronizing signal. The period of the free-run, τ, is considered to be the innate period of the rhythm. Also free-run, freerun.

frontal organ Stirnorgan; an extracranial organ, below the skin, lying in the median plane in some anurans, considered to be part of the pineal complex (it is not the pineal proper), served by the frontal nerve.

FSH Follicle stimulating hormone; glycoprotein hormone secreted by the pituitary gland that stimulates the gonads.

GnRH See LRH.

HIOMT Hydroxyindole-O-methyltransferase; pineal enzyme that converts N-acetylserotonin to melatonin with the methyl donor S-adenosylmethionine.

5-HIAA 5-hydroxyindole acetic acid.

5-HT 5-hydroxytryptamine; serotonin; precursor of melatonin.

5-HTOH 5-hydroxytryptophol.

hormone A chemical product of a ductless gland carried to its "target" via the blood; less rigorously used to denote any chemical messenger.

in vitro Outside the animal, as in organ culture, cell culture, or superfusion culture.

in vivo In the living animal.

ISO Isoproterenol.

isoproterenol An analogue of norepinephrine; may be more potent than norepinephrine.

LH Luteinizing hormone; interstitial cell stimulating hormone; glycoprotein hormone of the pituitary gland that stimulates the gonads (e.g., Leydig cells of testes).

LRH Luteinizing hormone releasing hormone; also abbreviated LHRH or GnRH.

LD 14:10 Light-dark cycle consisting of 14 hours of light in alternation with 10 hours of dark.

melatonin M, MT, MEL; methoxyindole hormone of the pineal gland.

melanophore A pigment-containing cell in the skin.

MIAA Methoxyindole acetic acid.

MSH Melanophore stimulating hormone or melanocyte stimulating hormone.

MT Melatonin.

5-MT 5-methoxytryptamine.

MTOH Methoxytryptophol.

NAT *N*-acetyltransferase; *N*-acetyltransferase activity, NAT is a pineal enzyme that converts serotonin to *N*-acetylserotonin and is distinguished by its marked circadian rhythm and sensitivity to light and dark.

nervi conarii Primary innervation of the pineal.

nocturnal Active in the nighttime.

NE Norepinephrine, a catecholamine that stimulates melatonin synthesis in some species.

parietal eye "Third eye" present in 60% of lizard genera; located in the midline of the dorsal head between the lateral eyes; may be covered by a transparent scale; part of the pineal complex (not the pineal proper).

photoperiod Light-time; length of the light-time; daylength.

photoperiodic Of phenomena that are responsive to daylength (or nightlength).

photoreceptor A structure that detects light.

phase Of a rhythm, "instantaneous state of an oscillation with a period, represented by the value of the variable and all its time derivatives"*

pineal Epiphysis cerebri.

pinealocytes One of the kinds of cells found in the pineal.

pineal recess Region of the third ventricle close to the pineal.

PMS Pregnant mare's serum, used experimentally for its gonadotrophic activity.

progonadal Promoting growth or function of the ovaries and/or testes.

PRL Prolactin; protein hormone of the pituitary gland related in structure to growth hormone.

puberty Period of sexual maturation.

rapid plummet Drop in *N*-acetyltransferase or melatonin that occurs in response to light at night with a halving time of 5 minutes or less.*

recrudescence Growth, increase in size, renewal of function (e.g., of testes); normal part of a seasonal cycle.

refractory period Portion of time including the late subjective night and early subjective day when melatonin synthesis (*N*-acetyltransferase) cannot be stimulated by placing the organism in dark.

* J. Aschoff *Circadian clocks,* pp. x–xix. Proceedings of the Feldafing Summer School. Amsterdam: North-Holland, 1965.

regression Involution, reduction in size, diminution of function (e.g., of testes); normal part of a seasonal cycle.

retinohypothalamic tract The nerve tract from the eye to the hypothalmus.

RIA Radioimmunoassay; a method of measuring a hormone or other molecule that involves binding characteristics of specific antibodies.

second messenger Cyclic nucleotide that acts within cells to convert information from receptor-hormone interaction to a sequence of enzymic steps.

Silastic® capsules Tubes with plugged ends filled with a substance (e.g., melatonin crystals); a means of administering a hormone continuously.

subsensitivity Reduced ability of melatonin synthesis to respond to stimulation (e.g., by isoproterenol); occurs after prolonged stimulation.

SCG Superior cervical ganglia; a pair of sympathetic ganglia located in the neck that relay neural signals to the pineal gland.

supersensitivity Increased ability of melatonin synthesis to respond to stimulation (e.g., by isoproterenol); occurs after stimulation deprivation (e.g., by denervation).

SCN Suprachiasmatic nuclei; bilateral region of the hypothalamus thought to generate circadian rhythm information which is conveyed neurally to the pineal gland in some species (e.g., rats).

synaptic ribbons Organelles found in the cytoplasm of pinealocytes in the vicinity of the plasmalemma; have daily cycles in some species; consist of an electron-dense rod surrounded by a layer of electron-lucent vesicles.

target Cells, tissues, or organs upon which a hormone acts.

transducer A mechanism for converting one type of signal into another type of signal (e.g., nerve signal into endocrine signal).

TRH Thyroid stimulating hormone (TSH) releasing hormone.

Annotated Bibliography

In science, there are a number of levels of information.

First, there is the direct knowledge of the scientist who actually did an experiment. The author, for example, has done pineal experiments with NAT assays which constitutes first-hand experience.

Second, there are the articles written by the scientists who did the experiments, the "primary literature." These articles usually contain descriptions of the actual methods used, the protocols used, and examples of the data that were obtained. References in these articles are usually to other primary articles.

Third, there are review articles. These articles consider, criticize, and compare the results of primary studies by many investigators. Review articles are particularly rich sources of references to the primary literature.

Fourth, there are chapters devoted to the specific topic of interest in textbooks that cover a broader subject area. Chapters on the pineal gland now appear in a number of endocrinology textbooks.

Fifth, there are books that are devoted entirely to the topic of interest. The books on the pineal gland are of different kinds. Symposium volumes are collections of papers (reviews and/or primary articles) presented by the scientists at a particular scientific meeting. Survey volumes are collections of invited chapters (reviews with some primary data) by various people in the field. Annual review volumes by a single author describe results of pineal research in a particular year.

In choosing references for the chapters in this book, the author included both primary articles and, where possible, review articles. These references, along with the citations in the review articles and the bibliographies provided in the books listed below, should lead to almost the entire primary pineal literature. Sadly, some of the older volumes are now out of print.

Fortunately, there is now a quarterly *Journal of Pineal Research* published by Alan R. Liss. The journal began publication in 1984 and is edited by R. Reiter, M. Karasek, and W. Quay.

ALTSCHULE, M. 1975. *Frontiers of pineal physiology.* Cambridge, Mass.: MIT Press. Nine contributions forming the proceedings of a conference under the auspices of the Foundation for Medical Research in Boston in 1970. 269 pp.

AXELROD, J., F. FRASCHINI, AND G. P. VELO. 1983. *The pineal gland and its endocrine role.* New York: Plenum. A compilation of papers presented at the NATO meeting in Erice, Sicily, in 1982. 604 pp.

BAGNARA, J. T., AND M. HADLEY. 1973. *Chromatophores and color change.* Englewood Cliffs, N.J.: Prentice-Hall. This book is an enthusiastic review (447 references) of the subject of skin pigmentation in lower vertebrates using the functional approach. It is well illustrated with photographs of pigment cells and with graphical illustrations and physiological data. 202 pp.

BARDASANO, J. L. 1978. *La glandula pineal.* Madrid: H. Blume Ediciones. A summary of what is known about the comparative morphology of the pineal gland. Paperback. 210 pp.

BARGMANN, W. 1943. Die epiphysis cerebri. In *Hdb. Mikrosk. Anat. Mensch.,* Bd. VI, 4, pp. 309–502. Hrsg. W.v. Mollendorff. Berlin: Springer-Verlag.

BIRAU, N., AND W. SCHLOOT. 1981. *Melatonin: Current status and perspectives.* Oxford: Pergamon Press. Contains 50 papers. Proceedings of an International Symposium on Melatonin held in Breman, Federal Republic of Germany, September 28–30, 1980. 410 pp.

BROWN, G, AND S. WAINWRIGHT. 1985. *The pineal gland: Endocrine aspects.* Oxford: Pergamon Press. Contains 50 contributed articles compiled as a result of a symposium in conjunction with the Seventh International Endocrinology Congress held in April 1984 in Digby, Nova Scotia. 367 pp.

GONZALES GONZALES, G., AND M. ALVEREZ-URIA, EDS. 1984. *La glandula pineal de los mamiferos.* Oriedo: Oriedo Press. Comprehensive review of the ultrastructural morphology of the pineal gland of mammals. In Spanish. 210 pp.

GUPTA, D., AND R. REITER, EDS. 1986. *The pineal gland during development: From fetus to adult.* Beackenham, Kent, Great Britain: Croom Helm Ltd. Twenty-six articles based on the papers presented at the International Workshop on the Pineal Gland During Development in Bad Urach, West Germany. 274 pp.

HADLEY, M. Endocrine role of the pineal gland. Chapter 20 in *Endocrinology,* pp. 466–487. Englewood Cliffs, N.J.: Prentice-Hall. This chapter (8 figures, 53 references) and bibliography cover pineal development and morphology, the melatonin hypothesis (biochemistry, regulation by light and dark, site of action, rhythms), and putative pineal hormones, proposed roles, and pathophysiology.

KAPPERS, J., AND P. SCHADE, EDS., 1965. *Structure and function of the epiphysis cerebri*. Progress in Brain Research 10. Amsterdam: Elsevier. Contains 37 research articles. The proceedings of an international roundtable conference under the auspices of the International Society for Neurovegetative Research at the Royal Netherlands Academy of Sciences in Amsterdam in 1963. 695 pp.

KITAY, J. I., AND M. D. ALTSCHULE. 1954. *The pineal gland*. Cambridge, Mass.: Harvard Univ. Press. A classic volume presenting early evidence concerning the function of the pineal gland, including an extensive 165-page bibliography of original papers. 280 pp.

MARTIN, C. R. 1985. The pineal and thymus glands. Chapter 20 in *Endocrine physiology*, pp. 847–886. New York: Oxford Univ. Press. The chapter combines consideration of the pineal (all but 2 pages, 6 figures) with that of the thymus because "Both organs were thought to provide protection against premature maturation of the reproduction system, to regulate water and electrolyte balance, and to be involved in the mechanisms for coping with neoplasia." The author covers pineal structure and innervation, "regulators" synthesized by the gland, control of enzymes, peptides, role in seasonal changes, influences on pigmentation, and other topics.

MATTHEWS, C. D., AND R. F. SEAMARK. 1981. *Pineal function*. Amsterdam: Elsevier/North-Holland. Contains 28 articles. Proceedings of the Satellite Symposium Sixth International Congress of Endocrinology Melbourne, Australia, February 1980. 271 pp.

MILCU, I. 1957. *Epifiza glanda endocrina*. Bucharest: Editura Academier Republicu Populax Romine. Review of the author's early work along with that of others. Paperback. 114 pp.

MILCU, I., AND L. NANU. 1979. *Glanda pineala ca organ metabolic*. Bucharest: Editura Academier Republicu Socialiste Romania. Update of the 1957 volume. 190 pp.

NEUWELT, E. A., ED. 1984. *Diagnosis and treatment of pineal region tumors*. Baltimore: Williams & Wilkins. Clinical pinealogy and some basic data. 393 pp.

NIR, I., R. J. REITER, AND R. J. WURTMAN. 1978. *The pineal gland*. Journal of Neurotransmission Supplementum 13. Vienna and New York: Springer-Verlag. Contains 24 contributions. Proceedings of an international symposium held in Jerusalem in 1977. 408 pp.

O'BRIEN, P., AND D. C. KLEIN, EDS. 1986. *Pineal and retinal relationships*. Austin: Academic Press. A collection of 27 papers from a Symposium on Pineal and Retinal Relationships held in Sarasota, Florida, in 1985. 442 pp.

OKSCHE, A., AND P. PÉVET. 1982. *Pineal organ: Photobiology, biochronometry, and endocrinology*. Developments in Endocrinology 14. Amsterdam: Elsevier/North-Holland. Contains 20 papers from the Second Colloquium of the European Pineal Study Group held in Giessen, Germany, in July 1981. 366 pp.

QUAY, W. B. 1974. *Pineal chemistry*. Springfield, Ill.: Charles C Thomas. A detailed analysis of pineal chemistry including the nonindole as well as the indole-related biochemistry and a comprehensive bibliography containing 1103 references. 430 pp.

REITER, R. J. 1977. *The pineal—1977*. Montreal: Eden Press. Second (following Relkin 1976) of a series of annual research reviews. 184 pp.

———. 1978. *The pineal 3—1978*. Montreal: Eden Press. Third annual research review. 236 pp.

———. 1979. *The pineal 4—1979*. Montreal: Eden Press. Fourth annual research review. 213 pp.

———. 1980. *The pineal 5—1980*. Montreal: Eden Press. Fifth annual research review. 234 pp.

———. 1981. *The pineal 6—1981*. Montreal: Eden Press. Sixth annual research review. 265 pp.

———. 1982. *The pineal 7—1982*. Montreal: Eden Press. Seventh annual research review. 240 pp.

———. 1981. *The pineal gland I: Anatomy and Biochemistry*. Boca Raton, Fl.: CRC Press. Eleven invited chapters presenting research endeavors of the preceding two decades. 320 pp.

———. 1981. *The pineal gland II: Reproductive effects*. Boca Raton, Fl.:CRC Press. Eight invited chapters presenting research endeavors of the preceding two decades. 227 pp.

———. 1982. *The pineal gland III: Extra-reproductive effects*. Boca Raton, Fl.: CRC Press. Nine invited chapters presenting successful research endeavors of the preceding two decades. 240 pp.

———. 1982. *The pineal and its hormones*. New York: Alan R. Liss. The camera-ready proceedings of an international symposium January 2–9, 1982, on the SS *Song of Norway*. 295 pp.

———. 1983. *Pineal research reviews I*. New York: Alan R. Liss. Six invited review articles by Karasek; Gern and Karn; Vivien-Roels and Pevet; Goldman; Vriend; and Brown, Grota, Pulido, Burns, Niles, and Snieckus. 264 pp.

———. 1984. *Pineal research reviews II*. New York: Alan R. Liss. Five invited review articles by McNulty; Korf and Moller; Quay; Kennaway; and Vaughan. 214 pp.

———. 1984. *The pineal gland*. New York: Raven Press. Eleven invited chapters by authorities in their subfields of pineal research. 382 pp.

———. 1985. *Pineal research reviews III*. New York: Alan R. Liss. Seven invited review articles by Zrenner; Welsh; King and Steinlechner; Pang; Arendt; Webb, Lewinski and Reiter; and Lehrer. 268 pp.

———. 1986. *Pineal research reviews IV*. New York: Alan R. Liss. Six invited review articles by Ebadi and Govitrapong; Pang and Allen; Heldmaier and Lynch; Jansky; Quay; and Lang. 254 pp.

———. 1987. *Pineal research reviews V*. New York: Alan R. Liss. In preparation.

REITER, R. J., AND M. KARASEK, EDS. 1986. *Advances in pineal research I*. London: John Libbey. An international volume of 23 chapters by 54 authors. 240 pp.

RELKIN, R. 1976. *The pineal*. Montreal: Eden Press. Seventeen research reviews and 100 pages of references for years up to 1976. First of a series of Annual Research Reviews in Biomedical Science. (See also Reiter 1977 and following.) 187 pp.

————, ed. 1983. *The pineal gland.* New York: Elsevier. Eight review chapters (three by Relkin). 311 pp.

SCHMIDEK, H. 1977. *Pineal tumors.* Masson Cancer Management Series 3. Masson Publications. 152 pp.

THIÉBLOT, L., AND H. LeBARS. 1958 *La glande pinéale ou épiphyse.* Paris: Maloine. In French. Paperback. 206 pp.

VOLLRATH, L. 1981. *The pineal organ.* New York: Springer-Verlag. Contains 190 figures (many photomicrographs) and 108 pages of references. Covers pineal morphology beginning in 1943 as a continuation of the monograph by Bargmann. 665 pp.

WOLSTENHOLME, G. E. W., AND J. KNIGHT, EDS. 1971. *The pineal gland.* London: Churchill Livingstone.

WURTMAN, R. J., J. AXELROD, AND D. E. KELLY. *The pineal.* New York: Academic Press. A summary of the state of knowledge as of 1968. 199 pp.

WURTMAN, R. J., AND F. WALDHAUSER, EDS. 1985. *Melatonin in humans.* Cambridge, Mass.: Center for Brain Sciences and Metabolism Charitable Trust. Contains 22 contributed papers representing the proceedings of the First International Congress on Melatonin in Humans held in Vienna, Austria, in November 1985. 444 pp.

Index

Abbreviations (*see* Glossary)
Acetyl coenzyme A, 57, 64
Adenyl cyclase, 66
Adrenal cortex, 145, 266
Adrenal medulla (*see*
    Catecholamines)
Aggression, 142
Amphibians, 23,
    128–35 (*see also*
    Melanophores)
Anolis (*see* Lizards)
Arginine vasotocin:
  daily cycle, 178
  function, 111, 147, 149
  in pineal, 66, 175, 176, 191
  seasonal cycle, 178, 179
  secretion, 177
  structure, 64
  synthesis, 177
  targets, 180
Aromatic-L-amino acid decarboxylase,
    60
Arrhythmia:
  blinding, 245
  constant light, 77
  pinealectomy, 116, 117
Autoradiography, 17
Auxin, 254

Beta-Adrenergic receptor (*see*
    Receptors)
Beta-carboline, 57, 182
Biological clock, 3, 95, 211,
    263, 265, 288
Blind, 84
Brain, 164
Bünning hypothesis, 104

Calcification (*see* Concretions)
Calendar, 271, 289

Carbohydrates, 66
Catecholamines:
  in pineal, 63
  systemic, 97, 148, 264
Catechol-O-methyltransferase, 65
Cat melatonin uptake, 57
Cattle, 65, 161
Cerebrospinal fluid, 5, 53, 157,
    161, 162, 175
Chicken:
  anatomy, 38, 41–46
  catecholamines, 23, 25
  comparative physiology, 243–45
  melatonin, 60, 74
  N-acetyltransferase, 61, 74, 76
  reproduction, 7
Chipmunk, 234
Chromatophores (*see* Melanophores)
Clock-gate model, 278
Color (*see* Melanophores)
Compensatory hypertrophy, 100, 112
Concretions, 16, 46, 158, 186, 188,
    203, 215, 233
Convulsions, 139, 198
Critical photoperiod, 103
Culture:
  cell, 25
  organ, 24
  superfusion, 25
Cyclic AMP, 64, 66, 94
Cyclic GMP, 66, 287
Cycloheximide, 62, 94
Cysteamine, 61, 64

Daily cycle, 8
Deep pineal, 38
Deer, 228
Dense core vesicles, 158
Depression, 198
Diurnal, 32
Duration, 108, 271

Es peptide of Neascu, 181
Endocrine glands, 167, 265, 267
Entrainment, 71, 117, 118
Enzyme clock model, 273–77,
    288, 289
Evolution, 35
Excretion, 161
Exercise, 197
Exhaustion, 93
External coincidence, 104, 109
Eyes (*see* Photoreceptor; Retina)

Fibers, 47
Fish, 136, 137, 251
5-Hydroxyindole acetic acid, 27, 73
Follicle (of pineal), 40
Follicle stimulating hormone,
    148
Frontal organ (*see* Photoreceptor,
    third eye)
Fur color, 134, 135

Gerbil, 36, 46, 52, 233
Glial cells, 44
Glycogen, 66
Goldfish, 47, 49, 252, 253
Ground squirrels (*see* Squirrels)
Growth hormone, 145
Guanylate cyclase, 66

Hamsters:
    Djungarian, 134, 221, 232
    golden, 23, 39, 100–113, 148,
        166, 216, 231
Headache, 198
Hibernation, 141
Histochemistry, 16, 158
Humans, 225 (*see also* Chapter 12)
Hydroxyindole-O-methyltransferase:
    assay, 31
    function, 62, 110, 111
    seasonal cycle, 77

Indole Separation, 27
Innervation:
    commissural fibers, 51
    parasympathetic, 51
    peptidergic fibers, 52
    sympathetic, 51
Inorganic constituents, 68
Insulin, 61, 149
Intermedin (*see* Melanophores)

Internal coincidence, 104, 110
Interval timer, 110, 278
Isoproterenol, 23

Jet-lag, 71

Lampreys, 251
Light:
    duration (*see* Duration)
    quality, 82
    safelight, 32
    sources, 32
Lipids, 66, 159
Lizards, 129–32, 247
Locomotor behavior, 118, 142
Lumen, 40, 50
Luteinizing hormone, 148

Macromolecules, 66, 93
Marmots, 141
Melanophores, 2, 7, 12, 28,
    128–34, 147, 156, 167, 168,
    170, 248, 251, 263, 289
Melanophore stimulating hormone
    (*see* Melanophores)
Melatonin:
    antigonadal properties, 106
    bioassays, 27
    blood, 159
    counterantigonadotrophic
        action, 107
    half-life, 157, 160
    hypothesis, 108
    radioimmunoassays, 28
    replacement, 22, 121–23, 195
    retinal, 59, 135, 136
    secretion, 158
    structure, 64
    synthesis, 158, 189, 206, 208, 214
    transport, 157, 160
Menstruation, 113, 196
Mice, 142, 221, 235
Microscopy:
    electron, 16, 40
    light, 15, 39
Microtubules and microfilaments, 170
Mitochondria, 48
Monkeys (*see* Primates)
Monoamine oxidase, 62

N-Acetyltransferase:
    assays, 30

comparative biochemistry, 225
daily cycle, 9
function, 60
inhibition, 62, 80
instability, 61, 79
location, 58
reinitiation, 81
stimulation, 61
Nerves, 47
Nerve terminals, 48
Nervi conarii, 2
N-Ethylmaleimide, 80
Neuroendocrine loop model, 269, 270
Neuroendocrine transducer, 3, 8, 264
Nocturnal, 32
Norepinephrine, 25, 64, 80

Oxytocin, 147

Pacemaker, 8, 71, 266 (see also
      Biological clock)
Parathyroid, 149
Parietal organ (see Photoreceptor,
      third eye)
Phase response, 71, 83, 84
Phosphodiesterase, 66, 94
Photoperiod, 3, 119, 213
Photoreceptor:
   cone elongation, 137
   development, 209
   disk shedding, 136
   extraretinal receptor, 8
   eyes, 82
   pineal, 2, 264
   third eye, 2, 7, 8, 142
Pineal:
   amino acids, 63, 65
   cell nuclei, 49
   cell types, 40
   definition, 1, 284
   discovery, 4
   dissection, 15
   evolution, 35
   homogenates, 26
   inhibition, 23
   lacking in, 38
   light perception, 95, 97
   location, 13
   peptides, 111
   pharmacology, 90, 195
   pinealectomy, 2, 4, 7, 17
      100, 106, 116, 194, 213, 215
   size, 222
   stimulation, 23, 95

target, 164
tissue handling, 26
transplants, 19, 119, 162
vascularization, 14, 50, 97
Pineal antigonadotropin, 181
Pinealocytes, 36, 42
Pituitary, 165, 180, 198, 266
Planaria, 254
Plants, 254
Plummet (see Rapid plummet)
Pregnancy, 196, 206, 211
Primates, 226
Prolactin, 145, 148, 166
Ptosis, 20
Puberty, 112, 196, 203, 212

Quail, 59, 60, 245

Rapid plummet, 79, 80, 81, 96
Rate limiting enzymes, 60
Rats:
   cell culture, 26
   daily cycles, 9, 73, 75,
      92, 229
   development, 209
   NAT blockers and stimulators, 91
   neural regulation, 87, 89
   pinealectomy, 60
   rapid plummet, 80
   response to catecholamines, 23, 25
Receptors:
   alpha-adrenergic, 287
   beta-adrenergic, 87, 90, 195
   down regulation model, 279
   melatonin, 168–70
Refractory period, 79
Reinitiation, 81
Reproduction:
   methods, 21
   pineal function, 100–113, 146,
      180, 196, 212
   target of melatonin, 166
Reptiles (see Lizards)
Resetting, 82
Retina, 9, 88, 111, 123, 124, 135,
      167, 248
Retinohypothalamic projection,
      86–89
Rhodopsin, 66, 82, 88
Ribonucleic acid, 93

S-Adenosylmethionine, 57, 64
Schizophrenia, 198

Scotoperiod, 3
Seasonal cycle, 8, 102, 104,
    105, 271
Season analog model, 271
Serotonin:
    daily cycle, 70, 73, 74
    function, 181
    inhibition by melatonin, 156
    seasonal cycle, 253, 262
    substrate for NAT, 31, 55, 56
Sheep, 226
6-Hydroxymelatonin, 57
6-Methoxytetrahydroharman, 64
Skeleton photoperiod, 101, 119
Skin color (see Melanophores)
Sleep, 197
Smooth endoplasmic reticulum, 48
Sparrow:
    HIOMT, 77
    pineal anatomy, 14
    pineal function, 23, 116–24,
        140, 246
    temperature, 140
Squirrels, 141, 234
Subsensitivity, 93
Superfusion, 162, 163
Superinduction, 91
Superior cervical ganglia, 20,
    47, 87, 89, 95, 105, 106,
    121, 195, 210
Supersensitivity, 91

Suprachiasmatic nuclei, 20, 86, 87,
    88, 89, 105, 121, 206
Sympathetic regulation (see Superior
    cervical ganglia)
Synaptic ribbons, 49

Temperature, 139–42, 248
Terminology, 5, 10, 71 (see also
    Glossary)
Theophylline, 91, 94
Thermoregulation (see Temperature)
Threonylseryllysine, 181
Thyroid, 146, 149, 180
Timekeeping, 95, 96
Timestick, 79
Toad bladder, 168
Torpor, 142
Tryptamine, 31
Tryptophan hydroxylase, 30, 60
Tumors, 194, 199
2-Deoxyglucose, 88

Vasopressin, 147

Weasel, 134, 135

Xenopus (see Amphibians)

Zeitgebers, 71